Mental Patient

Basic Bioethics

Arthur Caplan, editor

A complete list of the books in the Basic Bioethics series appears at the back of this book.

Mental Patient

Psychiatric Ethics from a Patient's Perspective

Abigail Gosselin

The MIT Press
Cambridge, Massachusetts
London, England

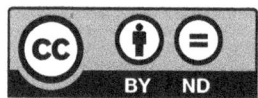
The MIT Press would like to thank the anonymous peer reviewers who provided comments on drafts of this book. The generous work of academic experts is essential for establishing the authority and quality of our publications. We acknowledge with gratitude the contributions of these otherwise uncredited readers.

This book was set in Stone Serif and Stone Sans by Westchester Publishing Services. Printed and bound in the United States of America.

Library of Congress Cataloging-in-Publication Data

Names: Gosselin, Abigail, 1977– author.
Title: Mental patient : psychiatric ethics from a patient's perspective / Abigail Gosselin.
Other titles: Basic bioethics
Description: Cambridge, Massachusetts : The MIT Press, [2022] | Series: Basic bioethics | Includes bibliographical references and index.
Identifiers: LCCN 2021052789 | ISBN 9780262544313 (paperback)
Subjects: MESH: Gosselin, Abigail, 1977– | Psychotic Disorders—psychology | Mentally Ill Persons—psychology | Professional-Patient Relations | Personal Autonomy | Therapeutic Alliance | Patient Compliance—psychology | Personal Narrative
Classification: LCC RC454 | NLM WM 200 | DDC 616.89—dc23/eng/20220209
LC record available at https://lccn.loc.gov/2021052789

10   9   8   7   6   5   4   3   2   1

To Rhea and Phoebe

Contents

Acknowledgments

I thank everyone who read early drafts of chapters while I was working on the book, including Jason Taylor, Karen Adkins, Becky Vartabedian, Anandita Mukherji, and Ron DiSanto. I extend a special thank you to Ted Zenzinger, who helped me conceptualize my project more clearly, and to several anonymous reviewers whose feedback on the manuscript greatly improved it.

Thanks goes to my colleagues named above for their encouragement and friendship, as well as to Dean Tom Bowie and Provost Janet Houser, whose support over the past several years has been pivotal in my success at work.

I thank the many clinicians who have worked with me over the years, including Dr. Samuel Clinch, Ethan Selvig, Dr. Michael Weitzner, Rebecca Baker, Dr. David Weiss, and the staff at Centennial Peaks Hospital. Special appreciation goes to John Romeo, who understood me in a way few clinicians have.

I am grateful to my parents, Deb and Marc Gosselin, and my sister and her partner, Joanne Gosselin and Jason Carter, for always being there for me. I extend special gratitude to my husband, Derrick Belanger, whose love and support over the many years has been tremendous, as well as to my children, Rhea and Phoebe Belanger, who are the greatest kids one can have.

Introduction

When I was receiving treatment for psychosis a few years ago, I underwent a huge fissure in my identity and experience. Here I was, a middle-aged, heterosexual, married White woman with children, a philosophy professor used to directing students and working with colleagues, now in the most vulnerable position I could imagine. I had lost my mind, my sense of self, my identity, my ability to interact with others and respond to the world appropriately. I no longer felt like a professional; I no longer felt like a grown-up. I felt lost and confused in my psychosis, and I felt like a child on the receiving end of treatment from mental health professionals, obligated to obey (to comply with treatment) yet feeling irrationally defiant, stuck in my sickness. Doubtful my situation could ever improve, I was unsure if I even wanted to get better. To go from being a professional, grown woman in charge of many things to feeling like a lost and confused child victimized by psychosis and at the mercy of others was a seismic shift in how I experienced the world and how I understood myself.

Feeling lost and bewildered, I had difficulty relaying to others what I was experiencing. My psychiatrist and I were often at loggerheads due to miscommunication and misunderstanding. My family and friends could tell something was seriously wrong with me, but they struggled to understand, and I found it difficult to express myself accurately. Confused in my own mind, I struggled to articulate to myself what I was going through by writing about my experiences; immersed in the strangeness of my experience, I was able to chronicle my symptoms but unable to explain their significance. This difficulty came partly as a result of lacking a broader framework within which to understand my experience and partly as a result of being unable to think clearly within my psychosis. As months passed, and then two years, my psychosis eventually receded, and I found it easier to think clearly and to read and write.

As reading and writing became easier, I did what good academics do: I tried to understand my experiences in academic terms. Immersing myself in various philosophical, psychological, and scientific literatures, I tried to understand how academics understood psychosis and recovery to see how this meshed with my own experience. The philosophical literature on hallucinations and delusions fascinated me; some of it gave me helpful new ways to understand my experience, while others of it seemed to be abstract theorizing with very little basis in reality. The scientific literature on effects of antipsychotic medication was educative and made me feel a little more reassured about the safety of my medication. The nursing literature on auditory hallucination simulations frustrated me, making assumptions about hallucinations that were narrow minded and problematic. The psychological literature on recovery from severe mental illness was illuminating and struck me as right on target.

The philosophy literature in general was rather limited. In the context of philosophy of psychiatry, I found that some philosophers seemed to have a good understanding of the experience of psychosis and the ways that psychosis constrains agency and autonomy, but others did not. While there is much written in scientific and psychological literatures on recovery (and much of it good), there is relatively little written in philosophy about the experience of recovery and what recovery requires, especially recovery from psychosis. What I thought was needed was a detailed understanding of the precise ways that psychosis can impair agency and autonomy and how this can make recovery so difficult. Many philosophers did not seem to understand the pull of psychosis, the way psychosis can feel like it has agency of its own and the way that this can hinder recovery. As a result, they did not have a clear understanding of how the quality of the therapeutic relationship is so central to recovery and how recovery requires engaging in epistemic and moral activities that increase agency and autonomy. In writing this book, I set out to articulate these themes as best as I could.

Equipped with academic frameworks with which to understand my experience, I also wanted to have an intelligible and respectable way to tell the mental health professionals with whom I worked what they were doing right and what they could do better. My experience with clinicians was mixed; at times, I felt deeply understood and respected by my clinicians, and I felt that I could trust them to guide me well. At other times, I felt greatly misunderstood by and experienced condescension from my clinicians, and I did not believe they could help me out of my sickness at all. When I was in the throes of psychosis, I had some very frustrating experiences working with clinicians who did not understand psychosis (probably at least partly because they had little experience treating psychotic patients). I wanted to write about my experiences as a mental patient in order to be able to articulate to clinicians some aspects of psychotic experience and recovery that they didn't seem to understand. In particular, I wanted to explain why psychotic patients sometimes feel ambivalent about recovery and struggle to stay committed to recovery, hoping that with this knowledge clinicians could do a better job treating recalcitrant patients.

This book is written with two motivations in mind: to explain my experience of psychosis and recovery in philosophical terms and to make recommendations to clinicians about what they should do to help patients like myself in recovery. I want both academics and clinicians to rethink some of their previous suppositions about psychosis and recovery, and I want them to learn some aspects of what it can be like to suffer from psychosis and what it can be like to be a mental patient at the mercy of those professionals tasked with treating them. This way, clinicians can do a better job at treating psychotic patients, and academics can better understand a condition with which they usually have little personal experience. Philosophy provides useful tools and frameworks for understanding the nature of psychosis and recovery, which can be used to improve therapeutic relationships between clinicians and patients and provide direction for treating psychotic patients; but, in order to be useful, these must be grounded in real-life experience. In providing a firsthand perspective of recovery from psychosis, this book grounds the philosophical discussion of psychosis and recovery in real-life experiences for the benefit of clinicians and academics alike.

Patients' experience with mental disorders can vary considerably, even among patients who suffer from the same disorders; thus, my experience may not be applicable to all people who have severe mental illness, or even all people who suffer from psychosis. I am more privileged than many who suffer from severe mental illness, as I have a stable job, a spouse, and a home, and I have never been subject to violence, abuse, or traumatic coercion in mental health treatment. Partly because of my privileged background, I have had more positive experiences with the mental healthcare system than negative experiences, which gives me more hope and optimism in the system and makes it easier for me to trust clinicians compared to many others with the same mental disorders. While my perspective is limited, and my experiences are particular to me, my experiences nonetheless probably share many similarities with those of many other patients and thus can be fruitful for understanding some aspects of psychosis and recovery, at least for some people. Throughout this book, I analyze my own experience in order to illustrate certain aspects of some people's experience with psychosis and recovery, especially in relation to agency and autonomy, situating my experience within the context of psychosis and recovery more generally.

This book is for anyone who wants to understand a perspective of what it is like to be working on recovering from psychosis and to be a mental patient being treated for psychosis. In using philosophical frameworks for thinking about psychosis and recovery, this book provides an academic examination of psychiatric ethics issues such as autonomy, paternalism, medicalization, trust, coercion, empathy, epistemic justice, and narrative approaches that arise in the process of recovering from psychosis. In connecting with personal experience of psychosis and recovery, this book grounds the academic discussion of psychiatric ethics issues in real-life experience to make it more relevant and less abstract. I explain some of the particular vulnerabilities that some patients experience due to their illness and to the way they are positioned as sick people needing treatment, and I highlight some of the particular difficulties that patients may experience with recovering from psychosis. In examining the patient experience, this book illuminates the complicated process of recovery from psychosis using philosophical frameworks from a patient perspective.

In this book, I explain one person's experience of what being psychotic is really like, showing how it can pull a person in and destroy their abilities to function in various life activities, to make choices that are truly their own, and to act with integrity. I also explain what one person's experience with recovery is like, demonstrating how much work recovery can involve and what kind of support a patient may need from mental health professionals. The book details some of the activities that a patient may need to do as they are working on their recovery in order to be successful, by practicing exercising their agency in various ways, with the support of clinicians who guide them to think more clearly and rationally and to value what is truly worth valuing.

In my experience, psychosis was personified: it had its own agency, autonomy, power, and persuasiveness, all of which overwhelmed the power that I had as an individual. Psychosis had the power to replace the values and goals that I had had before I was sick with values and goals of its own, supplanting my own vision of what a meaningful life consists of—formed through years of experience as a wife, mother, and professor—with its own view. It had the power to motivate me to adopt its vision of a meaningful life and to take the steps necessary to achieve this vision, despite the fact that this conception of a worthwhile life contradicted and thwarted my own view. This way of understanding psychosis as having power and agency of its own in framing what choices are available to a patient provides a unique perspective into what it can be like to have and to overcome psychosis.

From the vantage point of having overcome psychosis, with some distance between the time when I was psychotic and now in my present frame of mind, I can see that psychosis is not truly like a person and does not truly have agency of its own. But when I was in the midst of psychosis, it sure felt like psychosis had this power. Some of the way I talk about psychosis in this book assumes this personification and agency granted to psychosis because this is the only way I know how to convey what power it held over me.

Recovery from psychosis is often hard, harder than anyone who has not experienced it can know. In order to recover successfully, I needed treatment that would help me resist the vision, agency, autonomy, and persuasiveness of psychosis and help me reformulate a conception of a meaningful life independently of psychosis that could counter the goals dictated by psychosis. Medication helped me to perceive reality more accurately and to reduce the power of psychosis, while therapy helped give me the tools to reconceptualize what a worthwhile life consists of and to make choices and take actions that allowed me to pursue this more autonomous vision. Recovery was a struggle, however, because the psychosis wanted to keep me in its grip and prevented me from being able to accept treatment wholeheartedly. It took a lot of trust in my clinicians, in science, and in the promise of a better life for myself to be able to take my prescribed medication consistently and to do the work required in therapy. Through empathetic understanding, therapeutic alliance, and epistemic humility, the best clinicians I worked with helped me to deliberate more intentionally about what was important and about how to act on my values and achieve my goals. When clinicians empowered me to exercise my agency and to develop my autonomy, they gave me the tools to confront my psychosis and lessen its power over me.

The book proceeds as follows. Chapter 1 introduces the concept of a "mental patient," explaining what psychosis is and how it impairs epistemic and moral agency. Chapter 2 analyzes the way that psychosis impairs autonomy and autonomous choice. Examining the way psychotic experience is medicalized, chapter 3 explores what it is to be a patient receiving mental healthcare treatment from clinicians. Following this, chapters 4 and 5 examine two crucial aspects of a productive therapeutic relationship: trust, both the patient's trust in the clinician and the clinician's trust in the patient, and empathy, namely the empathetic understanding a clinician must have of their patient's experiences and perspective. The last three chapters explore three different activities that patients need to engage in as they work toward recovery in order to increase their agency and autonomy: giving testimony that is taken up by clinicians appropriately; making meaning of their experience by constructing a personal narrative about it and situating it within a larger framework of meaning; and making choices, especially choices to engage in treatment, but also choices to show up and participate in life activities more generally.

1 Psychosis

Introduction

I have been a mental patient, on and off, since I was fifteen years old. At that time, I developed anorexia, and two years later bulimia; I was also diagnosed with anxiety and depression. While in high school, I was hospitalized twice for anorexia and began seeing a therapist and a psychiatric nurse practitioner. I have been in the care of therapists and psychiatrists almost continuously since then. By the end of college, after seven years of being anorexic and bulimic, I finally overcame these diseases, managed my anxiety and depression, fell in love, and actually liked myself. Right after college, I got married; we immediately moved from New Hampshire to Colorado, where I was enrolled in the PhD program in philosophy at the University of Colorado in Boulder. For a couple of years, my husband and I settled into our new life together; I was happy. At this time, I was not on medication or under a psychiatrist's or therapist's care.

Then, when I was twenty-five, I had a manic episode and was diagnosed with bipolar disorder. While I was a graduate student, I suffered for three years with depressive, manic, and mixed episodes with very little break. After graduating, I moved to Moscow, Idaho, to teach at Washington State University in Pullman, about twenty-five minutes on the other side of the border, and I had my first child later that year. I believe that it was hormonal changes of pregnancy that finally relieved me of mania and depression. The following year, I got my second job at Regis University in Denver and did well for a while, exhausted with a newborn but mentally stable. But I had a hypomanic episode the year after that, and since being at Regis, I have had several manic, hypomanic, and depressive episodes (as well as one more child), luckily interspersed with periods of reprieve where I felt what I consider "normal."

This is the story I tell my students every year in my Philosophy of Mental Health class. I give them the opportunity to ask me questions, and they usually ask me about symptoms, self-awareness, my family, and such. That story changed in August 2017 when I had a psychotic episode without a corresponding mood change.

During that time, I had a psychotic break while attending a conference in Seattle. Experiencing a lot of stress while traveling, I disintegrated as soon as I arrived. I felt drawn by an invisible force to the docks by the water and walked the mile or so down there every time I had a break in the conference schedule. Something unseen and unknown was pulling me there. Pieces of me were dripping from me as I walked. I do not know what I mean by that, but that is what happened. There was little of me left when I sat in conference sessions. I was unable to talk to anyone except the friend with whom I was presenting a paper and unable to do basic communicative gestures I would normally be able to do like smiling or making eye contact. "I" was simply not there; "I" had dissipated. If I had been at the conference for one more day, I am convinced that I would have gone down to the water without returning and would have had to be hospitalized.

As it was, I made it home, in pieces, and somehow had to pull myself together to begin the new semester. When I started the school year, I had great difficulties talking and connecting with people and found myself paranoid, interpreting my colleagues and boss as being "out to get me" and thinking that some of them might be robots. This impacted the way I related to people, and more than one friendship became strained while others simply fell by the wayside. The world outside my mind lost much of its meaning and became more and more irrelevant. I was a shell of the person I used to be.

I knew something was wrong with me, and I wondered if I was psychotic, but I did not feel manic or depressed so I was not sure if I could be psychotic.

In October, I began hearing a voice telling me to kill myself. When I shared this with a friend, I reassured him, "You don't have to worry about me. I'm not suicidal; it's just the voice saying that." The following month I developed depression, and by December, I was suicidal *and* hearing a voice telling me to kill myself. Although I increased my antidepressant medication, it did not help enough. I lost many cognitive abilities. Constantly in a fog, not only could I frequently not understand what people were saying, but I could hardly even hear them. While keeping track of details is difficult for me normally, it became literally impossible. Reading and writing were at this point very difficult for me as my eyes would jump all around the page and I could only follow a train of thought by seeing its pieces and trying to fill in the rest. Teaching was torturous, and I could not complete some of my duties as chair of the philosophy department. Since I could not understand the context of things, everything felt disjointed. Having no memory at all, short term or long term, I lived in an everlasting present. Hardly able to follow a conversation, I frequently felt confused about what was going on around me. The more difficult being connected to the outside world became, the more I retreated to the world inside my mind. Here I felt solace and comfort, *and* had a voice telling me to kill myself, at the same time. It was a very confusing and scary place to be.

I finally got in to see my psychiatrist in early February, months after I had made the appointment. (He was booked solid until then.) He listened to me describe my symptoms and saw me shaking with agitation, and he considered hospitalizing me. Instead, he prescribed me ziprasidone (brand name Geodon), an atypical antipsychotic medication that also helps with depression. Upon taking it, I felt some reprieve, but only briefly. Hating the medication's side effects and being pulled by my psychosis to remain in its foggy world, I found it difficult to take the medication consistently as prescribed. The voice telling me to kill myself came back, and my despair increased. My coping methods—running, hiking, bird watching, and attempts at writing—ran out. Nothing gave me relief. I finally determined that I had two options: I could go to the crisis center and see what they could do for me, or I could take an overdose of drugs. I decided to try the crisis center first. On a Wednesday morning, after a restless hike, I walked into a crisis center and asked to be hospitalized.

This was my first time being hospitalized as an adult, and it was as positive of an experience as it could be. For the first three nights, I stayed in the intensive treatment unit (for patients who were psychotic and/or suicidal); for the last four nights, I stayed in a less intensive unit (for patients who mostly suffered from depression or anxiety). Even though it fit many stereotypes of psychiatric wards, I actually preferred the intensive unit because I felt like I could relate to other patients, who also suffered from psychosis, more easily. Because I had some insight and self-control, however, and because my psychosis was subsiding in the intense environment of the psychiatric hospital, the staff thought I would do better in the less intensive unit, which was focused less on simple safety management and more on learning better coping methods. Our days were highly structured with group activities, which were generally interesting and helpful.

What I hated most about the hospital was being vulnerable to and intimidated by the psychiatrists and staff, who held all the power for treatment and discharge decisions, making me feel utterly powerless over my situation. I also did not like having to ask for items like toilet paper, which felt demeaning; being cold all the time (I wore thermal underwear); and taking lukewarm showers. What I liked the most were my fellow patients and the food. The cafeteria always had tasty vegetarian options, which impressed me to no end. Relating to and connecting with fellow patients, I made many temporary friends on both units and got along well with my roommates. Listening to the advice of my fellow patients, I learned how to do hospital life from them and learned to do everything that was expected of me so I could be discharged as soon as possible. Summoning my inner teacher, I listened to my fellow patients' stories with deep interest and empathy and provided what one patient said was a calming influence on the unit. With other people in charge of me, and having fellow patients to whom I could relate and with whom I could connect, I felt more comfortable, less alienated, and safer in the hospital than I had felt at home for the past many months.

I stayed in the hospital for a week in April 2018 and came out more stable and less psychotic. Although I wanted to return to work immediately, I got only some of my responsibilities back. For a few weeks, I attended an intensive outpatient program (IOP) that met for three hours a day, three times a week. I was now on a higher dose of ziprasidone, and that helped the psychosis considerably but not the suicidality. For many months following, I struggled with constant obsessive thoughts of suicide and did not get relief from that until the following winter, when I was at a sufficiently high dose of mirtazapine, an antidepressant. I attended IOP again for months in the fall and then intermittently in the following spring. Through IOP, I learned useful skills related to mindfulness and distress tolerance.

My depression lifted in January 2019; since then, I have had at least two psychotic episodes without a corresponding mood change. When I tried decreasing the ziprasidone early in spring 2019, I immediately started hearing the voice, and it pulled me farther and farther away from shared reality into an idiosyncratic world of my own inside my head. With heightened awareness of physical sensations, I got lost in particular notes of songs and saw significance in random objects like garbage on the side of the street. Convinced there were secret messages all around me, I tried to decode hidden messages in various things. Strange ideas popped in my head; I was convinced that something was controlling what I said and did. I couldn't stand being around other people and thought they were stealing my soul. Sensitive to the quality of sunlight in the sky, I thought the sun was trying to kill me. I went into crisis again and nearly elected to be hospitalized, but I tried some medication changes instead and returned to IOP. Unable to maintain the medication changes, I stopped taking the antipsychotic medication completely. Within two weeks, I was lost in my inner experiences again and unable to read and write, or simply think, so I chose to go back on it. After reaching a high enough dose, I started to feel normal again.

I felt normal for about six weeks, and then in May 2019 my psychosis was triggered by a hearing test, where I could not tell which sounds were tinnitus, which sounds were psychotic, and which sounds were coming from the headphones I wore in the testing booth. The different levels of reality were overwhelming. Although my discomfort around the hearing test faded quickly, the psychosis did not. Unable to feel emotions, I felt like a zombie. My husband said it was like something else had taken over my body. I could not read or write or interact with people, nor could I make eye contact, and I spoke in a quiet monotonous mumble that was hard to understand. I was so confused much of the time that I felt like I had dementia. I knew that if things did not improve before the start of the fall semester, I would have to go on disability because there was no way I could teach like this.

For much of two years now, I had been struggling with psychosis, and now, even at my highest dose of ziprasidone so far, I was still ill. Losing hope, I went into deep despair. I heard messages in music and elsewhere to kill myself. Feeling like I had little control over what my body did, I feared the voice was going to take over and do it for me. As I felt so unsafe, I wanted to hospitalize myself, but my family was doing a lot of traveling and I was trying so hard to hold it together. Instead, I increased the ziprasidone again and added a smidgen of risperidone (brand name Risperdal) to my regular regimen. Within days of adding risperidone, I started to feel better, and then, as I increased the risperidone, I began to feel more or less normal. I now know that if I am not on a sufficiently high dose of antipsychotic medication, I will not only get nutty but sink into a dementia-like state. That terrifies me.

Staying on a sufficiently high dose of antipsychotic medication is not always easy, however. For well over a year after I was first prescribed an antipsychotic, I struggled with taking my medication as prescribed for reasons I do not fully understand but which I explore in this book. In brief, my illness was self-perpetuating. When I was psychotic, I thought I needed to stay psychotic. I heard a voice tell me constantly not to take my medication as prescribed, and every time I took my medication I had to fight with the voice and make a deliberate decision about whether to take my medication and how much of it I should take. I did not dare disobey the voice though I did sometimes negotiate deals with it. My psychosis wanted to keep me in its grip, and I felt powerless to counter its demands. If I were going to recover, I needed to learn how to talk back to the voice and how to value the life I had when I was not psychotic enough to be able to try to regain that life. Treatment had to involve relearning how to be an autonomous agent who could act in my own best interests of maintaining my health and well-being.

Being hospitalized in April 2018 began my adult career of being what one might call a "heavy service user" or what I think of as being a mental patient. For a decade and a half, I had been a mental patient to greater and lesser degrees when my bipolar disorder was active, interspersed with periods when I was well and merely consulted mental health professionals in order to stay on track. Once I began struggling with psychosis, I became a full-fledged *patient*, someone who was sick and needed treatment. I called myself a "repeat customer" because for months I was at my mental health clinic several times a week: attending IOP three times a week, getting individual therapy once a week, and seeing my psychiatrist every month or so. I became "known," not only to the clinicians I worked with but also to other clinicians who answered my calls to the crisis line or answered the emails I sent to my therapist or psychiatrist when they were out of the office. I became a "regular" with the reception staff; even the security guard knew me by name. I know that I was "known" in the clinic even by clinicians I had never met because one time when I spoke with a crisis team member, she said, "We haven't seen your name in our basket for a while." I was taken aback that she knew my name, but upon reflecting on my involvement with the behavioral health clinic, it made sense. With my continuous mental health problems over the past couple of years, I had become very much a mental patient.

In this chapter, I examine what it is to suffer from psychosis. First, I examine what the term "mental patient" means and argue that it is an appropriate term for the group of people this book is about. Then I explain what makes psychosis a mental illness and show some ways in which psychosis is psychologically debilitating. Examining various cognitive harms of psychosis, I show that being a mental patient who has psychosis can lead to extreme losses of epistemic and moral capacities, a loss of a sense of oneself as a subject of experience and as an agent, and losses in epistemic and moral agency. These must be addressed in recovery.

Mental Patient: A Word about Terminology

Let me acknowledge right away that the term "mental patient" is controversial among people whom this term covers. This is because it emphasizes people's sickness, presuming their[1] mental condition to be pathological, or medically problematic, and needing to be cured or managed through treatment. Some people view their mental condition as "mere difference," a deviation from the norm, but do not accept it as illness. Some people who hear voices, for instance, are opposed to the medicalization of their experience,[2] as I explain below. In addition, some people may be opposed to the passive stance implied by the idea of a mental patient. For some, the term "mental patient" suggests that a person is a passive recipient of treatments that are done to them by mental health professionals.

In order to avoid presuming that a person's deviating mental condition is pathological, and to avoid seeing a person as a passive recipient of healthcare services, alternative terms have been proposed. The recovery literature largely refers to people with deviating mental conditions as "service users" or "consumers" of mental healthcare, and sometimes "survivors." The former two emphasize a person's agency while the latter suggests that the person has been through trauma and has at least survived it. All these terms reframe the primary relevant issue.

"Service user" frames the relevant experience around the act of using mental healthcare services, as opposed to framing it around being sick, and it emphasizes the agency involved with "using" services rather than seeing the phenomenon as "receiving" services. The service user movement has been particularly strong in the United Kingdom, where service users have demanded that they be treated as collaborators in mental health research, education, and training.[3] In addition, they have fought to have conditions like hearing voices seen through a nonmedicalized lens.[4]

"Mental healthcare consumer" emphasizes the agency involved with choosing to get treatment and choosing what kind of treatment to get. It conceptualizes the person with mental illness as a partner in co-determining their mental healthcare treatment rather than being a passive recipient of it.[5] Rather than being sick, the relevant experience is regarded as the choices a person makes in responding to their mental health condition.

"Survivor" frames the experience of being in the mental healthcare system as one of trauma inflicted on a person by the mental health system and is typically used by people who were coerced into receiving mental healthcare or who were abused within the mental healthcare system.[6] This term does not seem to cover people who seek out mental healthcare and who have generally positive experiences with it. Those who are covered under the term "survivor" tend to have had mental healthcare inflicted upon them.

While the desires to emphasize the agency of people with mental health conditions and to not make presumptions about the pathological nature of their conditions are admirable, they are misplaced. I am personally opposed to the labels of "mental healthcare consumer" and "service user" because they emphasize the wrong aspects of the experience as relevant, and they understood the nature of agency involved incorrectly. "Service user" emphasizes the activity involved with getting treatment, not a bad term if one is put off by the passive stance suggested by "mental patient"; it does not, however, capture the way a person is situated in the therapeutic relationship in relation to clinicians.

"Mental healthcare consumer" does not just frame the relevant experience in terms of choice but puts it in a consumer framework as if one's decision to get treatment is like choosing what product to buy at the grocery store.[7] This treats mental healthcare as a commodity in a capitalist economy. But people do not make many choices about whether and what kind of treatment to get, especially those whose functioning is so severely impaired that they can be regarded as "sick." I am lucky to have a job that allows me to choose among two options for health insurance (a luxury that only some people in the US have), and I am lucky to be happy with the insurance I have. But many people in the US who are as sick as I am do not have health insurance or have only one option. Moreover, while I made a choice to seek help in being hospitalized, I had no choice in where I went, what help I got when I was there, or when I could leave. Many people who are as sick as I have been are placed in involuntary or forced treatment, which, I shall argue later in the book, is sometimes justified; these people make no choices about their treatment. Given my health insurance, I had a few options in choosing a therapist and psychiatrist; I feel fortunate to have gotten clinicians I like, but the options are nonetheless limited. Options are even more limited, if not nonexistent, for people who have worse or no health insurance. Choice is not predominant among those with severe mental healthcare needs.

The term "survivor" has only limited use, applying only to people who have been mistreated by the mental healthcare system. The term seems to view the mental healthcare system as an entity or agent that has done a person wrong by subjecting them to procedures to which they did not consent or over which they had no control, or that caused unnecessary pain and suffering. While this does describe the experience of some people who have been traumatized, abused, or otherwise harmed by the mental healthcare system, it does not describe the experience of all. Many people who receive mental healthcare treatment are grateful for it at least to some extent. Most people who enter the mental healthcare system do so willingly, seeking out care in order to feel better or to function better. Even those who do not enter the system of their own accord are often grateful for receiving care after the fact.[8] Many people, of course, have mixed experience with their mental healthcare treatment, perhaps dissatisfied with their particular treatment providers, wishing they could access more treatment or different modalities of treatment (for example, more therapy sessions than what is offered), or unhappy with the particular inpatient or outpatient therapies and programs offered. But most people, even those with mixed experiences, are grateful to have access to at least some form of mental healthcare treatment and find some benefit from it even if the treatment is not uniformly beneficial. While "survivor" describes the experience of people who have been traumatized, abused, or otherwise harmed by the mental healthcare system, it does not describe the experience of people who are benefitted by it.

The terms "consumer," "service user," and "survivor" are jargonistic terms popular in the academic literature; the former two are sometimes used in clinical settings, while the latter is sometimes used in informal peer support settings. They are not uniformly or perhaps even commonly accepted by either patients or treatment providers, however.[9] Treatment providers see themselves as professionals providing mental healthcare services to clients or patients in need. Most people receiving such services see themselves as having healthcare needs that must be tended to by professionals trained in helping their problems. If I queried people in the intensive outpatient program I sometimes attend, fellow patients in the hospital, or people attending the behavioral health clinic I go to for therapy or psychiatric care, few, I wager, would even be familiar with these terms; even fewer, if any, would identify with these terms. The average person receiving mental healthcare treatment sees themselves as a person with medical needs needing to be taken care of (a "patient"), or as a person with the kind of problems that can only be helped by a professional (a "client").

For all these reasons, I prefer the terms "client" or "patient." A client is one who consults medical or mental healthcare professionals for help with their problems in order to be able to feel better, framing the relevant experience as being in the care of treatment professionals; a client can consult with professionals without necessarily being *sick*. A patient, on the other hand, is one who is *sick* and in need of treatment in order to be able to function or at least not deteriorate.[10] A client consults professionals for help in the area of the professionals' expertise; mental health clients consult psychiatrists for medication and consult therapists for counseling. A patient is in the care of medical or mental health professionals and receives treatment through those relationships; mental health patients receive drug treatment from psychiatrists and receive therapies of various kinds from therapists. Clients seek out professional help through their own will; when patients receive treatment, on the other hand, they may do so out of their own choice (electing to be hospitalized or to receive outpatient services) or they may be forced to do so (through involuntary hospitalization or other compulsory treatment). Clients see professionals on an outpatient basis, consulting with professionals in their offices. Patients receive treatment either as inpatients in hospitals or other institutions, or through outpatient services of various kinds. In this book, I use "patient" as the more inclusive term to include all who receive treatment regardless of whether this is by choice or not and regardless of location of treatment (inpatient or outpatient setting), primarily because

I am referring to sick people in need of treatment, who are positioned as recipients of care vis-à-vis their clinicians.

Since patients are defined by their role in receiving treatment by medical or mental health professionals for a medical or mental health condition, they are defined in terms of their relationship to clinicians. I use the term "clinician" as a broad term that includes all treatment providers from whom a mental patient may receive treatment. Clinicians include doctors (including psychiatrists); nurses (including psychiatric nurse practitioners); psychologists and social workers providing counseling and psychological therapies (such as cognitive behavioral therapy and dialectical behavioral therapy); and other therapists of various kinds (including not only counselors, but also those providing services such as occupational, art, music, and movement therapies). (The words "therapy" and "therapist" are broad terms encompassing a wide range of services; the specific meaning of the term must be gleaned from the context in which it is used.) "Patient" is thus a relational term that can only be understood in context. The patient role must be understood in relation to the specific kinds of treatment patients receive and the medical and mental health professionals whose services they receive.

In addition to these considerations, I like the term "mental patient" as a way of reclaiming a label sometimes used pejoratively, similar to the way LGBTQIA+ people have reclaimed the term "queer" as an expression of pride. People who have been the recipients of mental healthcare should be proud to affirm their identity and experience as something not to be ashamed of, but rather as something to embrace and explore. We often cannot help being sick people in need of treatment, but we can accept this as a part of our identity and learn and grow from it.

Now that I have established that my focus in this book is on mental patients, and one patient's experience and perspective as a mental patient in particular, let us unpack what this term means. The term has two components. The "mental" aspect refers to the way a person's problems are experienced as mental rather than physical, affecting cognition, perception, affect, volition, and/or behavior. These mental impairments diminish a person's ability to function in various life domains because they diminish agency and autonomy. The "patient" component reflects the way a person is situated as a sick person, subject to the will of others through medical and mental healthcare treatment, and embodying a sick role that affects a person's identity, agency, power, and relationship with others. In this chapter and chapter 2, I examine the "mental" aspect of mental patient experience; in chapter 3, I look at the "patient" aspect of mental patient experience.

The "Mental" in "Mental Patient": Mental Illness

The "mental" part of mental illness has to do with the way abnormal mental processes can make someone severely ill, causing mental impairments that impede their functioning as well as create significant distress. A mental patient is one who is made ill by their mental condition. Mental patients, in general, have mental disorders, though not all people who have mental disorders are mental patients. Let me explain.

A mental disorder is a diagnostic category used to identify a set of experiences and behaviors ("symptoms") that are considered abnormal, pathological, impairing, and/or distressing. Mental disorders are categorized in North America in the American Psychiatric Association's *Diagnostic and Statistical Manual* (DSM) and in Europe in the *International Classification of Diseases*, and they are diagnosed by psychiatrists who must identify specific disorders in order for health insurances to pay for treatment. The DSM defines a mental disorder as "a syndrome characterized by clinically significant disturbance in an individual's cognition, emotion regulation, or behavior that reflects a dysfunction in the psychological, biological, or developmental process underlying mental functioning." The DSM goes on to say that "mental disorders are usually associated with significant distress or disability in social, occupational, or other important activities."[11] Mental disorders are thus best understood as delineating clusters of symptoms that hang together in some relevant way.

A mental illness, in contrast, is a state of being made "ill" or sick by one's mental disorder.[12] All mental illnesses are caused by having a mental disorder; not all mental disorders make a person ill. For example, deficient focus and attention capacity can be impairing enough to be diagnosed as a mental disorder (attention deficit/hyperactivity disorder), but they do not usually make a person *sick*. A mental disorder is a deviation from the norm in some area(s) of mental functioning, such as cognition, perception, affect/mood, volition/will, social functioning, or behavior; a mental illness, in contrast, is a gross deviation that causes major functional impairments. A person who has a mental illness has major impairments that affect functioning in various life domains such as work, school, family life, friendships, interactions with others, and personal hygiene. When severe enough, difficulties with functioning can lead to many losses, including losses of employment, housing, family relationships, and friendships. People who are made "ill" by their mental disorder experience severe impairment and often (though not always) distress. In my analysis of what it is to be a mental patient, I am concerned with people who are seriously impaired by their mental condition and thus vulnerable to significant losses.

Mental disorder and mental illness are both objective concepts, in that they have external criteria that occur independently of subjective feelings of distress, and that are observable by others. These criteria constitute the symptoms associated with a particular mental disorder. When these symptoms are severe enough, they cause functional impairment that is observable by others, and that occurs independently of subjective feelings about the condition. This constitutes mental illness. While people may be distressed by their mental disorder or mental illness, distress—which is a subjective quality of experiencing pain or suffering—is neither a necessary nor a sufficient condition of either. A person may possess a cluster of relevant symptoms warranting diagnosis, regardless of whether they are distressed by these symptoms; they may be impaired in some significant way without necessarily feeling distress by that impairment. While impairment may (but does not always) cause distress, distress may (but again does not always) also cause impairment. People who are distressed severely enough may become impaired by their distress when it interferes with their ability to function in certain ways. This compounds whatever impairment they also experience from their mental disorder symptoms. Thus, people may be harmed through impairments caused by their mental disorder as well as through the distress they feel as a result of their symptoms. Impairments due to either cause constitute objective harms, as they involve functional limitations that are observable by others and that negatively impact one's quality of life.

Some mental disorder symptoms are more generally impairing than others, and some are impairing more consistently. One set of symptoms that are especially impairing are those associated with psychosis. Psychosis interferes with agency and autonomy in a broad way, affecting all life domains. Impairments caused by psychosis, such as those I described above as having personally experienced, are objective harms that drastically reduce a person's quality of life.[13]

Psychosis

People who experience psychosis are often regarded as having the most severe mental health problems because psychosis can interfere with all aspects of functioning in ways and to degrees that are unparalleled by other mental health problems except perhaps severe (suicidal) depression. People with psychotic illnesses are the heaviest users of mental healthcare services, requiring more frequent and intensive treatment. They are more likely to be in the kind of crisis situations requiring first responder attention, emergency room care, or crisis stabilization services such as hospitalization. They are more likely to be unemployed, as they may be incapable of working a steady job in the employment of others, and homeless, as they may be unable to afford or maintain a home. They are more likely to be unable to take care of themselves and get their basic needs met without the help of others. In addition, they are more likely to appear disheveled and behave bizarrely in ways that mark them as "Other" and make the general public uncomfortable.

People with psychotic illnesses generally have more severe needs than people with other mental health problems because of the way psychosis has a global effect on how people think, feel, behave, and relate to others. Psychosis refers to thought disorder, in contrast to mood disorders like bipolar disorder or major depression; anxiety disorders like generalized anxiety, social phobia, or obsessive-compulsive disorder; attention disorders like attention deficit/hyperactivity disorder; and developmental conditions such as autism. The umbrella term used to describe most psychotic disorders is "schizophrenia," although both bipolar disorder and major depression can have psychotic features, and psychosis can also occur in anxiety, dissociative, and personality disorders. The range of psychotic disorders found in the DSM—which include schizoaffective disorder, delusional disorder, schizotypal personality disorder, schizophreniform disorder, and brief psychotic disorder—are often referred to as "schizophrenia-spectrum disorders."[14]

Psychosis can be understood as impairment in one's connection to reality or as global distortion of meaning. Psychosis has both "positive" symptoms—symptoms that are added to a person's experience and personality—and "negative" symptoms—symptoms that subtract from a person's experience and personality—as well as cognitive symptoms that affect how a person thinks. The most notable symptoms of psychosis are the positive symptoms of hallucinations (perceptions without external causes), delusions (bizarre ideas believed despite counterevidence), and paranoia (a pervading sense of fear, often experienced as the feeling that others are "out to get" a person). Negative symptoms of psychosis include flat affect (having little or no emotional expression and possibly little or no emotional feeling), monotonous voice, social withdrawal, apathy, low energy, disinterest, lack of motivation, and catatonia (inability to move) or muscle rigidity. Psychosis also includes cognitive or disorganized symptoms, which involve problems with logic and reasoning, confusion, arbitrary word or symbol associations, faulty attribution of meaning, and incoherent speech. Disorganized thinking leads to bizarre behavior as one relates to the world and to other people in unorthodox ways and an inability to take care of oneself or one's personal hygiene (hence the unkempt appearance of some psychotic people). Phenomenologically, psychosis causes a loss of a core self so that a person no longer experiences themselves as a subject of experiences and an agent who performs actions, leading to loss of a sense of first-person subjectivity and agency and making a person feel radically disconnected from the world and from oneself.

Some aspects of psychosis may be experienced as positive, while others are usually experienced as negative. In particular, positive symptoms may be experienced as beneficial, harmful, or both, while negative symptoms and cognitive symptoms are usually experienced as simply harmful.

Hallucinations and delusions can be experienced as beneficial because they can provide people with a sense of meaning, significance, and purpose; this results from the ways psychosis assigns objects with salience and directs attention to them.[15] Hallucinations, delusions, and paranoia can fulfill various functions for people. For example, voices can provide advice, encouragement, information, reassurance, comfort, and companionship, as well as a sense of specialness.[16] Voices can mitigate against loneliness, which people with mental illness commonly feel; they also provide motivation and influence agency and identity. In addition, delusions and paranoia fulfill functions in helping people deal with the stresses of their environments by offering ways for people to interpret their experience so it makes sense to them.

While the positive symptoms of psychosis can appear meaningful, interesting, and comforting, they can also be distressing, of course. People can find their voices scary or feel beaten down by them; they can feel profound confusion about what is reality when the distinction between their hallucinations and the shared reality others experience is not clear. When paranoid, patients typically feel great fear of other people. They may also feel a generalized sense of fear about "everything" that somehow gets localized onto specific objects (such as law enforcement or aliens); this is a form of the uncanniness that people commonly feel in which seemingly random objects appear salient and get assigned meaning.

While positive symptoms of psychosis may be experienced as either beneficial or harmful, or both concurrently, both negative symptoms of psychosis and cognitive symptoms are more consistently distressing and impairing. Social withdrawal, disinterest, apathy, lethargy, flat affect, and monotonous voice do not fulfill particular functions; they are not enjoyable, interesting, or meaningful. Confusion, disorganization, and sensory disintegration impede functioning and can be rather frightening. Negative and cognitive symptoms of psychosis unequivocally reduce a person's quality of life. They typically lead to distress, a loss of meaning, and a loss of hope, and sometimes to suicidality.

Negative, positive, and cognitive symptoms of psychosis lead to many harms. These include subjective experiences that are internal to the person such as distress and loss of meaning and hope, but they also include many objective losses that diminish functioning. Psychosis can cause losses of various cognitive capacities, memory problems, fatigue, apathy, disinterest, a sense of passivity, communication difficulties, and an inability to complete the activities of daily living.[17] Pulling a person into an idiosyncratic private mental world of their own, psychosis causes a person to disengage from others and from shared reality[18], leading to the loss of social relationships and of interpersonal contact. This also results in losses of practical and emotional support.[19] People lose competence in their capacities, confidence in themselves, and credibility in the eyes of others. People also lose their sense of security, respect by others, autonomy, and physical health.[20] The cognitive problems caused by psychosis lead to diminished engagement in work, education, family life, and other spheres of activity, resulting in losses of employment, housing, hobbies, family relationships, and friendships. These losses constitute some of the objective harms that people with mental illness experience due directly to their illness. I shall return to this idea in chapter 3.

Disorganization and Loss of Agency

If I were to characterize psychosis in terms of only one symptom, it would be thought disorganization. Thought disorganization involves changes in meaning structure and loss of order of ideas and events. Most other symptoms of psychosis are connected to this one; it is responsible at least in some way for most of the losses a psychotic person experiences due to their illness.

A person who has disorganized thinking cannot see how ideas connect to each other and so cannot follow a train of thought well. They have difficulty thinking through their own ideas, cannot follow conversations well, and struggle to make sense of texts (not only reading material, but also visual texts like movies). They cannot see the context for ideas, so ideas seem to be isolated and random rather than developing from other ideas or fitting within larger structures. Perception is changed, too, as sensations are perceived as all-consuming yet disconnected and cannot be easily distinguished, made sense of, and put into context. This can feel very overwhelming. Elyn Saks describes the overwhelming nature of disorganization vividly:

> My awareness (of myself, of him [her father], of the room, of the physical reality around and beyond us) instantly grows fuzzy. Or wobbly. I think I am dissolving. I feel—my mind feels—like a sandcastle with all the sand sliding away in the receding surf. . . . Consciousness gradually loses its coherence. One's center gives way. The center cannot hold. The "me" becomes a haze, and the solid center from which one experiences reality breaks up like a bad radio signal. There is no longer a sturdy vantage point from which to look out, take things in, assess what's happening. No core holds things together, providing the lens through which to see the world, to make judgments and comprehend risk. Random moments of time follow one another. Sights, sounds, thoughts, and feelings don't go together. No organizing principle takes successive moments in time and puts them together in a coherent way from which sense can be made. And it's all taking place in slow motion.[21]

Disorganization severs a person's connection with reality so they no longer can see or experience the world the way others do. Thought disorganization is ultimately a profound loss of meaning and coherence.

Disorganized thinking is connected to many other symptoms, including hallucinations, delusions, cognitive dulling, and memory loss, all of which occur due to the changes in meaning structure that disorganized thinking causes. Thought disorganization is evidenced in a variety of speech patterns and behaviors in which a person's inner experience does not seem to make sense. Some examples of disorganized thinking include poverty of thought; seeing meaning where others do not; connecting ideas in ways that appear to others to be random; an inability to recognize existing structures such as rules, roles, boundaries, and customs; and an inability to recognize the normative force of social norms, moral principles, or justificatory reasons.

The cognitive problems involved with disorganization cause many epistemic impairments. People who are psychotic struggle to comprehend readings and speech. They have difficulty formulating ideas and questions. They tend to assign salience to objects and ideas that others do not perceive while failing to recognize what others find meaningful. They struggle to make relevant distinctions, and they have difficulty understanding, never mind analyzing or assessing, ideas. Because they have difficulty understanding and evaluating reasons and evidence, it can be hard or impossible to weigh evidence or compare reasons. Psychotic people tend to lack the logic that would allow them to determine what conclusions reasons and evidence support, often leading them to form beliefs in faulty ways. Other epistemic capacities that can be compromised include the ability to organize information in meaningful ways and the ability to associate relevant concepts together. These epistemic impairments create major constraints on a person's epistemic agency, or their ability to act as a knower.

Agency is the power to choose and to act based on reason. Epistemic agency involves the capacity to act as a knower, guided by reason[22], while moral agency involves the capacity to act in a moral context by making decisions about how to act based on reason.[23] In addition to impairing epistemic capacities, disorganization impairs moral capacities, negatively impacting moral agency. Psychotic individuals struggle with determining what is of value, often assigning meaning arbitrarily, unable to provide reasons for what they value and choose that are intelligible to others. Lacking a meaningful valuation system, they struggle to formulate desires and make rational choices. This negatively impacts their decision-making capacity and their ability to act based on rational choices grounded by values. In short, psychosis creates significant constraints on people's epistemic and moral agency, making it difficult for them to participate meaningfully in normal epistemic and moral practices.

Other symptoms easily impair epistemic and moral agency as well. Hallucinations and delusions can colonize a person's mind, shaping the person's sense of reality and imposing a meaning structure on things and events that does not reflect the shared meaning that others find intelligible. By taking over a person's mind, hallucinations and delusions diminish a person's epistemic agency so they cannot have access to accurate knowledge about the world, only access to mistaken and confusing beliefs. Hallucinations make the world "feel" a certain way to a person, and this feeling feels like it constitutes knowledge, but it actually just constitutes delusory views of the world; hallucinations do not tend to convey much real knowledge of what the world is like. Cognitive dulling can further diminish a person's epistemic agency as it makes it so that a person cannot understand what is happening around them and thus cannot respond to it or interact with it in a meaningful way. When psychotic patients "lose touch with reality," this disconnection occurs just as much from the cognitive dulling that destroys knowledge and understanding of the world as it does from the delusions and hallucinations that change a person's meaning structure.

Hallucinations and delusions can impede not only knowledge about the world, but also self-understanding, too. In changing the meaning structure of a person's experience, they can change what a person can know about themselves. Psychotic people typically become preoccupied with their unusual experiences so that the hallucinations and delusions become not only the most interesting, but also the most dominant things in their subjective awareness. A psychotic person will come to ignore other aspects of experience as they pay most of their attention to the delusions and hallucinations they experience, which severely limits their understanding of themselves as a self and limits what self-awareness they have of themselves.

These limitations on epistemic agency also diminish moral agency, as lacking access to knowledge about the world and lacking self-understanding makes it so that a person cannot make informed decisions. A person cannot choose what to do if they cannot understand what is happening around them, to them, and within themselves. When patients lose memory, they lose their connection to themselves in the past and through this lose an important aspect of personal identity and sense of selfhood; when they lose the ability to imagine themselves in the future, they lose the ability to set meaningful goals for which to strive and lose motivation and interest in doing things. As their cognitive separation from the world around them makes it impossible to connect to the world sufficiently to be able to be moved by it or interested in it, psychotic patients can lose motivation, energy, interest, and ability to choose and act. Patients with severe psychosis can become catatonic as they literally become unable to choose or act.

In addition to impairing epistemic and moral agency, psychotic symptoms can also impair a person's ability to see themselves as a subject of experience and as an agent who acts. Disorganization often causes a shift in a psychotic person's sense of self and agency, so they no longer experience thoughts, feelings, and actions as their own. Hallucinations and delusions reinforce this loss of a sense of self and agency as individuals focus disproportionately on their unusual experiences and ascribe them to fanciful causes. Some theorists propose that schizophrenia is best understood at a phenomenological level as a disturbance of self-awareness and of one's experience of oneself as a subject and agent.[24] In this ipseity disturbance model of schizophrenia, the primary problem of schizophrenia is seen as an alteration of consciousness or a change in one's sense of subjectivity and agency whereby a person no longer recognizes themselves as being the origin of their thoughts, feelings, and actions. They experience hyper-reflexivity, where they have exaggerated self-consciousness, directing their attention toward mental and physical processes and phenomena that are normally in the background of awareness. What is normally implicit and backgrounded becomes explicit and foregrounded. For example, a person may pay undue attention to bodily sensations or sensory perceptions that normally people would not notice. This is accompanied by diminished self-reflection, where a person has a decreased sense of existing as a subject of awareness of an agent of action, and a disturbed hold or grip on the world, where they have difficulty distinguishing between different kinds of experiences (such as perception vs. memory vs. imagination). The loss of core self or ipseity that occurs with schizophrenia leads to a loss of a sense of agency, where a person's thoughts, feelings, and actions are experienced as happening *to* them, but not *by* them.[25] This makes a person lose their ability to take ownership of their experience and to authorize their choices.

Losses of epistemic and moral capacities and the loss of a sense of oneself as a subject and agent impact self-understanding, creating further epistemic impairments. These limitations make it hard for individuals with psychosis to access epistemic resources that would allow them to understand their condition better. Epistemic impairments can make it difficult for individuals to understand the ideas and theories surrounding their illness, and the loss of a sense of subjectivity and agency can make it hard, if not impossible, for individuals to be self-reflective about their experience. Oftentimes psychotic people lack insight, meaning they do not realize they have an illness. When deficits in epistemic and moral capacities cloud a person's self-awareness, they are not able to see that certain ideas such as illness concepts apply to them. Lack of insight further hinders self-understanding as it makes it so that a person loses the broader context for understanding what is happening to them; they fail to recognize they are sick because they lack the context that would make that knowledge meaningful.

Finally, deficits in epistemic and moral capacities and the loss of a sense of self that psychotic individuals experience can make it very hard for them to interact with others, which prevents them from being a participating member of an epistemic or moral community. Thus, psychosis can lead people to lose both capacities and a community in which they could participate and exercise their capacities. In addition, to the extent that psychotic individuals are self-aware of their deficits, they typically develop a lot of uncertainty and anxiety around them, which diminishes their confidence. Realizing that they do not always see the world or understand ideas accurately, they may lose faith in their ability to interact with the world appropriately and retreat into a mental world of their own. This social withdrawal further separates them from others and removes them from an epistemic or moral community in which they could participate in epistemic or moral practices with others.

As I explain in chapter 2, the loss of epistemic and moral capacities and the diminishment of a sense of oneself as a subject and agent that occur with impaired epistemic and moral agency can lead to further losses of competence and voluntariness, thereby diminishing autonomy, or the ability to deliberate about ends and to choose actions based on one's conception of the good. Psychotic symptoms can interfere with a person's ability to act as a knower and a chooser and consequently to make choices that can be reflectively endorsed. Thought disorganization and its many related symptoms thus can create many losses for individuals that impair their agency and autonomy.

Conclusion

What is so debilitating about psychosis is that it can profoundly impair agency and, as I shall explain in chapter 2, autonomy. Although psychosis typically leads to a lack of epistemic and moral agency and a lack of the sense of oneself as a subject and agent, these are essential for patients to be able to live a life that is not dominated by their illness. Thus, it is crucial that patients develop these in the process of recovery. Developing moral and epistemic capacities, a sense of oneself as a subject and agent, and actual agency requires that patients participate actively in the recovery.

Patients only develop capacities and agency if they have the means to practice these so they can get better at them.

Recovery from psychosis required me to participate actively in the processes of recovery in a variety of ways. In order to claim ownership of my experiences, seeing them as belonging to myself, I had to learn to recognize my thoughts and behavior as my own. I had to reclaim my voice by describing my experiences as I understood them and by being treated as a credible and reliable witness to my experience. Part of this involved developing a narrative about my experiences that made them make sense to me and situate them within larger frameworks of meaning. I had to learn to recognize what was in my best interests and to value these as part of a worthwhile life. Moreover, I had to develop the ability to conceptualize myself in the future so I could make meaningful goals for my future, including treatment goals, that gave me something to strive for. Finally, I had to practice making decisions about my treatment that furthered my best interests of health and well-being rather than promoting the psychosis.

Using my voice, making sense of my experiences, and making choices of my own were crucial processes for me to engage in. I had to be given opportunities to participate in these practices through the process of recovery. Having positive therapeutic relationships with my clinicians, based on trust and empathy, was essential for allowing me the opportunities to engage in these practices in meaningful and productive ways. Recovery involved a lot of hard work. The foundations had to be in place for this work to be successful. This book analyzes what foundations may be needed for recovery from severe mental illness to be successful, showing that patients often must have positive therapeutic relationships based on trust and empathy, and often must be given opportunities to practice exercising their agency, in order to be able to recover. In the next chapter, I examine the way psychosis can interfere with autonomy and show that one of the main goals of the therapeutic relationship has to be to increase patient autonomy and agency.

2 Autonomy

Introduction

While I was on the phone with a nurse on the crisis hotline one evening, my youngest daughter, who was then eight years old, drew a picture of a smiling face with the caption "Don't forget to smile!" and left it under my door. I found it when I finished the phone call. Wanting to be touched by her concern for me, I wanted to be able to mobilize that concern as a resource that I could draw upon in helping me make positive choices. I wanted to be able to think to myself, "I've got to get better so I can be present for my family." But I couldn't. Not consistently anyway. I would try to remind myself how much my family loved and cared about me, but I felt so disconnected from the world outside my mind that I could barely register their concern. When my husband hugged me and told me how much he cared about me, I felt like he was talking to someone I used to be but no longer was, and I was unable to respond. Feeling like a zombie, a shell of the person I once was, I could not understand why my family wanted me to be better when "I" no longer existed. Their concern for me seemed misplaced. Because I couldn't connect with it, I couldn't use it as a motivation to get better. The psychosis pulled me in and took hold of me, and no amount of concern from others could keep me outside of it.

Within my psychosis, the only thing that mattered was the psychosis. I was consumed by my inner experience, losing myself in a song, in a sensation, in the thoughts that chaotically coursed through my mind, in the incessant noise I heard in my head. Nothing else felt real, so nothing else mattered. My imperative was to pursue the only thing that felt real, my inner experience. It was hard to try to care about the external world, and even harder to try to make decisions that would keep me in the external world. All I wanted to do was to escape into the internal world, where I could let go and not have to fight so hard.

The distance between my inner world and the outer world was profound and impossible to bridge. When I was in situations that called for me to respond, like conversations with my husband, children, or colleagues, I would try to pay attention, trying desperately to understand what they were saying, and then give up. I became adept at making responses that sounded like I was tracking the conversation even though I wasn't. Most people, most of the time probably thought I was participating in conversation. But I was not participating; "I" was not there; I was in my own head, hearing noise that no one else could hear, finding that noise the only thing I could pay attention to. I could hardly even hear people speak over the noise in my head; even harder was trying to understand what they meant. My husband could see through my attempts to respond to conversation that I could not follow, and he knew something was terribly wrong but did not know how to help me. He said that I had no emotional tone at all. He said that talking with me was like talking with something that had taken over my body but wasn't me. That was exactly what it felt like.

In this zombielike state, setting goals to get better and making choices that would keep me in the external world were impossible. On one hand, I had few desires and little motivation. I did not want to get better, because getting better was inconceivable. I did not want to take action that would keep me in the external world because paying attention to and understanding the world around me was too hard. Therefore, I did not feel motivated to engage in conversation with others, to make plans, to try to accomplish something; I certainly did not feel motivated to take my medication as prescribed. There were things that I "had" to do: I had to teach in order to keep my job, and I had to do basic caretaking of my children. Doing the bare minimum, I wasn't sure if I could maintain sufficient work standards to keep my job, nor did I feel like my caretaking was adequate. My husband picked up a lot of slack, participating in my children's lives in a way that I, barely able to go through the motions, couldn't. I knew I was doing a terrible job with carrying out my home and work responsibilities. Although I felt a little bad that I was letting the people around me down, since I could not feel much of anything, I did not feel terribly bad; mostly the fact that I was letting the people in my life down seemed irrelevant. Everything seemed irrelevant. I felt profoundly untethered from reality.

On the other hand, I was in distress. Frequently the world felt "creepy" to me, like I was in a waking nightmare. The strange ideas in my head (like the idea that the sun was trying to kill me or that my colleagues were out to get me) made me feel confused and persecuted. The incessant noise in my head distracted me from the world outside my head and made paying attention to and understanding what was happening around me nearly impossible. Periodically I heard a voice telling me to kill myself, and as time went on it became harder and harder to ignore. Sometimes when I was trying to interact with others, the voice would narrate what was "really" happening so that I would reinterpret what other people were saying and doing; I could take nothing at face value because everything that I could understand of the world outside my head had other meaning behind it (for example, thinking that other people were stealing my soul). This further distracted me and made me feel more disconnected to the world outside my head. Feeling so much distress, I did have one desire: to feel less distress. I kind of knew that treatment should help, but, immersed in the psychosis, I felt ambivalent about treatment.

Consumed by my inner world, a big part of me was not interested in trying to become less psychotic, so I was not able to take my medication as prescribed consistently. Pained by my disconnection with reality, however, and both suicidal and hearing a voice telling me to kill myself, part of me was in great distress, and this motivated me to seek *some* treatment—to make an appointment with my psychiatrist; to try out a new therapist and, when that didn't work, a second new therapist; to take some of my prescribed medication; to call the crisis hotline repeatedly; eventually to go to the crisis center and ask to be hospitalized. The hard part was being consistent, following through on what my psychiatrist and therapist advised, doing the work that recovery requires. I wanted to suffer less, but I wanted to stay in my inner world—to stay psychotic—too. I did not recognize that I could not have it both ways. Unable to reason properly about what I desired or what I valued, I couldn't see that suffering less was inconsistent with staying psychotic.

Psychosis for me was both self-perpetuating and debilitating. While I was psychotic, I wanted to remain psychotic, even when I was suffering immensely from it. But psychosis destroyed my ability to determine the direction of my life. Thinking about the future and past were impossible, so I was unable to imagine a future life for myself and unable to form desires about what my future life should be like. Being so disconnected from reality, I was unable to recognize what I had once valued as belonging to me. Although I was in distress, I could not imagine what it would be like to not be in distress, never mind how to get there. Unable to determine what was of value or to set goals for myself, I could not deliberate about ends at all. In this state, I was too incompetent to make decisions about my future. I could not formulate goals. I did not value anything in a deep way except the experience of psychosis, and I only valued that because it was the only thing that felt real to me. Of course, I valued my family and my job in an abstract way, but I felt so distanced from these things that they felt like they belonged to, and were valued by, someone else; I recognized that I had once valued these things, and that I ought to value these things, but they no longer felt relevant or real. Lacking a sense of myself as a self, I did not possess a sense of agency. In short, I lacked both the reasoning capacity and the voluntariness required for autonomy.

With a deficient capacity for autonomy, I struggled to make autonomous choices, and since making choices was so difficult, I tried to avoid doing so wherever I could. Finding it easier to just "go with the flow," I went along with whatever the people around me were doing and followed along as if I understood and wanted to do the same. Really, it was the path of least resistance. Lacking self-direction, it was hard for me to do anything on my own. Fearful of not being able to figure out where I needed to go or what I needed to do to get there, I stopped driving anywhere that was outside of my regular daily or weekly routine. Unable to form a desire about what to do, I spent a lot of time either pacing or lying around, covering my ears as if that would quiet the noise in my head. Afraid of not being able to understand what people said and of not being able to figure out how to respond to them, I stopped socializing completely. Unable to be in charge of myself, I experienced extreme stress when I had to be in charge of my kids, especially if we were supposed to go out somewhere. Everything felt so hard, stressful, and scary.

This intense lack of self-direction led to a serious lack of self-trust: I didn't trust myself to be able to figure out what was going on around me and to figure out how to respond to others or what to do in a given situation. This lack of self-trust made me feel very uncertain and ill at ease all the time. Everything I did manage to do was tentative and wavering; I was always on the verge of giving up trying and often did.

Unable to determine what I wanted or to make choices about what to do, I developed a deep dependence on my husband. He is a very self-directed person, always able to figure out what a situation demands of him and always able to rise to the occasion and respond appropriately. He is always able to take charge in a situation, problem-solve, and make determinations with decisiveness. As he was the complete opposite of myself, I relied on him heavily to make the decisions for both of us, to determine what a situation called for and to respond appropriately. Whenever there was a choice that had to be made, I let him do it. Whenever there was something that had to be taken care of, I asked him to do it. Even my regular chores became too overwhelming to do, and he took over some of these (like doing dishes and helping our daughters get ready for bed). If there was a problem that needed fixing (like a broken appliance), I had to ask him to deal with it. In social situations, I had to stay by his side so he could respond to people since I felt incapable of doing so; when he couldn't attend social gatherings (such as some of my work functions), I found myself unable to do so as well. I am well aware of how this dependency fit a stereotype of mentally ill women being needy and dependent on men, but I couldn't help it.[1] I just couldn't organize myself enough to figure out what to do and to make myself go out and do things. Instead, I relied on my husband's self-directedness to direct me as well.

The changes to a person's meaning structure that psychosis often causes can make it very difficult to make choices, especially autonomous choices. In my experience, psychosis created many losses of abilities that are involved with autonomy and decision making, including the abilities to see my choice and action as having an effect on the world, to see myself in the future, to care about the future, to formulate values, to set goals for myself, to figure out how to realize goals, and to form desires that reflected my values. I believe this is true of many people who struggle with psychosis, when their psychosis involves disorganization and loss of meaning structure. Psychotic patients in such a situation often experience significant losses in competence and voluntariness, which make them unable to make choices that can be reflectively endorsed.

Moreover, the self-perpetuating nature of some psychosis exacerbates this difficulty. Living in an ever-present reality of intense internal experiences can make a person too disconnected from the world around them to be able to interact with it and respond to it in a meaningful way. This can interfere with the person's ability to value things that they ought to value and to use that as motivation to act. Psychotic people do make choices and act, of course, as well as form desires and values, but all of these occur *within* psychosis, and within the idiosyncratic meaning system that psychosis creates, and often serve to perpetuate the psychosis rather than to help the person find their way out of it. Stuck within their psychosis, psychotic patients may have difficulty with stepping outside of their present reality to be able to reflect upon that reality and to make judgments about the nature of their circumstances. If they lack the abilities to reflect, judge, and endorse, they cannot develop or maintain a valuation system in which they formulate what is worthwhile based on reasons that they can share intelligibly with others. Thus, while they can make choices in the sense of opting one course of action over another, they sometimes struggle to make autonomous decisions in which they deliberate about what is of value. They may need assistance to develop the autonomy required to make meaningful decisions.

This chapter analyzes the way psychosis can interfere with autonomy and proposes that certain kinds of paternalistic action, namely those which increase a patient's overall autonomy, are often justifiable. First, I explain what autonomy is and what comprises autonomous choice. Then, I show how psychosis can diminish competence and voluntariness, making autonomous choice very difficult, and how the epistemic and moral impairments caused by psychosis can interfere with a person's ability to reflect rationally about ends (values and goals), threatening the general capacity for autonomy. Finally, I argue that when a person cannot act with sufficient autonomy, paternalistic interference is justified as long as the interference increases the general capacity for autonomy. The most justifiable form of interference is when clinicians educate and guide patients to make better choices that further their best interests (including health and well-being), helping patients to develop autonomy by helping them to practice the skills of autonomous decision making through guided choices.

Autonomy

In some circles, the idea that psychosis threatens autonomy and moral agency is uncontroversial. Psychotic illnesses are commonly regarded as potentially exempting a person from moral responsibility because of the way they impair understanding, the formation of beliefs, and rational capacities.[2] In other circles, however, this is not taken as fact. Some philosophers argue that psychosis rarely if ever impairs rationality sufficiently to impair autonomous decision making. For example, George Szmukler claims, "The vast majority of people with a mental illness, even those with a diagnosis of 'serious mental illness,' have capacity for all or most decisions, all or most of the time."[3] Other philosophers argue that the capacity for choice is such an important good that a patient's wishes regarding treatment should be respected at all times, not only when they are rational and sane; Dan Egonsson, for example, argues that it would be "offensive" to heed a person's hypothetical rational desires at the expense of their actual desires even if these are irrational.[4] Advocates of deinstitutionalization and defenders of the "civil rights" of mentally ill patients who unconditionally oppose compelling psychiatric patients to receive treatment against their will argue that psychiatric patients' choices should always be respected, no matter the quality or condition of their choices.[5] In all of these contexts, the choices of mentally ill patients, even psychotic patients, are seen as having significant moral standing that ought to be respected more than they are, and sometimes unconditionally. In these contexts, the choices of mentally ill patients are seen to be sufficiently autonomous to entail respect, regardless of the nature of the choices. Either that or advocates of patient choice in these contexts simply do not care whether patients are autonomous in making their choices. In this chapter, I argue that autonomy is of great importance, but that psychotic patients sometimes lack the conditions required to have significant autonomy. The quality of a person's choice matters, and nonautonomous choices should not always be respected.

Autonomy is self-rule or self-determination: deciding for oneself what kind of life is worthwhile, making choices based on what one finds worthwhile, and taking actions in accordance with these choices. Jodi Halpern defines autonomy as "a psychological capacity to make decisions that reflect one's own goals and an ethical ideal of individual self-determination."[6] Autonomy involves deliberating about ends—about what is valuable and what is worth doing—in a way that is guided by reason.[7] Marina Oshana characterizes the self-determination of autonomy as self-directedness, which involves having the authority to make choices that impact the course of one's life and the power to take action in accordance with these choices.[8] Choices and actions involving health, relationships, career, and civic engagement are examples of areas in which a person tries to direct their life. Being self-directed involves setting goals for one's life based on what a person values, which a person tries to accomplish through their own action.

Autonomy and moral agency[9] are closely related. Autonomy can be understood as the establishment and pursuit of ends (desires, values, and goals) that are truly one's own, inasmuch as they are guided by reason and thus formulated independently of undue external influences. Moral agency is the power to make choices and to act based on reason. Implementing autonomous choices and action successfully requires agency, as a person must have the power to make choices and to act based on reason in order to satisfy their desires and to accomplish goals. Autonomy and agency can come apart, of course: a person can make voluntary and competent choices, which are thus autonomous, that are not actionable when the person lacks the power to implement those choices; and a person can have the power to act and choose based on reasons yet make a nonvoluntary choice based on undue external influences. In general, however, possessing autonomy increases a person's agency, as being able to make choices that are truly one's own enables a person to act in ways that are based on reason, and having agency increases a person's capacity for autonomy, as being able to choose and to act based on reason increases the voluntariness of a choice.

Certain capacities related to moral agency are required for autonomy, including self-efficacy (the belief that one can act successfully to accomplish one's goals or desires) and the capacity to imagine goals in the future.[10] In order to exercise self-efficacy, a person must be able to see that the future is not wholly determined and that the world is responsive to their agency. In addition, in order to be able to choose and act based on a conception of value, a person must be able to conceptualize for themselves future goals that embody what they believe a good life consists of; in order to be successful at this, they must be able to see that their own immediate future is tolerable, and they must be able to imagine implementing their goals efficaciously. Both moral agency and autonomy involve practical reason: agency requires the ability to give reasons for one's choices and actions, while autonomy requires the ability to give reasons for what one values and the ability to justify one's conception of the good life in a way that makes sense to others.[11] If a person can't give reasons that are intelligible to others for their choices, their choices may be unresponsive to counterincentives, in which they lack agency, or they may be unduly influenced by external forces, in which they lack autonomy. Through the regular exercise of autonomous choice, a person develops their character, gives their lives meaning, and exercises moral agency.[12]

Philosophers distinguish between global autonomy, which involves having the general capacity for self-determination, and local autonomy, which involves making specific autonomous choices.[13] These two ideas come apart: a person can have the general capacity for autonomy but fail in certain instances to make autonomous choices; or they can lack the general capacity for autonomy yet make particular choices that are autonomous. Psychotic people sometimes lack the general capacity for autonomy because their psychosis impairs the epistemic and moral capacities required for reflection and valuation. Their choices may be autonomous to different degrees, depending on the degree of competence and voluntariness they have in a given choice; but if they experience epistemic and moral impairments and lack of a sense of agency, this frequently prevents them from making choices that are truly autonomous. In this chapter, I refer mostly to autonomous choice, except in places where it is clear that I am referring to the general capacity for autonomy.

Autonomous Choice

Not just any choice is autonomous. Autonomous choices are those choices that are up to us, that come from our own wills. In order for a choice to be autonomous, it must be adequately voluntary, and it must be made while competent. Competence involves the capability of performing a particular task effectively[14] or having the practical wisdom to carry out certain actions.[15] Competence is assessed within specific domains, so people can be competent at some tasks but not others. In a psychiatric context, the domain of competence that is normally assessed has to do with decision-making capacity, usually regarding treatment. (Competence is sometimes understood as a legal notion of having adequate decision-making capacity, while "capacity" refers to decision-making capacity in a medical context.[16] Philosophers use both words, sometimes interchangeably; because I use the word "capacity" to refer to particular kinds of mental abilities [namely in the context of epistemic and moral capacities], I use the term "competence" here instead of "capacity" or specify that the kind of capacity to which I am referring is decision-making capacity.) If a person is competent, they have adequate decision-making capacity. A person must be competent in order for their choice to be considered autonomous.

Decision-making capacity (or competence) involves many abilities.[17] A person must have the ability to understand, in other words to comprehend intellectually the object of deliberation. They must have the ability to appreciate, meaning that they can apply the relevant facts to their own situation; this involves forming beliefs about how the facts apply. They must have the ability to value, creating a motive for action that, when the relevant facts are applied to their situation, leads to a decision. Finally, they must have the ability to reason, which involves a set of process-related abilities involved with such things as thinking through consequences, seeing how conclusions follow from premises, and thinking through means and ends relationships. Competence is a threshold concept, so a person must possess these abilities to an adequate degree in order for them to be considered to have competence.

In addition to possessing competence, a person must make the choice with sufficient voluntariness in order for the choice to be autonomous. We choose voluntarily when our choices come *from us* and are not coerced by any force external to our will (whether that be a source internal to our bodies, like psychosis, or external to us, like manipulation). As Joel Feinberg says, "Such persons assume a risk in a fully voluntary way if they shoulder it when fully informed of all relevant facts and contingencies, with their eyes wide open, so to speak, and in the absence of all coercive pressure. In the ideal case, there must be calmness and deliberateness . . . no distracting or unsettling emotions, no neurotic compulsion, no misunderstanding. To whatever extent there is compulsion, misinformation, clouded judgment (as for example from alcohol), or impaired reasoning, to that extent the choice falls short of perfect voluntariness."[18] Voluntary choices, in other words, are those that are decided upon through rational deliberation.[19]

Feinberg notes that few if any of our choices are perfectly voluntary, but most of our choices are voluntary enough. Voluntariness, like autonomy and competence, is a threshold conception; people can choose and act with different degrees of voluntariness, but above a certain threshold, we just designate a choice as voluntary regardless of the degree of voluntariness. However, we can still make distinctions between low-voluntary choices, where a person makes a choice based on a first-order desire and so is to some extent one's own, but which is constrained nonetheless by influencing factors that shape the desire and so not fully one's own, and high-voluntary choices, where a person's choice is made under conditions closer to perfect voluntariness, through rational deliberation. When a person is incompetent, their choices are nonvoluntary (if they do not reflect the person's desires) or at most low voluntary (if they do reflect first-order desires). This is because a person who is incompetent is unable to understand, appreciate, value, and/or reason adequately; these impairments make the deliberation required for voluntariness nearly impossible and act as a coercive force that inordinately shapes a person's choice.

Lack of coercion is evidenced by the ability to deliberate about one's choice rationally. The rational deliberation required for autonomous choice can be understood as reflective endorsement. Gerald Dworkin characterizes this reflective endorsement in terms of alignment of lower-level desires and preferences with higher-level desires, preferences, and values, defining autonomy as "a second-order capacity of persons to reflect critically upon their first-order preferences, desires, wishes and so forth and the capacity to accept or attempt to change these in light of higher-order preferences and values."[20] Similarly, Harry Frankfurt defines a free will as the state of having one's first-order desires cohere with one's second-order volitions.[21] Reflective endorsement cannot consist of mere alignment of lower-order and higher-order desires, however. As Gary Watson points out, reflective endorsement must also involve evaluating one's desires according to one's valuational system.[22] A person must be capable of assessing the desires they have based on whether the desires cohere with, and in a sense stem from, their values and goals. They must be capable of affirming their desires as their own by considering whether their desires reflect what they value.

Simply having values and goals that one's desires are based in and that therefore provide some direction to one's life when enacted through choice is not sufficient for autonomy, however. As Danny Scoccia notes, values and goals can fail to be autonomous;[23] if these are nonautonomous, then the desires we form based on these lack autonomy as well. Thus, a person must be capable of reflectively endorsing their values and goals, along with their desires, in order for these to be autonomous. These values and goals need not be acquired through substantive procedural independence, in which they are acquired without any influence from external sources; true procedural independence is nearly impossible to achieve because we are always influenced by a multitude of sources. Moreover, as Gerald Dworkin points out, procedural independence is inconsistent with other values we hold, such as loyalty, objectivity, commitment, benevolence, and love.[24] What is key is that a person can recognize the various influences that affect their choices and reflect on the power of these influences and whether they ought to be followed or not. In the end, a person must be capable of affirming or rejecting values and goals while recognizing the influences that lead a person to have these and revising their choices and behavior based on assessment of their values and goals.

Reflective endorsement may be hypothetical; it need not be actual. Oftentimes people do not in fact trace the sources of their desires, values, and goals and do not deliberate consciously on these. But they must be capable of doing so if they have a reason to do so, for example if something in their experience indicates that it is worth checking to see how autonomous these desires, values, and goals really are. A person must be disposed to endorse their desires, values, and goals if they are to reflect on what they value.

Reflective endorsement involves not just endorsement—affirming the importance of what one values—but also reflection—being able to give reasons for what one desires and values. Not just any reasons will do; reasons based on idiosyncratic meaning, as sometimes occurs in psychosis, are insufficient for this kind of reflection. Reasons must be intelligible, meaning that they *make sense*. Making sense is a relational notion: reasons make sense when they are intelligible *to others*. A reason that makes sense only to oneself does not really make sense. Intelligibility thus involves accountability: it requires that a person can give an account to others that makes sense to those to whom one gives an account. Others do not have to agree with one's views and choices, but they must be able to understand the person's own reasons for why they have these views and make these choices given the particularities of their situation.

Reflective endorsement requires not only the capacity to *give* reasons, but also the capacity to respond to others' reasoning. Andrea Westlund argues that autonomy involves answerability: a person who is autonomous is answerable to others for their choices.[25] Being answerable to others means that one is sensitive to reasons given by others, able to explain why they reject alternative viewpoints and courses of action and able to revise their beliefs and choices when others' reasoning warrants it. Westlund argues that a person must be sensitive to the considerations of others in order to ensure that they are not in the grip of some force that is external to their will. Recognizing reasons given by others, responding to these reasons in an appropriate way, and being willing to change one's views and choices based on these reasons is necessary for a person to be truly reflective about their choices. Through being answerable for their choices, a person is able to authorize their choices as their own and thus reflectively endorse them.

Objecting to this thicker account of the rational requirements of autonomy, Marina Oshana contends that reasons-responsiveness is not necessary for autonomous choice, that the rational conditions for moral agency and autonomy are different.[26] While moral agency requires normative competence, she argues, autonomy requires only prudential or instrumental reasoning. While I agree that full normative competence may not be necessary for autonomy, being receptive to reasons in general is. A person does not need to understand and appreciate the normative dimensions of their choice and the moral norms that they are expected to follow in order to be able to choose autonomously, but they do need to be receptive to different kinds of reasons that have bearing on their choice and to be answerable to others for their choice. Being sensitive to the considerations of others is an important aspect of reflective endorsement, for without the abilities to recognize alternative reasons for action and to be open to revising one's choices based on those reasons, a person cannot truly authorize a choice as their own. Being both answerable to and accountable to others are important aspects of reflectively endorsing a choice as one's own.

Psychotic Constraints on Autonomy

Psychosis can interfere with reflective endorsement and rational deliberation about ends in a number of ways. First, the changes in meaning structure and cognitive dulling that commonly occur with psychosis can lead to losses of epistemic and moral capacities, which in turn create a loss of competence. Epistemic and moral impairments can create difficulties with understanding, appreciating, applying information to oneself, reasoning, and valuing. These impairments can interfere with a person's decision-making ability. Decision making requires forming beliefs: believing that certain things and not others are good. Forming beliefs requires being able to discern, understand, and access the relevant information that beliefs are based upon. If a person's epistemic capacities are impaired, they may have difficulty forming beliefs based on evidence and reason, maintaining beliefs when warranted, and revising beliefs when evidence or reason demands this. If their cognitive capacities are impaired, they may have difficulty with determining what is salient, comprehending relevant information, selecting information based on what is required by a situation, accessing information so that it is available and usable, and recognizing influences that bear on their values and choices. If their rational capacities are impaired, they may not be capable of giving reasons for what they value or capable of being able to engage with other people's reasoning appropriately. Moral impairments may make it impossible for a person to figure out what is worth valuing and what constitutes a good life.

My psychosis certainly impeded my abilities in these areas considerably. Incompetence is contextual: people with psychosis can be incompetent to different degrees and in different ways, depending on the extent to which they possess these abilities in a given context. I was competent to make decisions about what to eat for breakfast but not about whether to participate in treatment. In some cases, I was competent enough to make decisions about what to do in my daily life—I did manage to continue teaching during much of my psychotic period, after all—but in other cases I was not, and this is where I became deeply dependent on my husband for direction in my life.

Second, the loss of a sense of agency that can occur with psychosis creates a loss of voluntariness. Making a choice that is uncoerced by sources external to the will, such as psychosis, requires the ability to deliberate rationally about the object of one's choice and to endorse reflectively what one ultimately chooses. Rational deliberation requires having sufficient epistemic and moral capacities to be able to reflect and value. The impairments identified above all impede rational deliberation.

Rational deliberation about ends also requires that a person has a sense of themselves as agents: that they are able to see that what happens is not wholly determined and that their action has some effect on what happens in the world. They must be able to imagine a future self for which they can formulate future possibilities and be able to envision different goals as possibilities for themselves. They must be able to imagine that states of affairs can be different from the way they currently are, that change is possible, and that their action can enable change. A person cannot deliberate about ends when they do not perceive themselves as a locus of reflection. They cannot be self-reflective when they have no sense of self, and they cannot endorse choices as their own when there is no self that can authorize. Moreover, psychosis can divorce a person from their own desires, so even their first-order desires seem not to come from them. Choices and actions, and even sometimes desires, that occur under these conditions do not stem from a person's will because the person does not experience themselves as having a will; instead, they stem from the psychosis.[27] Because psychotic patients typically lose their sense of subjectivity and agency, they are often unable to deliberate rationally about ends and unable to be self-reflective about what they choose and value, and sometimes unable even to identify first-order desires as their own.

When they lack a sense of themselves as subjects of experience and agents, a psychotic person experiences many of their choices and actions as determined for them by something else. Certainly, I did, as I felt as though experiences and events were happening *to* me rather than feeling that they were something in which I participated actively. If a person is delusional, they might attribute their choices and actions to some other agent, such as the FBI; if the person has some degree of insight, and they recognize they have an illness, they might attribute their choices and actions to their illness. I usually recognized that I had an illness, but I often felt as if something other than myself was making me think, speak, and act in certain ways. Personifying my illness, I attributed the agency of these thoughts and actions to the illness as if the illness had a self of its own that controlled me. Some of my actions were nonvoluntary because they seemed to emanate from a force outside myself that controlled me.

In addition, the way that a patient is situated as a sick person needing treatment can further erode autonomy. When a patient is under the care of clinicians, they are subject to the power of their clinicians in various ways. Being in such a position of vulnerability puts constraints on their agency, narrowing their options for action, and shapes a person's desires and values in a sometimes inordinate way as a patient reacts to their vulnerability and to the power clinicians have over them. In hospitals, where patients are arguably the most vulnerable to the power of others, patients suffer severe constraints on their agency and autonomy as the institution dictates the details of their daily life and, through this, shapes how a person sees and reacts to the world and what they desire and value.

Deliberation is necessary for both autonomy, the establishment of ends of one's own, and agency, the power to choose and to act based on reason, as it is necessary to help a person determine what is of value and set goals for themselves as well as to develop the steps necessary to reach those goals and to act on what they value. In order to have both autonomy and agency, a person must have the ability to give reasons to others and to be willing and able to make adjustments in their choices and action in light of dialogue with others; they must be able to give reasons for what a meaningful life consists of, and they must be able to give reasons for the choices and actions they undertake in the pursuit of their conception of the good. Psychosis can hijack the process of dialogue by posing as the "other" with whom one dialogues, persuading the psychotic person to adopt the vision of the good life that the psychosis dictates and convincing the person to reset their values and goals and the means undertaken to achieve these goals and to act on what is seen to be of value.[28] In this way, psychosis can interfere with both autonomy and agency.

Psychosis can be seen as an encumbrance that piggybacks on a person's will, shaping and changing the person's desires and values in accordance with the dictates of the psychosis.[29] A psychotic person may be able to formulate first-order desires, but these desires may reflect the demands of the psychosis and not necessarily the will of the person independently of their psychosis. By limiting what options are available to a person—what shows up on their deliberative screen, so to speak—the mental impairments caused by psychosis can have a coercive influence, shaping a person's choice unduly and making it hard for other options for action to appear plausible and salient.[30] When psychosis changes the meaning structure of a person's experience of reality and dulls cognitive capacities, it causes impairments in epistemic and moral capacities that diminish a person's competence and voluntariness. When psychosis makes a person lose a sense of themselves as an agent and a subject of experience, it further erodes voluntariness. In these ways, psychosis can cause significant impairments to the capacity of autonomy and make autonomous choice very difficult.

Respecting the Choices of Psychotic Patients

In recognizing that psychosis at least sometimes exempts mentally ill people from moral responsibility, many philosophers accurately understand the way psychosis constitutes an encumbrance or an external force that shapes a person's desires. On the other hand, philosophers, civil rights lawyers, and others who take a psychotic patient's choice at face value and argue that we need to respect any such choice, no matter the content, fail to recognize the way psychosis can impede the reasoning and valuation and sense of agency involved with autonomous choice. Or if they do not fail to recognize it, they fail to think it matters. But it does matter.

When my psychosis told me to not accept more intensive treatment because it did not want to be made to go away, my psychosis was acting upon my will, giving me first-order desires to refuse to participate in certain kinds of treatment that did not cohere with what I would have willed if I had not been psychotic. These desires did not express what I would have willed, if I had been unencumbered, and they did not express what I did will, because, when my psychosis was active, my inability to reason and value appropriately and my inability to experience my desires as coming from myself (stemming from my lack of a sense of self at all) made it so I did not even have an active will. Unable to formulate a conception of the good and unable to deliberate about ends while I was psychotic, I lacked an effective will.

I think I have made it clear that psychosis can interfere with valuation and reflective endorsement in significant ways and thus can undermine a psychotic person's autonomy. We might then ask whether we ought to respect a psychotic person's choices when such choices are not their own in an important sense. My answer is a qualified "yes": under certain circumstances we ought to respect a psychotic person's nonautonomous choices, though under other circumstances we ought not to. We ought to respect a person's nonautonomous choices when they are low-stakes choices and at least to a small degree voluntary, but we ought not respect a person's nonautonomous choices when they are choices in which something highly important is at stake—such as their health. Thus, I support a version of a sliding scale of voluntariness and competence, where the more significant the issue about which one is deliberating, the greater degree of voluntariness and competence is needed for the choice to be respected, at least when the consequences of respecting the choice can be negative and serious. This is because we want to make sure that a person is fully competent before we allow them to accept significant negative risks.[31]

Low-voluntary choices should be respected when they have consequences that are not significantly negative, for in these cases a person is not taking a significant risk with their choice. There is little cost to respecting low-stakes choices, so there is little lost when someone makes a bad choice. Low-voluntary choices on issues of significant consequence, however, should not always be respected, particularly when their consequences are gravely negative and the harm is immediate and avoidable. In areas of great consequence, there can be high costs to making bad choices. Sometimes that cost is not worth the good of respecting the choice. As Danny Scoccia recognizes, commonsense morality dictates that autonomy and beneficence can each trump the other in certain circumstances.[32] In cases of low-voluntary choices on high-stakes issues that have potential negative consequences, concern for a patient's welfare outweighs the value of respecting their choices. Low-voluntary choices should be respected when they are of little consequence, such as choices about what to eat for breakfast or when they have significant positive outcomes, such as choices not to harm oneself, but not when something grave is at stake that can have serious negative consequences, especially where the harm is immediate and avoidable, such as choices to seriously self-injure oneself or to commit suicide. Some of the most serious negative consequences involve choices that restrict freedom of choice by impairing a person's capacity for autonomy.

Some of the significant choices that a psychotic patient makes regarding their recovery are choices about whether to engage in treatment and choices about whether to be present to the shared reality experienced with others. The choice not to engage in treatment can be a choice that is of great significance, since accepting or refusing treatment can make the difference between health and illness. It can have serious negative consequences, some of which may be immediate and avoidable, especially for psychotic patients. Not getting treatment can prolong a patient's psychosis, creating harm to the patient and to the people around them, leading to more uses of crisis and emergency services, causing significant distress, and even causing suicidal behavior. It is important to note that not only does the choice not to engage in treatment impact a person's welfare, but it also can reduce a person's autonomy by allowing psychosis to fester, thus further impairing the person's epistemic and moral capacities and decreasing their sense of subjectivity and agency. Depending on the particular circumstances related to the acuity and severity of the patient's need for treatment, and the immediacy and avoidability of harm, the choice to refuse treatment can be a high-stakes choice with potentially grave consequences.

The choice not to engage in treatment can be voluntary to different degrees. When a person refuses treatment based on intelligible reasons, such as finding side effects of medication intolerable, the person may be making a choice based on values and can reflectively endorse their choice. If the person is sufficiently autonomous, they may be sensitive to others' reasoning about their choice, able to respond to others' reasoning and willing to change their choice if warranted. When a person refuses treatment based on idiosyncratic meaning, however, such as out of a need to obey a voice that tells them not to accept treatment, the person's choice is unduly influenced by their psychosis. The choice does not reflect what they value; they might not even know what they value; but, in any case, they are not capable of reflectively endorsing the choice and thus it is nonautonomous. If the choice reflects a first-order desire, the choice is a low-voluntary choice, but if the choice goes against a first-order desire, or if the person is too detached from their desires to claim the choice as their own (because they lack a sense of subjectivity and agency), the choice is nonvoluntary. In either case, such a choice is nonautonomous; when it can result in significant harm, it ought not be respected.

It is not only choices about engaging in treatment—taking medication as prescribed, participating in therapy, practicing the skills learned in therapy—that matter, but also the everyday choices about whether to be present to the reality surrounding a person. Recovery involves choosing over and over again to show up and be present and to participate in life activities, to not get swept up by the strange sensations and special meanings that psychosis brings, and to resist voices that tell a person what to do. Recovery involves constantly making choices about how to perceive and construct one's reality and how to respond to and interact with that reality. Participating actively in recovery requires a person to make these choices deliberately and intentionally. Choices to succumb to psychosis are nonvoluntary or low voluntary, shaped by the psychosis itself, and must be addressed in therapy so the person can learn how to make more voluntary, and thus more autonomous, choices. Choices to resist psychosis require a person to exercise their reasoning, appreciating, and valuing capacities to a greater degree than they might have thought possible. Strengthening one's ability to resist psychosis thus requires increasing one's autonomy.

Increasing Autonomy

Autonomy is intrinsically valuable because it is partly constitutive of what it is to be an agent, to have a character, and to be a person.[33] Respecting autonomy is paramount because it is a way of respecting the dignity of persons.[34] Respecting autonomy involves respecting the authority a person has "to demand that they be allowed to make their own choices and lead their own lives," as Stephen Darwall says.[35] Even when people make bad choices—choices that do not further their best interests, choices that do not reflect what they take to be their good—as long as these choices are to some extent voluntary, these should be respected to the extent possible because this is an important aspect of respecting individuals as persons.

When people make choices that are not autonomous, it is harder to see why these should be respected. Choices that do not reflect a person's will or that do not reflect any reflected-upon values at all cannot be authorized by a person, and thus these choices cannot be considered an expression of the person's character. Low-voluntary choices—those that reflect a person's desires but may be heavily constrained by a force external to the will, such as psychosis—may be worth respecting because they express some of the person's desires, even if they cannot be reflectively endorsed. In such cases, the patient's welfare and the good of respecting their low-voluntary choice must be weighed, and choices that do not significantly impair their welfare should be honored, while choices that do significantly damage their welfare should not be. Nonvoluntary choices—those that do not reflect a person's own desires—need not be respected because they do not come from the person in a meaningful way. Honoring these choices would therefore not be respecting the person making them. When a person is not capable of making sufficiently voluntary choices—choices that are voluntary enough to constitute autonomous choices—in some important area of their life, such as their health and well-being, paternalistic interference may be necessary to help the person increase their autonomy.

Since directing one's life in the way one desires is such an important part of being human, autonomy should be increased wherever possible so that people have greater control over the various areas of their life that matter to them. According to a maximization principle of autonomy, decisions are good when they promote greater autonomy.[36] For people who lack autonomy, such as psychotic patients, increasing overall autonomy may require paternalistically interfering with a person's low-voluntary choices in order to put the person in a better position to be able to make more and better choices in the long run.

Some of a psychotic patient's choices can severely limit the patient's free-dom by prolonging their psychosis, so the psychosis has greater influence on their choices and there is less room for the patient to develop their own freely willed desires about what they want; choices that keep the patient psychotic, such as choices not to participate in treatment, maintain the coercive influence of psychosis on the patient's will in this way. Choices that severely limit the patient's freedom by exacerbating psychosis are arguably low-voluntary or nonvoluntary choices: made under the coercive influence of psychosis, whether or not they reflect first-order desires. When others interfere paternalistically with a psychotic patient's low-voluntary or non-voluntary choices to prolong psychosis, the patient's low-level freedom is curtailed in the short term by short-circuiting their low-voluntary or non-voluntary choices; in the long term, however, such interference gives the patient the opportunity to increase high-level freedom by increasing volun-tariness and by enabling the patient to develop the capacity for autonomous choice. As Danny Scoccia argues, it is better to have one's high-autonomy desires be satisfied than have one's low-autonomy desires be satisfied.[37]

It is justifiable to interfere paternalistically with a person's low-voluntary or nonvoluntary choice, such as a choice not to engage in treatment, when such interference increases overall autonomy and allows the person to make choices with greater autonomy. Paternalistic interference when a person is incompetent or cannot make sufficiently voluntary choices constitutes soft paternalism.[38] Paternalistic interventions that cause a patient to take medi-cation as prescribed, for example, can help the patient think more clearly; over time, being able to think more clearly will help the patient to increase their epistemic and moral capacities, and thus increase their competence and voluntariness, thereby increasing their autonomy. When a patient can think more clearly over the long-term, they increase their ability to value, developing capacities to evaluate different goods, weigh different values, and formulate a conception of the good that provides reasons for action. Then they can make treatment decisions that reflect a valuation system and that can be reflectively endorsed, for which they can give intelligible reasons and about which they can engage with other people's reasoning. Through this, they can be receptive and responsive to clinicians' reasoning about the value of engaging in treatments that promote their health and well-being. They can consider valuing health and well-being themselves and make decisions in accordance with these values. Such choices are truly autonomous choices. Paternalistic interference can be critical in helping patients develop the autonomy to make autonomous decisions about their treatment.

What kind of paternalistic interference is employed matters. Paternalistic interference can include everything from educating and guiding patients to make informed decisions to coercing patients through incentives, negative consequences, or even force. The danger of paternalistic interventions is that they can thwart a person's autonomous choice when their choice is autonomous, or they can subject a person to epistemic injustice when such interventions are not based on reasons that would be intelligible to the person if the person were competent. When the goal is to increase overall autonomy, paternalistic interventions should be the least restrictive means of getting a patient to change their behavior as possible,[39] and they should be decided upon based on reasons the person, if competent, would be able to endorse or at least understand. This means that clinicians should use education, guidance, and encouragement to help patients make better decisions about their well-being rather than forcing patients to take medication, to show up to life activities, or to otherwise engage in treatment, at least most of the time. Clinicians should teach patients to do the reasoning and valuing involved in making autonomous choice and guide patients to formulate their own conceptions of the good and to make choices based on this. Through education, skills building, guidance, and encouragement, clinicians can help patients develop the internal motivation to remain engaged in treatment, based on a recognition of this as furthering their own good over the long term. Helping patients to participate actively in their treatment helps patients to stay committed to their recovery and to make decisions continuously that further their health interests.

Patients learn to do the reasoning and valuing involved in making autonomous choice by practicing these. For this reason, it is important to allow patients to make choices wherever possible, in a range of areas in their life, so they can practice the act of making a choice. Respect for low-voluntary choices whenever little of significance is at stake (low-stakes choices) or when the consequence of such a choice is positive is important for all of the reasons that autonomous choices are important, including that it makes a person feel happy or fulfilled to have their desires satisfied and that it allows a person to have more control over their life. But it is also important for another reason: respecting low-voluntary choices helps people to develop greater voluntariness and autonomy. When people make choices that are respected by others, their act of choosing and the freedom involved with that choosing is validated and encouraged. It is important that people continue to make choices because it is through the process of exercising the capacities involved with making choices—including reasoning and valuing capacities—that people get better at using these capacities and so learn to make better, more autonomous choices. As Aristotle pointed out millennia ago, we develop virtues and capacities by practicing them.[40]

Practicing making autonomous choices is necessary for developing greater autonomy, but it is not sufficient. We can make low-voluntary choice after low-voluntary choice and never develop enough epistemic and moral capacities and sense of agency to be able to make highly competent and voluntary choices. In addition to having the opportunity to practice making autonomous choices, therefore, we must have some guidance on how to make such choices. A psychotic person may be unable to develop reasonable beliefs without someone showing them the unreasonableness of their delusions. They may be unable to break out of their inadequate reasoning capacities unless someone helps them to recognize reasons, to see means-ends relationships, and to follow a logical argument. They may be unable to sit back and reflect on what they value, forming desires based on whims, impulses, or perceived coercion (for example, based on a voice telling them what to do), until someone helps them to discern what they value, based on reason, and to use what they value as reasons for action. Patients need guides to help them practice these capacities *well*. This is one of the most crucial roles that mental health professionals play in the therapeutic relationship: acting as guides to help patients practice the various capacities involved with autonomous choice so they can learn how to make autonomous decisions and so they can develop greater autonomy.

Developing autonomy is important not only for being able to make treatment decisions and practical decisions that further one's best interests, but also for addressing some of the existential aspects of recovery. Recovery from a chronic, severe illness is usually not a linear process of treating the illness and then becoming better; often, recovery is a circular or spiral process of getting better at times but also getting sick again at other times and having to deal with some of the same issues repeatedly. For many patients, recovery involves putting psychosis into remission for a while until life circumstances or changes in brain chemistry unleash it again. Because I have lived with bipolar disorder for most of my adult life, I regard my own sickness to be episodic as I cycle through periods of illness and wellness. One of the central questions that patients face in recovery, therefore, is how to live a good life despite the possibility of remaining sick, or of getting sick again.[41] Being able to address this question requires being able to determine what is of value and to deliberate about how to live a worthwhile life given one's constraints. Possessing the capacities involved with autonomy is necessary to be able to do this kind of deliberation.

Developing the capacity for self-directedness and self-determination requires practicing making choices so that a person can develop their capacities for competence and voluntariness, and ultimately for reflective endorsement, more deeply. When people become better at making choices that reflect their values, for which they can give intelligible reasons and which are responsive to the considerations of others, they become better at deciding how they want to live their lives and directing their lives to be the way they want their lives to be. They are better able to set goals for themselves and to figure out what to do to realize their goals. Paternalistic interference when patients lack the capacity to make autonomous choice is justified but only for the sake of increasing autonomy so patients can make better decisions on their own. The kind of interference best justified in this context is education and guidance. Clinicians play an important role in guiding patients to make autonomous choices that reflect their best interests.

Conclusion

When I was psychotic, I lost my ability to be an autonomous adult. This made me feel alien within my roles as professor, spouse, and parent. Although I inhabited roles that involved being in charge of things, I was not capable of being in charge of myself. I was supposedly in a position of authority with respect to my students and my children, but I could not authorize my own actions. While the symptoms of my psychosis made it hard for me to teach, interact with my colleagues, and take care of my children, being alienated from my social roles exacerbated this difficulty. It is hard for a person to teach and work with colleagues when the person avoids interpersonal interactions or when they cannot follow conversations easily.

It is even harder when they lose the capacity for self-determination and do not feel like their actions are their own.

The deep dependence on my husband that I had developed changed the dynamic of our relationship: I was no longer an equal partner to my husband. He did not like this, but he knew it couldn't be helped. He took charge of the things I needed him to take charge of and supported me as best as he could. My husband has an infinite amount of patience to be able to deal with long periods in my life when I have not been okay, or anything close to "normal," and somehow, he always waits patiently for the real me to come back. After struggling with psychosis for many months, I despaired that the real me would never reemerge, and that I would be a shell of a person for the rest of my life. He had enough faith and trust in the world, and in my ability to deal with my problems, to believe that things could get better.

It was not until I was on sufficient antipsychotic medication that the gap between my mind and the external world could be bridged, and I could interact with others normally again. Once my perception of reality changed, I was able to see more clearly what my needs and interests were and see that health and well-being were important goods to strive for. When I could see this more clearly, I was able to make choices about what to do that were in my best interests, and it became easier to ignore the voice that told me to go down on my medication and stay committed to treatment. As my reasoning and valuing capacities improved, I became better at deliberating about what I ought to do, and my choices became more autonomous. After several months of taking a sufficiently high dose of antipsychotic medication, I could make choices that felt like my own. Years of being psychotic left me distrusting my ability to be self-directing, however. It was only after a full year of recovery that I started to trust myself, having faith in my ability to follow conversations, to interact with people appropriately, to deal with problems, and generally to know what to do in whatever situation I found myself. Only after a year of feeling better was I able to take charge of more aspects of my life and do activities without leaning so much on my husband. Finally, I was able to exercise some self-directedness.

Being able to direct our lives in the way we desire is an important aspect of being human. Psychotic patients who do not know how they want their lives to go because they cannot formulate ends of their own or who cannot direct their lives in ways that they value lose out on an important aspect of being human. For this reason, one of the goals of treatment should be to restore autonomy in psychotic patients. Psychotic patients need to learn how to formulate ends for themselves and to practice valuing and reasoning so they can choose values, goals, and desires and reflect on their choices in a way that allows them to endorse or revise their choices. Developing positive therapeutic relationships in which patients can do this psychological work is important. Having the right kinds of relationships with one's clinicians and actively participating in treatment enables the development and exercise of agency and autonomous decision making that promote one's health and well-being.

Clinicians play an important role helping patients to develop these capacities within the context of a positive therapeutic relationship built on trust and empathy. I explore these in chapters 4 and 5. Patients learn to develop these capacities in part by engaging actively in various practices related to recovery, including giving testimony, making meaning of their experiences, and making choices about their treatment. I explore these in later chapters. In the next chapter, I explore the basis of the therapeutic relationship by looking at what it means to medicalize mental illness and to be in the sick role.

3 Patient

Introduction

Being hospitalized was a game changer. Up until that point, I was struggling with symptoms that I didn't understand, wondering if I was psychotic but not having a framework to make sense of my experiences. I was not yet a mental patient: I was a client who consulted mental health professionals, as if my problem was something that could be resolved with periodic consultations. But my problem was too deep to be resolved at that level. More intensive treatment was necessary.

Before hospitalization, I felt like I was on the lam, running away from something that was pursuing me and trying to get away with living with my psychosis unabated. Part of me did not want the psychosis to go away. Immensely compelling, the psychosis dominated my life: it colored all of my experiences and opened the door to a mesmerizing world of strange sensations and special meaning; it told me what to do; it shaped my experience, feelings, thoughts, and actions. By living with my psychosis, I felt like I was getting away with something that I knew I ought not to be getting away with; holding onto and pursuing my psychosis felt illicit, and thus exciting.

But at the same time that I was having a thrilling adventure, I was utterly falling apart. The voice telling me to kill myself, the incessant noise in my head, my general confusion about what was going on around me, my difficulty understanding people—these were all untenable. It got to the point where I simply could not go into the classroom, and I just could not take care of my children. My suicidal ideation grew acute, and I realized I needed serious help, or I was going to make an attempt on my life. Scared of what changes this would bring, I went to the crisis center and asked to be hospitalized.

I knew that once I turned myself in, there would be no more running on the lam. There would be no more days watching the sun's rays cascading across the sky and setting my internal experience according to the quality of sunlight that emanated down. There would be no more days of hiking, looking for birds, trying to outrace and calm down the jumbled, speedy, confusing thoughts in my head. There would be no more days of seeking out secret messages embedded within songs and obeying their commands. Once I let myself receive more intensive treatment, my pursuit of psychotic experience was going to have to stop. Medication would dull my experiences, and intensive medical attention would dominate my time and energy, replacing the force of the psychosis. Finding solace in the very thing that was trying to kill me, I was scared to let go of the way psychosis dominated my life and scared to enter a new chapter of experience. But it was bound to come to an end anyway, as had I not sought out more intensive treatment, I surely would have made a suicide attempt.

Once I was hospitalized, the experiences of strange sensations and special meanings became firmly medicalized. I was given a diagnosis (bipolar I disorder, depressive episode with psychotic features) that for the first time used the word "psychotic" to describe my experiences. All of my wondering about what I was experiencing became encapsulated in a word: "psychosis." During some of my previous manic and depressive episodes, I had had what I consider psychotic experiences, but no one had ever used that word to describe them. Even when I asked my psychiatrist and the first therapist I saw briefly in early spring if I was psychotic, they would not confirm this. The therapist said I had too much insight to be psychotic. My psychiatrist focused more on the depression. But they only saw me when I was struggling with the psychotic depression. Since I never saw any mental health professionals during the fall after I had my initial psychotic break in August 2017, no one saw what I was like before I became depressed, so they did not see the psychotic episode that did not accompany a mood change. It was easier to focus on the depression and anxiety than to concede I had psychosis. And so, when I was finally given a diagnosis that used that word, it felt like a huge relief to finally have a framework to understand my experiences, and, at the same time, it felt overwhelming. "Psychosis" is not a word we use lightly; I wondered what the significance was of identifying my experiences as psychotic.

Why were my clinicians reluctant to identify my experiences as psychotic? I suspect it was because they were not ready to medicalize my experiences. Labeling my experiences as psychotic would make my experiences seem much worse and more significant than not labeling them this way would. It would open a whole new set of treatment options, including antipsychotic medication (instead of just mood stabilizers) and various crisis management tools. It would potentially subject me to more intensive treatment, including hospitalization and intensive outpatient therapy. It would position me more firmly as a mental patient and not simply as a client who sometimes consulted professionals. I suspect that the fact that I am moderately successful in my life—being a professor, wife, and mother—made clinicians reluctant to assign a label to me that is usually reserved for people too sick to have these kinds of successes. I did not seem sick enough, at least not consistently. When they saw me as a professor, they were biased against seeing me as a sick person. It was just too hard to imagine that someone who was a professional could be that sick.

And yet I was. I don't know how I managed to continue to function so well despite my illness. The fact that my job is extremely flexible helped a lot. There were only certain hours when I had to be organized enough to be able to be in charge: just while I was in the classroom or in meetings. During other hours I could, and frequently did, fall apart. Even as I was falling apart, somehow, I was able to do most of what was expected of me despite the fact that I was having strange sensations and obeying orders. The fact that my psychosis wanted me to hide it helped. It often told me to try to act normal so no one would know it was there. It wanted to stay in control, and it knew it could only do that if no one knew it was there. The psychosis caused too many problems with my cognition, understanding, and reasoning to stay completely hidden; it bled out when I reached the limitations of what I could do. But it allowed me to function to some extent, so it was easy to fool people into thinking I was not that sick. My general success in functioning is probably what made mental health professionals reluctant to identify my experiences as psychotic for so long.

Hospitalization positioned me incontrovertibly as a sick person. Once I was hospitalized, I was no longer a client who sometimes consulted with professionals for help with a problem; I had a problem that took over my life and needed intensive treatment to try to resolve. Hospitalization in no way cured me, and I needed to continue intensive treatment in order to continue addressing both the suicidal ideation and the psychosis. Hospitalization, and the serious diagnosis I was given, opened the door for further intensive treatment, including the intensive outpatient program in which I participated on and off for months. My diagnosis opened the door to different medications to try. In medicalizing the extraordinary experiences I had been having, hospitalization and a new diagnosis changed the orientation of my life so I was no longer on the lam trying to get away with being psychotic for as long as possible but now trying to address the psychosis and suicidal ideation so it would not rule my life. The medicalization of my experiences put new meaning on my experiences, locating them within a medicalized framework that changed the way I was living and opened doors to more effective treatment.

In this chapter, I explain how mental illness experience is often medicalized, positioning patients as recipients of mental healthcare treatment by their clinicians. I argue that psychiatric disability in the context of certain types of psychosis should be viewed as both medical and social, because patients often experience objective harms that make it an appropriate target of medical treatment, and patients also experience harms caused by the way their illness is treated by society. Patients tend to occupy a sick role in which they are relieved of certain responsibilities, but these are replaced with the primary responsibility of trying to get better. I explore the way that patients' situatedness as sick people affects their identity and how treatment can help increase the agency and autonomy that illness hinders. Medicalization can thus be very helpful to at least some patients.

Medicalization of Mental Illness Experience

The concept of a mental patient is controversial because it frames a person's experience firmly in biomedical terms, regarding mental illness experience as symptoms of a disorder: pathological and in need of treatment. It also presumes a level of passivity in being a recipient of treatment. In framing a person's experience in biomedical terms, the concept of a mental patient supports a medicalized view of mental illness as sickness.

The idea of mental illness experience as sickness comes into existence as a result of medicalization, or putting behavior, experience, or bodies under medical control. By designating certain people as sick, the medical system exercises social control. Some of the ways that medicalization exercises social control is through medical ideology, collaboration, technology, medical excusing, and medical surveillance.[1] Medical ideology in a mental health context means conceptualizing psychological distress in terms of mental disorders: disorders of the brain that are abnormal and pathological and in need of treatment. Collaboration occurs when medical professionals work together to produce and disseminate medical knowledge as they carry out their roles within the medical or mental health system. Medical technology includes the use of psychotropic medications to change brain chemistry and the use of technologies like electroconvulsive therapy, deep brain stimulation, and digital medicine; medical technology can even involve the use of therapies such as cognitive behavioral therapy, dialectical behavioral therapy, and acceptance and commitment therapy. Medical excusing concerns the way mental health conditions can excuse people from various responsibilities, which I shall explain more below in discussing the sick role. Medical surveillance involves the way medical professionals adopt the medical gaze to examine all aspects of the relevant health condition, even if the aspects are only indirectly relevant. Mental health professionals practice medical surveillance when they suggest that patients make lifestyle changes to promote their mental health, such as exercise, or when they ask patients to track their experience, such as through a mood journal, or when they assess the impact of patients' various activities on their mental health condition.

We often use the term "medicalization" in a normative context to refer to problematic cases of medicalization, namely overmedicalization or inappropriate medicalization, when conditions are wrongly regarded as pathological and requiring medical treatment. Conditions such as depression,[2] chronic fatigue syndrome,[3] premenstrual syndrome,[4] autism,[5] eating disorders,[6] and attention-deficit/hyperactivity disorder[7] have been critiqued as overmedicalized or inappropriately medicalized. In many cases, this inappropriate medicalization has the effect of obscuring the social and political conditions that lead to the condition or that cause the condition to be interpreted as pathological.[8] The motives for such overmedicalization or inappropriate medicalization are typically capitalist, involving the creation of industries devoted to addressing these conditions as problems of the individual rather than as social problems. In viewing conditions solely as problems of the individual rather than as social problems, medicalization can obscure the social problems that lead to these conditions, for example the oppression of women in many cultural contexts that leads to experiences of depression.[9] This obscuration has the potential to perpetuate oppression of marginalized groups of people whose voices are typically ignored, such as women or children,[10] and exploitation and domination of people who have relatively little power, such as people with developmental disabilities. Medicalization is often critiqued through a normative assessment that analyzes the problematic power relationships and dangerous social control that occur in the process of medicalization.

While medicalization is a term often used in a negative context, implying that medicalization is always bad, it is in fact morally neutral and refers simply to the process of treating behavior, experience, or bodies as pathological and requiring medical treatment. There is nothing inherently wrong with "medicalization"; many behaviors, experiences, and bodies are rightly regarded as pathological and needing medical treatment. Medicalization can in fact be beneficial in many ways.

First, medicalization can be epistemically beneficial, providing a useful framework for understanding experience as well as a way of dealing with its adversity.[11] Rather than obscuring power relations and methods of social control, medicalization can be a way of naming experience, of identifying it as a thing and giving it a conceptual framework that enables one to make sense of it. This increases understanding of the experience, which can lead to better means of addressing it, including opening the doors to more effective treatment. Other benefits of medicalization are that it can provide connection and access to resources. In naming and identifying experience, a person can find others who share the same or similar experiences and connect with others on that basis. Medicalization also enables a person to have access to resources to address the experience—such as through medical treatment—that they did not have before. In addition, medicalization can help secure other types of resources such as government aid or access to opportunities such as accommodations that enable participation in the workforce.

Moreover, medicalization can be beneficial in providing social power to people. Medicalization can "demarginalize" groups of people who have had trouble with access to resources and social support.[12] While medicalization can perpetuate injustices when it obscures social and political problems that result in the health conditions that get medicalized, it can also create justice for previously marginalized people who gain recognition, a voice, legitimacy, and authority through medicalization of their condition. For some people, recognition of their condition as pathological can confer legitimacy to their experience, granting them epistemic credibility and moral authority in areas related to their condition. While medicalization can sometimes be harmful, therefore, it can also sometimes be very beneficial.

Consider the effects of diagnosis. While some people diagnosed with a mental disorder object to their diagnosis, not wanting to be "labeled" or not wanting their experiences to be "categorized" ("put in a box"), others find some relief in being diagnosed. For these people, diagnosis is a form of recognition and confers legitimacy to their symptoms.[13] By providing hermeneutical resources to patients, it gives them a framework for understanding their experience, enabling hermeneutical justice, or the epistemic justice that results from being able to understand one's situation. Diagnosis externalizes the problem that a person is experiencing, giving them epistemic credibility regarding their condition,[14] and makes it clear that the person is not responsible for it.[15] Furthermore, diagnosis offers a way to address their symptoms through treatment. Diagnosis can be both empowering and disempowering: while it can invite stigma, it can also confer legitimacy, provide epistemic benefit, and grant access to treatment.[16]

In my own experience, receiving a diagnosis for my psychotic experiences was a huge relief. A year after hospitalization, the diagnosis I received in the hospital became inadequate. That diagnosis identified what I was going through at the time as an episode of bipolar disorder with psychotic features. But months later, I was struggling with psychosis without corresponding mood change. Neither depressed nor manic, I did not find the diagnosis of bipolar disorder to capture what I was going through. After struggling with psychosis for the better part of two years, I knew the psychosis was not part of my bipolar disorder but something else. I wanted my psychiatrist to recognize my experience for what it was, so I didn't have to feel like I was constantly trying to convince him of what I was going through. By this time, I believed that I had schizoaffective disorder, which means that on top of manic, depressive, and mixed episodes, I also have episodes of psychosis without corresponding mood change. He did not think I "look like" I have a schizophrenia-spectrum disorder, however. (I am not sure what he meant by that, but I believe he meant that I am too high functioning.) Since my psychiatrist did not think my symptoms fit any of the standard psychotic disorders, he diagnosed me with psychotic disorder not otherwise specified. Knowing that the bipolar disorder did not explain the psychosis, I was relieved to have this diagnosis as it provided a framework for understanding my experience, however vague it was. It allowed me to say, "I have a psychotic disorder" rather than saying (as I had been) "I think I have schizoaffective disorder" or "I have been struggling with psychosis the past two years" and wondering if my psychiatrist thought I was making the whole thing up. Having a diagnosis was a form of recognition of my symptoms and conferred legitimacy to my experience.

Some people who have experiences and behaviors typically viewed as mental illness symptoms object to the medicalization of such experience, arguing that rather than viewing mental health differences as necessarily pathological and requiring treatment, we should instead understand them as "mere differences,"[17] nothing more than deviations from a socially constructed norm. This view has its roots in the neurodiversity movement, which regards features of autism as "mere differences" in functioning rather than as impairments,[18] and the antipsychiatry movement, which regards treatment of mental illness to be more detrimental than mental illness itself. Some of the peer support movement for experiences like voice hearing supports this view, too. Some advocates for the Hearing Voices Network, for instance, argue that hearing voices is natural, not pathological, and that people are distressed by their voices primarily because society dictates that they should not be hearing voices.[19]

The idea that mental health differences are "mere difference" fits the social model of disability, which sees disability as problems of functioning caused by the way social structures are organized.[20] This is in contrast to the medical model of disability, which sees disability as biological impairments that ought to be fixed or ameliorated. In a psychiatric context, the social model of psychiatric disability sees problems of functioning as the result not of illness symptoms, but rather of social structures that make it hard for people with mental illness symptoms such as psychosis to gain or maintain employment, housing, and social relationships.[21] According to this view, if we were to arrange social structures differently to support people with severe mental illness symptoms more effectively, they would be able to function better. In addition, the social model of disability views psychological distress as deviation from socially constructed norms about how we should feel and experience the world, such as norms around feeling happy or calm, or being productive. According to this view, if we were to change our norms about what we should experience and feel, we would not view distress as disabling or find ourselves disabled by our distress. Advocates of a social model of disability object to the norming that occurs in a medical model of disability that regards some ways of being as inherently impairing and to the power and control this model grants to the medical establishment.[22]

While the social model of disability helpfully recognizes the limitations society puts on people with mental illness, it is inadequate by itself to account for and address certain types of harm many people with severe mental illness experience. The medical model of disability better accounts for and addresses this harm by recommending medicalized responses like medication and therapy that more directly address this harm. In contrast to the social model of disability, the medical model of psychiatric disability views problems with functioning as resulting directly from mental illness symptoms and views distress as a symptom or a natural reaction to one's symptoms. The idea that society should be organized in a way that supports people with severe mental illness is wholly consistent with this model as an effort to ameliorate people's impairments.[23] Unlike the social disability model, however, this model does not view social structures as the primary *causes* of people's impairment. Rather, the causes of impairment are the problems with biological and/or psychological functioning that constitute mental illness symptoms.[24] Impairment is thus seen as objective harm.[25] In this model, treatment is essential, commonly consisting of both medication and therapy, in order to treat the biological aspects of mental illness and the psychosocial factors that both contribute to and arise from illness. Thus, having expert care and a positive relationship with clinicians who can help increase the patient's agency, autonomy, and level of functioning, and help the patient make meaning of their experience and participate in their own recovery, is critical.

Objectively harmful impairments occur independently of how a person feels about their mental illness symptoms, and many of them are caused directly by illness, not by social structures. Some people who do not feel distress at hearing voices, for example, nonetheless lose the ability to engage with others meaningfully, deeply, and consistently. Regardless of how people feel about their voices, and whether they are distressed by them or not, for many people voice hearing is part of a larger distortion of meaning that removes a person from shared reality into their own private, idiosyncratic world, making social interaction difficult and impairing functioning of various kinds. This constitutes objective harm independently of how they feel about it (whether they feel distress about it or not). This loss is due directly, at least in part, to a person's mental illness symptoms, regardless of how they are treated by others or how society is structured. People with mental illness in fact experience many losses constituting objective harms due directly to their illness, as noted in chapter 1. The medical model of psychiatric disability can account for and address this objective harm in a way that the social model cannot.[26]

According to some in the neurodiversity movement, a mental illness like schizophrenia is not necessarily harmful when it is integrated into a person's identity and so is not necessarily pathological and in need of treatment. Robert Chapman argues that when an illness is integral to a person's self-identity, it should not be seen as harmful dysfunction but rather as mere difference. But the logic behind this argument is unclear. Our personal identity and sense of self change all the time in relation to what happens to us; why should we preserve the schizophrenic self if we can flourish better with a different self? Even if a person suffering from psychosis somehow identifies with their psychosis, and even if they like their psychosis, this is not enough of a reason to hold onto the psychosis if the psychosis is also causing significant objective harm. If a person's identity and sense of self change with the alleviation of psychosis, such change is not necessarily a bad thing if the person can consequently live a better life. What matters is what kind of life a person has with or without their psychosis. It is better to have a life that includes meaningful relationships and activities than one that is dominated by illness, if one has a choice.

The psychiatric disability associated with certain types of psychosis is best understood through both medicalized and social lens. The social model of disability helpfully points out that some of the difficulties that individuals with severe mental illness face have a social basis and must be addressed through social means. Social factors like poverty and marginalization[27] can play a role in contributing to psychosis by creating high levels of stress to which some people react by becoming psychotic. In addition, the ways that other people interact with individuals who are vulnerable to psychosis can trigger symptoms in them: people feel despair and distress when they are misunderstood and when their needs and interests are not taken into account; such distress can trigger or exacerbate psychotic symptoms. As the social model of disability recommends, social structures should be arranged differently to promote the flourishing of people with severe mental illness, such as through fostering greater social interaction between those with severe mental illness and the general population.[28] For those who experience objective harms caused directly by their mental illness symptoms, however, medicalization of their condition is also appropriate. The psychiatric disability involved with certain types of psychosis is best addressed both medically and socially.

Medicalization, Power, and Vulnerability

Medicalization of mental illness experience is important and necessary in many instances, but it also carries great risks. It can be empowering, enabling the patient to receive treatment from experts who can discern what treatment is appropriate to a particular patient's situation so the patient can get better and live a normal, healthy life. At the same time, it positions the mental patient at the mercy of clinicians who determine what treatment is appropriate, sometimes treatment that the patient does not wish. In positioning patients this way, medicalization creates a power dynamic in which the clinician holds considerable power over the patient and the patient holds very little power (and often perceives themselves to hold no power) in the relationship. This makes the patient vulnerable in many ways.

In subjecting patients to the power of mental health professionals, the medicalization of mental illness makes patients vulnerable to the various uses of power by clinicians. Medicalization is inherently paternalistic, in that the clinician role requires clinicians to act in their patients' best interests, ideally with the patient's consent, but sometimes not (when patients are unable to give meaningful consent). Clinicians have ultimate say in what kind of treatment patients are allowed or not allowed to have (at least within a medical context), so patients are subject to whatever treatment options are made available by the provider. By circumscribing patients' choice in this way, clinicians have control over what happens to patients. Patients often feel powerless in relation to this, particularly when they are given little or no opportunity to voice their opinion about their situation. Clinicians can exert pressure on patients to comply with their treatment recommendations; when this happens, patients may feel coerced into going along with their clinicians' decisions. With this pressure, patients can feel as if they are subject to threats or punishment if they do not comply with what is expected of them. While the threat of punishment is more likely a matter of patient perception rather than a fact about what clinicians do, it shows the vulnerability patients feel in response to the power clinicians have over them.

Some of what happens in the clinical encounter constitutes what outside of the clinical encounter would be an invasion of privacy. This infringement on privacy is justified as part of the way the clinician has to get to know the patient as a patient, but it nonetheless makes patients very vulnerable. Patients have to reveal the inner workings of their minds for clinicians to see what is happening to them internally; sometimes this involves sharing information about oneself one would rather keep private, even secret. In some clinical encounters, patients have to expose their bodies by disrobing. While this is less common in a mental healthcare context than in an ordinary healthcare context, it still sometimes occurs. For example, when I was hospitalized, I had to disrobe completely during the intake session so nurses could check my body for markings and scars. I felt utterly vulnerable.

Patients are also vulnerable to experiencing a loss of credibility and authority in relation to clinicians and are vulnerable to being misunderstood by clinicians. Clinicians have automatic credibility and authority by virtue of their professional role. In relation to this, patients have very little credibility and authority and often have to prove themselves to be credible because the default assumption about mental patients in particular is that they are discreditable by virtue of their mental illness. Because they are typically viewed as unreliable reporters and as incapable of participating meaningfully in many epistemic activities, mental patients are often not taken seriously by clinicians and their needs and interests are not taken into account sufficiently. Moreover, because their mental illness symptoms can affect their communication abilities and style, they are easily misunderstood. When clinicians do not make the effort to understand the perspective and experiences of their patients, they risk misunderstanding their patients, making patients feel as if they are not being seen or heard. I discuss this more in chapter 6.

Patients may experience a range of responses to the power differential between them and clinicians, including enthusiasm, willful compliance, reluctant obedience, confusion, resistance, and active defiance. Patients who trust medical professionals and trust the medical system in which they operate might lean toward enthusiasm or willful compliance. Patients who feel pressured to go along with clinician recommendations but who are distrustful or skeptical of clinicians may obey reluctantly. Patients who do not understand the nature of the relationship between clinician and patient and the role of power may experience confusion. Patients who distrust medical professionals and/or the medical system and are unmoved by the power they can exert may resist clinicians' recommendations. Patients who resist in the appropriate context, when they have good reasons to be distrustful of medical professionals and/or the medical system (such as when they have experienced abuses of power or are especially vulnerable to experiencing abuses of power based on how they are socially situated) may express the virtue of defiance.[29] Personally, at different times, I responded to clinicians in different ways, covering most of these responses at one point or another.

Being Sick

People who have mental illness—people who are made sick by their mental disorder symptoms (see chapter 1)—occupy to some extent what Talcott Parsons identified in the 1950s as the "sick role."[30] The sick role is an institutionalized role that positions people within power relations with respect to the medical system. Here people are positioned within the mental health system by virtue of their role as psychiatric patients. They encounter and engage with mental health professionals through that role. Mental health professionals are also positioned within the mental health system by virtue of their role as (broadly speaking) medical professionals. The roles of medical professional and sick patient set up the conditions for engagement between the two, circumscribing what form encounters take and what outcomes can result from those encounters.

Certain expectations and obligations attach to, and detach from, the sick role. People who are sick are sometimes excused from normal social responsibilities because their illness impedes with their ability to carry out such responsibilities. Mental illness that impairs cognitive, perceptual, rational, affective, volitional, or social capacities makes carrying out certain obligations difficult; when mental illness impacts behavior, it may incapacitate a person so that carrying out certain responsibilities is actually impossible. The sick role defines parameters of when it is and is not appropriate to expect someone to carry out responsibilities.

While being sick excuses a person from many obligations, it does entail a different responsibility, namely the responsibility to work on their own healing. When a person is sick, we expect that they will make efforts to improve their condition. Even if the person had no control over getting their illness, we expect that they will do what they can to receive appropriate treatment and to adhere to their treatment plan. This expectation is part of the "bargain" that we strike with people who inhabit the sick role: they will be excused from many responsibilities, but only on the condition that they are working to get better. They therefore have one major responsibility they must fulfill in order to be permitted to not carry out other responsibilities. When people fail to live up to this expectation of working on their healing, such as by not taking medication as prescribed or not following through on doctor or therapy appointments, we deem them "undeserving" of the sick role: undeserving, at least, of the benefits of the role, namely of being excused from many responsibilities.

When someone is in the sick role, we think it is unfair to expect that they can simply pull themselves together and get well by a simple change in attitude or a simple decision to do so. We recognize their illness as creating external constraints on them that are not subject to their will. Philosophers debate about the extent to which people with mental illness have sufficient free will to exert over their condition or whether they are subject to determination as their illness in some sense rules over them.[31] What seems most reasonable to say is that different mental illnesses impair agency in different ways and to different degrees and at different times, so in some cases people with mental illness act on free will despite their mental illness and in other cases people's actions are heavily shaped if not determined by their illness.[32] As I have explained in chapters 1 and 2, psychosis can significantly impair both agency and autonomy because of the way it tends to constrain epistemic and moral capacities and often leads a person to lose a sense of themselves as an agent and subject. Psychosis can thus shape people's actions in profound ways, ruling over them by overpowering their agency and autonomy.

In addition, being situated as a sick person can also decrease agency because it can induce a sense of passivity and powerlessness. When a patient is seen as the beneficiary of healthcare services, they are expected to comply with treatment recommendations; their biggest act of agency is simply to obey, not to develop their own goals and the means to achieve them.

When a patient sees themselves as sick, they may adopt a sick identity in which all of their experience seems to reduce to the experience of being sick and in treatment; their self-conception narrows so they no longer feel like they have an identity outside of being a sick person. They may become consumed by their sickness, and they may learn to feel like they are stuck in the present reality they are in and come to believe that their reality will never change and that they will never be able to get better. Unable to see themselves under different conditions, they may come to feel powerless, unable to change their circumstances. They may believe they have few or no options to act to make their situation different, and this belief actually constrains what they are able to do. In this way, feeling passive and power-less, they experience their agency diminish.

When I was sick, I could not see myself in any way other than as a sick person. When I was a patient receiving intensive treatment services, I believed that I would always need such services. I could not imagine myself as having a future that was different from the present. Perhaps this was a failure of imagination, or perhaps there is something about the sick role that makes a person entrenched within that identity. Surely my psychosis contributed to this. Psychosis makes a person live in an everlasting present, making it difficult to remember a past or imagine a future. It detaches a per-son from the psychological states that connect a person to a temporal iden-tity. But my identity as a mental patient probably also contributed. Being a patient situates a person within an institutional system that subjugates the person's own understanding of their needs and interests to clinicians' understandings of their needs and interests. In subjugating a person's self-understanding, the system encourages a dislocation of agency and conse-quently of autonomy. A patient learns to feel stuck. They develop a sense of powerlessness, feeling that how they are right now is how they will always be, and there is nothing they can do about it. Combatting this sense of powerlessness is important for a person to regain agency and autonomy by participating actively in treatment.

It is important to note that while mental illness (especially psychosis) and being sick can create significant constraints on free will, it does not eliminate free will entirely. It is only because there remains *some* room for agency that treatment is possible: a person can draw on and strengthen what little agency they have and exert control over some areas of their life, making it possible to exert control over other areas of their life. This is why engaging in practices involved with recovery such as giving testimony, making meaning of experience through narrative, and making decisions about treatment is so important: engaging in *some* practices of recovery to *some* extent helps a person to develop the capacity to engage in these practices more deeply, meaningfully, and autonomously. Interestingly, belief about having free will helps give patients more control: when patients *believe* they have free will in a situation, they are better able to exercise choice and control and consequently better able to manage their symptoms.[33]

The fact that mental illness can severely constrain agency but does not wholly determine people's actions underlies our attitudes toward people who are sick. We often recognize the injustice of expecting someone to do something that they do not have sufficient capacity to do. We do, however, expect them to *try*: to do what their doctor or therapist advises, with the hope that it will be conducive to healing. Even if the recommended action turns out not to have the results we desire (healing), we expect that someone in the sick role attempts that action. We also expect that the person *wants* to get better and is willing to do whatever actions their professional clinicians recommend as potentially leading them to get better. When a person inhabiting the sick role fails to try, and/or seems not to want to get better, we get very frustrated with them and regard them as "undeserving" of the sick role.

Sometimes their lack of trying and seeming lack of wanting to get better can be understood as symptoms of their illness: for example, these may result from apathy or delusion caused by depression or psychosis. When we can understand a person's lack of trying and seeming lack of wanting to get better as symptoms, or as signs of pathology, we can be more forgiving of them. In such a case, we regard their inaction as a sign of how sick they really are—so sick they are unable to help themselves—and when they are that sick, they appear to lack autonomy. When they are that sick, they seem incapable of making choices in their own best interest. Then we justify paternalistic and even coercive actions that try to save a person from themselves by acting on behalf of their interests. In other words, the general expectation of a person in the sick role is that they will work on getting better; when they seem incapable of doing this, however, we act on behalf of their interests in order to, in a sense, "make" them work on getting better.

Sometimes we do believe that people who have mental illness should simply find the determination within themselves to do something about their situation and, because we believe that people can and ought to do so, we blame them if they do not improve their condition. When we hold this view, we see the person as "undeserving" of the sick role, assuming that they are not *really* sick but only appearing to be sick. With this view, we make negative assumptions about the person with mental illness—believing they have a character flaw like weakness of will or a motive such as manipulation, for example—and thus perpetuate mental illness stigma. Certain stigmatizing attitudes, therefore, such as the belief that people with mental illness have a character flaw or are manipulative, constitute a rejection of the idea that the sick role applies to mental illness. Other stigmatizing attitudes, however, such as the view that people with mental illness are incompetent and need to be taken care of, endorse the sick role as applying to mental illness. What stigmas we hold affect what beliefs we hold about the appropriateness of the sick role applying to any given case of mental illness.[34]

The Patient Identity

Once someone—whether it is the sick person themselves or the people around them—determines that a person is sick, their role positions them as needing the services of the medical professionals whose role is to aid the sick. People who are deemed mentally ill are positioned to need the services of the mental health professionals whose role is to treat people with mental illness. With this, the person with mental illness enters the mental health system. They become a *patient* of the mental health professionals who treat them. Once a person enters the mental health system, they are defined always in relation to their need for treatment. Whether they accept or reject treatment, the perceived need for treatment is what designates them in their role.

People who are positioned in the sick role often adopt that role as part of their identity. They learn to see themselves as they are positioned: as needing treatment and as having that need for treatment define the parameters of their role and the boundaries of what they can or cannot do. It is very hard for a person to receive treatment in a clinic or hospital and *not* see themselves as their treatment providers do, and as they are positioned by virtue of their treatment: as a mental patient.

Even when a person rejects the sick role for themselves and denies their need for treatment, their denial is in relation to the perceived role: what expectations others hold for the person who is perceived as sick have already been set out for them by virtue of the sick role and, whether the person perceived as sick accepts or rejects the expectations, the expectations remain present. So even if a person rejects the sick role, once others perceive them in that role their rejection becomes part of how they carry out their role. In the case of mental illness, this is often seen as lack of insight (not recognizing one needs treatment) or noncompliance with treatment (refusal to accept treatment such as medication). People who are seen to need treatment are expected to accept the sick role and may be "punished" in various ways if they do not (for example, through harsher and more restrictive treatment or through negative judgment and negative attitudes by clinicians).

The more that a person engages with the mental health system, the more firmly that they tend to adopt the sick role and the more that it can become part of their identity. This means that the longer that a person is sick, the more they embody the role; in addition, the more acutely they are sick and need treatment, the more entrenched the role becomes. When people receive intensive levels of care, their identity as a psychiatric patient crystallizes; their day-to-day lives become structured around their treatment, for example in hospitalization, partial hospitalization programs (PHPs), and intensive outpatient programs (IOPs). Once a patient needs this more intense level of care, treating their illness involves not merely a weekly therapy appointment, but a daily commitment of time and energy that overtakes other interests so that a person actively maintains their treatment but little else in their life. At first this is disorienting, but over time it comes to feel normal, and the activities that once interested a person no longer seem very important compared to receiving mental health treatment. What a person cares about and how a person defines themselves relative to their interests changes.[35]

Both being sick and experiencing psychosis can change a person's identity or sense of self. While Jennifer Radden notes that some disunity in one's sense of self is common—with various life events leading to fragmentation, multiplicity, and discontinuity between psychological states—the disunity brought on by certain forms of mental illness and by the process of being sick (especially when one is sick for a long time) can be profound.[36] This can lead a person to feel like they are a completely different self when they are sick versus when they are well, or when they are in certain mood states or episodes of experience (such as psychotic episodes) versus when they are not, because they have dramatically different psychological states during some periods compared to others. This profound disunity can lead to a sense of disorientation and alienation from oneself. Someone who has been sick for a long time can forget what they were like before they were sick.

As a person receives more acute care, the parameters of the sick role expand relative to that level of treatment, so that the options for what kind of care a person needs changes. When a person has been doing weekly therapy and gets sick enough to warrant IOP or PHP treatment, IOP or PHP treatment is now always an option, whereas it may never have been one, or have been perceived as one, before. After a person becomes hospitalized once, hospitalization is always an option where it would not have been previously. Before I was hospitalized, hospitalization was never a treatment option on my horizon; after I was hospitalized, hospitalization was always an option (or a threat). Once I became a heavy user of the mental health-care system, intensive therapies such as IOP and other group therapies and support groups were always available to me, and I returned to them again and again when I was in need. Before being involved in these intensive therapies, they were barely on my radar; I saw them as being only for "sick" people. Once I became a heavy user of the mental healthcare system, however, I identified myself as a "sick" person eligible for these treatments. The range of possible options changes, and more intense levels of treatment always open the door to increasingly intense levels, but rarely the opposite. What it means to be sick changes, and with acute levels of care, the sick role becomes even more entrenched.

The danger of the entrenchment of the sick role comprises one of the reasons why critics object to the medical model of psychiatric disability that regards mental differences as pathological and in need of treatment. Advocates of the social model of psychiatric disability that views mental differences as natural rather than pathological are worried, among other things, about people becoming ingrained in the sick role and subsuming the sick identity. They want people to rebel against the expectations of the role and ultimately reject the role because it is bad for them to regard their experience as inherently negative (in need of treatment or amelioration) and to see themselves as inherently sick.

I am sympathetic to this concern, but I am also quite sure that advocates of the medical model of psychiatric disability want the same thing for patients. They do not want patients to adopt a sick identity; they want patients to overcome the sick role and transcend the expectations that correspond with it. They want patients to use medical and mental health resources when they need it, when they truly are sick, but to be able to leave those resources behind them as they get better. They do not want people to be perpetual patients or to see themselves as inherently sick. Part of the recovery process, after all, is to make a life for oneself that goes beyond the sick role and transcends mental illness experience. The sick role is a dangerous place to be because of the way that it can be reductive and negate other aspects of a person's identity and interests. At the same time, however, it is a helpful place to be for people who can benefit from mental healthcare services. Advocates of the social model of psychiatric disability are right to worry about the power of the sick role, but they are wrong to want to dismiss it entirely. Proponents of the medical model of psychiatric disability, on the other hand, see the sick role as serving a useful function in people who need it though it should not be the end goal or a norm.

Being a mental patient is an appropriate identity for people who benefit from receiving mental healthcare services. But mental patients should also try to be engaged in a process of recovery that allows them to transcend the parameters of that role and expand rather than restrict their identity and interests. To be positioned as a mental patient is to be in what ought to be a transitory role that helps a person move from one state—being sick, and sometimes being stuck in one's sickness—to another—being engaged in activities that promote one's health and well-being.

Agency, Autonomy, and Treatment

Because mental patients have diminished agency and autonomy, as well as decreased unity of self, due to their illness, increasing agency and autonomy should be some of the primary goals of treatment. Treatment can either support or undermine agency and power, depending on its goals and means. Outpatient treatment generally tries to increase patients' agency because this is conducive to treatment goals. Outpatient treatment aims to increase patients' ability to manage or prevent their symptoms; this requires patients to develop the power and agency that allows them to do this. In an outpatient setting, it is important to increase opportunities for patients to participate in epistemic and moral practices such as interpreting and understanding their experience, giving testimony, creating narratives of their experience that fit their experience into larger frameworks of meaning, asking questions, reflecting on their needs and interests, determining treatment goals, and making choices related to treatment. Patients are often encouraged to engage in these practices as part of the work they do in therapy; patients often participate in these practices in both therapy and psychiatry outpatient appointments. Clinicians both invite patients to engage in these practices and guide patients to engage in them productively. In an outpatient setting, patients are generally treated as credible participants in practices such as meaning making and decision making, whose contributions are not only valuable, but also necessary.

Engaging in epistemic and moral practices related to treatment helps patients develop competence because they exercise epistemic and moral capacities related to reasoning, cognition, and decision making, and through this exercise they develop these capacities more deeply, so they are better able to form and maintain beliefs, reason, and make choices. Engaging in these practices helps patients develop their sense of agency because, through this, they can be taught to see themselves as the source and locus of these activities. By reflecting on their needs and interests and reflecting on what they value, they can develop their sense of voluntariness, and both create goals for themselves based on what they value and determine the best means to achieve these goals. In increasing competence, voluntariness, and a sense of agency, engaging in these practices also increases patient's autonomy, allowing them to make choices that support their health and well-being and that they can endorse reflectively.

When patients have more agency and autonomy, they are able to recognize when their choices and behaviors support or undermine their interests and make informed decisions about what to do that advance their interests. This helps patients recognize their symptoms and learn to manage them effectively. Moreover, this is good for patients' long-term health: when patients have more agency and autonomy, they can develop a health-oriented disposition in which they recognize that their health and well-being are important goods that they ought to promote as much as possible and in which they consistently make choices that do in fact promote these. Engaging in an array of epistemic and moral practices in the context of outpatient treatment—such as by creating resourceful narratives[37] that enable patients to learn, grow, and heal from their illness—helps patients develop the agency and autonomy that allows them to develop this disposition. Through this engagement, patients can learn to manage their symptoms better and thus satisfy one of the important goals of treatment. For all these reasons, outpatient treatment generally tries to increase patients' agency.

Inpatient treatment, on the other hand, tends to restrict patients' agency. This is because inpatient treatment has different goals than outpatient treatment. The primary goal of hospitalization tends to be crisis management and safety promotion. People who enter a psychiatric hospital are very sick—sick enough to warrant hospital admission—and many of them, especially those on an intensive treatment unit, are a danger to themselves or others. Limiting their power in certain ways is necessary to create a safe environment in which people cannot hurt themselves or others. Limiting power may also be conducive to treatment when power could create obstacles to healing such as by creating responsibility one is not capable of managing or by creating conflict one cannot easily resolve. While choice and control are sometimes exalted as intrinsically valuable, and limitations on these are sometimes seen as necessarily bad or harmful, there are contexts in which limits on freedom and power can be beneficial and are justifiable. The psychiatric hospital is one of those contexts.

While restrictions on power and agency are justifiable in hospital settings in which such restrictions are conducive to the hospital's goals of safety and crisis stabilization, such restrictions put patients in a position of considerable vulnerability. Psychiatric hospitals are examples of what Erving Goffman called "total institutions": institutions that achieve their goals by managing people in ways that tightly schedule their day, require them to participate in activities with other "inmates," and collapse the normal boundaries between various spheres of life (work, sleep, and play) so these all occur in the same space. As total institutions, psychiatric hospitals achieve crisis stabilization and ensure patient and staff safety by managing mental patients in a totalizing way, dictating nearly all aspects of their life. Restrictions on freedom, power, and responsibilities brought about through this management help keep patients (and staff) safe and prevent patients from going into crisis. But the cost of this is diminished agency, and patients are put in a position of great vulnerability to the power of clinicians and staff in the institution.

In a hospital setting, patients usually are subject to the power of clinicians and staff in a way that is pervasive and nearly all-encompassing. The structure of the hospital dictates what patients do, and when, as well as what information they can know or share, and with whom. Patients may be permitted very few venues to share with staff how they are doing or what they are experiencing; they may be given very little information about their treatment plan and what the course of their stay will be. Clinicians make all the treatment decisions, often with little if any input from patients. Patient and staff interaction and communication may be minimal and may consist mostly of staff telling patients what to do. When patients have few opportunities to communicate with staff and little power in what they do, they lose the power they have as knowers and agents, and this can erode their epistemic and moral capacities as well as diminish their credibility. While restrictions on agency and power are justifiable in a hospital setting, they are also harmful: they make patients vulnerable to the power and dictates of clinicians as well as vulnerable to a loss of capacities and diminished credibility.

The goals of hospitalization are in tension with the goals of outpatient treatment. While the goal of increasing agency in outpatient treatment is not appropriate as a primary goal for hospitalization, it is valuable nonetheless as it helps patients in the long term. In the short term, patients in a hospital need to be safe; in the long term, they need to learn how to deal with their symptoms. To whatever extent a hospital experience is able to foster the long-term goal of increasing agency, it can be useful for far more than its most immediate effects of safety and crisis stabilization. To whatever extent the structure of the hospital can support patients' participation in epistemic and moral practices, therefore, it can have a lasting positive effect on patients' well-being. While certain restrictions on freedom are justifiable to achieve goals of hospitalization, hospitals should be designed to increase patient agency in certain other ways, such as by seeking out patient testimony, encouraging and guiding patients to make meaning of their experiences by putting it within a larger framework of meaning, and including patients in decision making. In this way, inpatient treatment can support the goals of outpatient treatment, making it a more useful mode of treatment.

In addition to increasing agency and autonomy, treatment should also focus on increasing unity of the self. Because unity of the self is necessary for a person to possess many moral goods, an important role for treatment, especially therapy, is to create more unity by addressing fragmentation, multiplicity, and discontinuity.[38] Learning to take responsibility for actions that a person has done is one way of addressing these forms of disunity. Through therapy, a person can learn to take responsibility (which I discuss in chapter 8) and, through this, make their different aspects of self cohere by identifying with actions they have done while ill and by responding appropriately to bad actions they have done with agent regret.[39] Constructing a narrative that tries to make sense of their experience, which is often done in therapy (as I discuss in chapter 7), is one helpful way for patients to identify with actions they have done and provides a way for patients to respond to their actions, enabling them to see the actions committed by them in different psychological states as belonging to a single self. When such narratives are resourceful, giving patients tools to use in helping to manage and grow from their illness, they increase agency, autonomy, and self-unity.

Conclusion

When I asked to be hospitalized that fateful day in April 2018, little did I realize that I was changing the trajectory of my mental health career. No longer would psychosis be a way of life, a dominating force that conditioned all of my experience, something that I actively pursued. Now mental health treatment would be my way of life. Rather than letting the psychosis determine how I would spend hours in my day, I would let the mental healthcare system determine how I spent my time. With hospitalization, my time was turned over completely to the treatment designated by the hospital structure, especially the group activities that constituted much of the day. After hospitalization, my time was structured by the intensive outpatient therapy I was in. Attending IOP for three hours a day, three days a week, for different weeks at a time, took up a good portion of my waking hours for many months. Practicing the skills I was learning in IOP took up more time. For months, I also saw my therapist weekly and my psychiatrist monthly. All of these appointments in the behavioral health clinic monopolized the time I spent outside of work. The hours I had once devoted to psychotic pursuit I was now devoting to mental healthcare treatment. I came to see myself as being very sick and saw my identity constituted chiefly as a mental patient. Other parts of me receded into the background as I focused my time and energy on treatment.

Medicalization had many benefits for me. It validated my experiences as being "real" and conferred legitimacy to the meaning framework that I used to make sense of them. It opened doors to new treatment options and gave me access to resources, such as consultations with crisis team members at my behavioral health clinic. Medicalization also made me vulnerable to the power of the clinicians who treated me. It allowed clinicians to infringe on my privacy; it sometimes made me feel coerced into accepting treatment I did not necessarily want; and, in positioning me as a patient, it diminished my credibility and authority and the tendency of others to take me seriously; it put me in a position where I was easily, and very frustratingly, misunderstood by some clinicians. In addition, medicalization restructured my time, refocused my energy, changed my future direction, impacted my future goals, and changed the way I saw myself.

Medicalization situates a patient into the sick role, where the patient's main responsibility is to work on getting better. Depending on how the patient views their own situation, and how much control they have over their experiences and behavior, they are able to carry out this responsibility to different degrees. The more debilitating a patient's illness is, the less control they have over changing their behavior, and the more they are subjected to the power of clinicians. While increasing agency is often a goal of outpatient treatment, so that a person can learn to manage their symptoms and cope with difficulties better, different treatments increase or decrease agency to different degrees. Giving patients opportunities to participate actively in treatment and encouraging them in this way helps patients to develop the agency and autonomy required for them to stay committed to their recovery and to continue working on getting better. In later chapters, I show how giving patients opportunities to participate in activities like giving testimony, making meaning of their experiences, and making treatment decisions is crucial for recovery.

Being able to navigate successfully the challenging role of being a mental patient is a key aspect of recovery. Having a positive therapeutic relationship with one's clinicians makes a big difference in how successfully a patient can address their mental illness. In chapters 4 and 5, I explain the importance of trust and empathy in the therapeutic relationship for helping patients to achieve the agency and autonomy required for them to be able to succeed in their recovery.

4 Trust

Introduction

When I was in IOP (intensive outpatient program), I always had homework. It was never expressed to us this way, but we were encouraged to try applying what we were learning in class to our daily lives. When we learned about mindfulness techniques, we were encouraged to practice paying attention and being mindful in our daily activities. When we learned about distress tolerance, we were encouraged to practice looking at difficult situations with an objective, open mind, seeing it from different perspectives so we didn't automatically go into crisis mode. A good student, I always tried to practice these things as best as I could. Sometimes I was not very successful, but sometimes I was. Practicing what I was learning was a choice I made. It was a form of participating in treatment.

My clinicians trusted me to participate in my treatment as best as I could. They encouraged me to at least try to do the things they recommended. They trusted me to value my health and well-being enough to work on my recovery. Sometimes I did, and I was able to use this valuation as motivation to act. Sometimes I did not, and I actively resisted what they recommended. At times, I would go down on my medication against their advisement, but then my psychosis would resurface and torment me. At these times, I would email my psychiatrist and therapist in distress, begging for help, even though I knew it was help I did not want.

When I did this, my psychiatrist was not happy with me. He felt frustrated because he wanted to see me get better. I felt frustrated because I didn't feel like I had control over what I was doing in reducing the medication, and I didn't understand why I was doing it. There seemed to be multiple motives behind decreasing my medication: I felt like I did not deserve to get better; I wanted to pursue the strange sensations and special meaning psychosis brought on; I felt obligated to obey the voice that told me to go down on the medication. More than anything, the psychosis was compelling me to decrease my medication so it could stay in power. Moreover, I felt frustrated because, in my psychosis, I could not make my psychiatrist understand what I myself did not understand. I wanted my behavior to make sense to him, so that it could make sense to me, and so that we could work together to try to help me deal with it. But, although he tried, he did not understand, and he probably felt like a broken record repeating to me the necessity of taking my medicine as prescribed. Caught in the grip of my psychosis, I felt helpless to change my behavior, and I felt hopeless that my situation could improve. Despite his frustration, however, and despite my feelings of helplessness and hopelessness, my psychiatrist maintained an attitude of optimism both that I would get better and that I would be able to make good decisions that would help me get better.

Depending on how competent I was, I was able to follow through on working on my recovery to different degrees at different times. Even when I was not able to follow through and did not do what they advised, my psychiatrist and therapist did not let go of their trust of me. Even when I actively resisted them, such as by playing with my medication or by not doing my homework, they trusted that I would be able to choose to act differently. They knew that recovery involves making choices, over and over again, to engage in the practices necessary to regain health and well-being. Despite sometimes not making this choice, my clinicians nonetheless trusted that I would be able to make better choices in the future. They did not let go of their optimism for me.

As I lacked the conditions of autonomy, it would have been justifiable if my psychiatrist or therapist had determined paternalistically that I needed more intensive treatment than I was getting at the time and if they had coerced me into receiving that kind of treatment. My psychiatrist could have determined that I needed to be hospitalized so that I would be forced to take my medication as prescribed, in order to alleviate my psychosis for long enough for me to recognize the reasons why I needed to take the medication as prescribed and for me to be able to use those reasons as motivation to do so. My therapist could have determined that I needed to participate in more intensive therapy than once-weekly or biweekly appointments in order to force me to recognize the reasons why I needed to work on getting better and to be able to use those reasons as motivation for doing that hard work. But they did not.

Since I began receiving treatment for psychosis, my clinicians have always given me the choice about what treatment I should participate in; even when I did not feel capable of making a decision, I had to do so. When I would start to have major problems with functioning in my daily life, my clinicians would ask if I wanted to go to IOP. Sometimes I said "yes," and sometimes I decided I could stick it out on my own. When I was in crisis—suicidal or hearing a voice telling me to kill myself—they would ask if I thought I needed to be hospitalized again. I always said "no," because I didn't *want* to be hospitalized again, but I didn't feel like I was making that choice for myself; I felt like my illness was in control of me, making a choice that would allow it to perpetuate itself. The illness did not want me to receive treatment that would make it recede; it wanted to stay present and alive. Thus, when my clinicians presented these choices to me, I didn't feel capable of making that decision for myself, and I was angry at my clinicians for not seeing this. But rather than deciding for me, my clinicians wanted to leave that up to me, because they wanted me to retain control over my treatment and ultimately over my mental illness. While my clinicians saw that I was not making choices that served my best interests, they rarely coerced me into doing so; instead, they gave me opportunities to try to act autonomously even though I lacked the conditions to actually be able to do so. They knew that by practicing making choices for myself, I could eventually develop actual autonomy. They trusted me to make decisions about my treatment because they knew that by making those decisions, I was exercising my agency and practicing being autonomous.

Participating actively in recovery involves making choice after choice to value health and well-being, to act on the recommendations of one's clinicians, to remain committed to recovery no matter how hard it is. Recovery is not simply a single decision to work on getting better; it is a constant, never-ending series of decisions to do the work required. Stuck in my psychosis, I often made choices to further my psychosis rather than to promote my health. Convinced I could never have a life that was different than the one I had, I gave up many times as I was working toward recovery, giving into the psychosis and following its dictates instead, or feeling immobilized by distress and tempted by suicidal ideation. But my clinicians—my therapist, my psychiatrist, and the social worker who ran IOP—never lost their hope and optimism for me, and they were able to hold it even when I couldn't. While it would have been justified if they had determined I needed coercive treatment, they never went that route, preferring instead to trust me to make good choices even though I clearly was not capable of doing so adequately.

In this chapter, I examine the role that trust plays in recovery, examining the nature of trust in the clinician-patient relationship. I argue that just as patients must be able to trust clinicians in order to have a successful working relationship, so must clinicians trust patients. Returning to the issue of paternalistic treatment brought up in chapter 2, I examine the justifiability and appropriateness of coercive treatment in the context of trust. I argue that coercive treatment is sometimes justified when a patient is too incompetent to make rational decisions about treatment but that it ought to be avoided as much as possible since it impedes internal motivation and self-efficacy. Instead, under most circumstances, clinicians should trust patients to make reasonable decisions about their treatment; this trust helps patients develop more self-efficacy in their decision making and thus helps develop autonomy.

Building Relationships of Trust

Instilling self-efficacy and restoring agency and autonomy in patients is often crucial for recovery. Self-efficacy is a person's belief that they will be successful in engaging in specific activities;[1] it involves having control over what they do, recognizing that they have this control, and having confidence that they can enact this control. Self-efficacy is thus a form of agency and often is an expression of autonomous action. Since psychosis typically produces a strong sense of passivity and feelings of being controlled externally, clinicians must do what they can to help patients see themselves as agents who have control over what happens to them. One way to encourage patients to exercise agency and self-efficacy is through trust. Trust builds self-efficacy in both directions of the trusting relationship: when clinicians trust patients to participate in their own recovery by engaging in treatment, they create the conditions that allow patients to do so; and when patients trust clinicians, they feel more invested in their recovery and are thus more willing to do the work involved with treatment.

Trust is thus one of the social conditions that enables active participation in recovery. Let us look at what trust is, and then we will examine both sides of trust in the therapeutic relationship.

Trusting someone means having faith in them and in their ability to fulfill our expectations of them. Trust has both cognitive and affective dimensions: it involves holding certain beliefs about the person, namely that they will carry out expectations regarding the thing that they are entrusted to do,[2] as well as having certain feelings toward the person and reacting emotionally when they either do or fail to do what they are entrusted with doing. Jessica Miller describes the trust belief in terms of the fidelity principle, which involves doing what one has promised to do.[3] While promises are often explicit statements of what can be expected, trust may be either based on explicit expectations that have been specifically identified or implicit expectations that are assumed by one or both parties though never specifically articulated, such as the expectations associated with one's social role. Clinicians and patients, for example, trust each other by holding certain expectations of each other that are relevant to their roles, as I explain below.

The belief that one will carry out expectations can be understood in terms of commitment: trusting someone involves relying on someone to meet a commitment that we believe they have or ought to have.[4] Distrust occurs when we do not believe that they will meet a commitment that we believe they have or ought to have. Trust is related to agency, in that it is generally appropriate to assume that others have certain commitments and to rely on people to meet those commitments, only when we believe they have the capacity to do so as agents.[5] Trusting someone appropriately thus typically requires that the person is competent in certain ways.

Trust can also be understood as an attitude of optimism that the person one trusts has good will and competence to carry out the activities with which we trust them.[6] This attitude is not a *belief* that the person will act as trusted, but rather a lens through which we see the person. Having trust in a person colors the way we interact with the person, including how we interpret their actions, and consequently our relationship with the person. When we trust someone, we are more likely to interpret their action benevolently: negative outcomes are seen as mistakes, while positive outcomes are seen as intentional and praiseworthy. When we distrust someone, we are more likely to interpret their action negatively: positive outcomes are seen as accidental, and negative outcomes are seen as the product of malevolent intent or negligence. This affects how people respond to us. Being trusted makes a person want to live up to that trust and respond positively to the person trusting them; when a person is not trusted, they feel resentful or dismissive of the person who doesn't trust them, and they respond negatively.

In this way, trust breeds more trust, while distrust sows more distrust. While trust involves seeing someone in an optimistic way as being inclined to fulfill certain expectations, distrust involves seeing someone in a pessimistic way as lacking good will in their interactions. Trust breeds trust because trusting someone creates conditions that allow a person to fulfill what is expected of them; when a person is viewed in such a hopeful way, they have motivation to try to live up to that hope and fulfill expectations. Similarly, distrust breeds distrust, as holding a pessimistic attitude toward someone can make the person feel a loss of worth and esteem, and they often react to this loss by interpreting others' expectations of them in negative ways and acting in ways contrary to expectations.[7] Trust and distrust are thus self-fulfilling, in that how we view a person creates the conditions for what kind of a person one becomes. This is why trusting patients to participate in their own recovery is so important: it encourages them to live up to the hope clinicians have in them and to fulfill expectations.

Since trust involves holding expectations about what someone will do, and being optimistic about their ability to fulfill those expectations, it is forward looking, reaching into an unknown future and formulating a hypothesis about what will happen.[8] Trust occurs in conditions of uncertainty.[9] If we had certainty about what people would do, we would not need to trust them; we would simply have knowledge. We need to trust people because we do not know for certain what they will do, yet we must take a risk and form a belief about what we think they will do or an attitude about what we expect or hope that they do. Trusting is a way of firming up uncertain futures,[10] not by cementing what is believed to be the case into certain knowledge—trust cannot do that—but by creating goalposts that the truster and trustee can use as a guide while wading through uncertain waters. Trust does not settle uncertainty through belief and prediction, therefore, but rather through an attitude of optimism and hope. As an affective attitude, trust is more like hope than like prediction, for we do not need to believe that our trusting will result in a positive outcome (the fulfillment of our expectations) in order for us to be able to trust.[11] When clinicians trust patients to participate in their own recovery, they do so under conditions of uncertainty; they put their faith in the patient and hope that the patient will work on their recovery. When patients trust clinicians to act in their best interests and promote their health and well-being, they put their faith in the clinician and hope the clinician will carry out expectations.

Sharing the same goals is important to build trust, as it is easier to trust someone when they have the same values and aims that we do: when we are able to assume that someone is motivated by the same values, goals, and interests that we have, it is easier to have optimism about what we think the person will do. Usually, in the medical context, there is a shared basis for vulnerability and trust, as both clinician and patient presumably want the same goals: effective treatment and ultimately health and well-being of the patient.[12] After all, patients frequently seek out clinicians when they are in distress because they believe clinicians have the knowledge, tools, and power to help alleviate their distress. When patients agree with their clinicians about the goals of treatment and means of attaining them, they have therapeutic alliance. Sometimes patients do not share the same goals as their clinician, however, and in such cases, it is more difficult to build trust. I discuss this below.

Trusting someone involves significant risk[13] and puts us in a position of vulnerability:[14] we are vulnerable to being disappointed and to being subject to harms that may incur if the person we trust does not follow through on what we trust them to do. When we trust someone, we are taking a risk that our expectations may be disappointed, that the person will not follow through on what we trust them to do. When we have hopes about what we expect them to do, their failure in not doing it may feel like they are letting us down. In some cases, if a person fails to do what we expect them to do, we also suffer a loss of what would have been the outcome had they done what they were entrusted to do, and we may also be outright harmed if they act wrongly. Trusting someone while knowing they have the ability to let us down thus requires us to be willing to endure disappointment as well as whatever consequences follow from the person not carrying out what is expected of them.[15] Because of the asymmetrical power relation between patients and clinicians, patients are much more vulnerable in trusting clinicians than clinicians are in trusting patients, and they have much more to lose. Let us look at both sides of the trusting relationship.

What Patients Trust in Their Clinicians

Trusting clinicians is beneficial to patients. As Jessica Miller points out, "Patients who trust physicians are more likely to seek care at the first sign of trouble, to communicate important information about their symptoms and feelings, to reveal any fears or concerns that could sabotage treatment, to comply with medical recommendations, and in general, experience less anxiety around issues of health."[16] Trust thus enables patients to access healthcare, to accept their vulnerability in the clinical encounter (when their bodies and/or minds are exposed for the clinician to examine), to feel confident about clinician recommendations, and to follow treatment protocol.[17] When the patient has trust in their clinician, this fosters many goals of therapy, including strengthening the patient's sense of self, providing opportunities for meaning and hope, creating new perspectives, decreasing the impact of hearing voices, and strengthening connections with others.[18] Trust helps create therapeutic alliance,[19] which increases adherence to treatment.[20] When patients can trust their clinicians, they feel more invested in their recovery and are more willing and able to put in the necessary work to participate in their recovery.

Most patients trust their clinicians.[21] This trust is based on many factors. To some extent we trust clinicians based on their expertise, which is acquired through training and experience.[22] We know that they have relevant, specialized knowledge that makes them especially capable of addressing specific health concerns. In addition, because the role of clinician is characterized by being essentially about promoting patient health, managing or curing illness, and ameliorating pain, we assume that clinicians share the same goals and values that many patients typically have: to improve the health and well-being of the patient.[23]

In addition to trusting clinicians based on their expertise and shared goals and values, we trust particular clinicians based on the archetype of their clinical specialty. Our trust in physicians partly comes from the positive stereotypes we have about what it is to be a doctor, stereotypes that include positive attributes such as benevolence, expertise, confidence, self-assuredness, and optimism that present states of affairs can be improved. Our trust in nurses partly comes from positive stereotypes of nurses as warm, empathetic, and caring. Our trust in therapists involves similar stereotypes. We assume that the particular individual with whom we are interacting fits the positive stereotype we have of members of their profession, and we feel trust toward them as a result.

Patients' trust of clinicians is based on many other factors as well. We trust clinicians who appear to us to be trustworthy, having demonstrated their reliability at following through on things they are trusted with in the past. Confident or at least comfortable with other people's judgments, we are more likely to trust clinicians when other patients speak positively of them and trust them as well. We often trust clinicians out of a sense of optimism; hopeful for a positive outcome of the clinical encounter, we put faith in clinicians that they will be able to provide helpful treatment. We also trust clinicians based on interpersonal factors such as warmth of personality, positive demeanor, respect for the patient, empathetic and caring disposition, and being a good listener. Making eye contact, moving closer to the patient (and away from the computer), leaning in while listening, asking questions, and repeating back what patients say are all important in interactions with patients. When clinicians show through their body language and tone of voice that they take us seriously, care about our concerns, and are capable of providing helpful treatment, we bestow them with trust.

The patient trusts the clinician as a professional who is obligated to carry out the responsibilities attached to their role. Part of being a professional involves having specialized knowledge that one uses for the good of the client.[24] Patients trust clinicians to have goodwill toward their patients and professional competency in their practice.[25] Patients trust that clinicians will make their best medical judgment and prescribe the best treatment that the clinician believes will be effective. Patients should be able to trust that their clinician is acting in the patient's best interests and that the clinician will not make treatment decisions based on self-interest or other nonpatient factors such as kickbacks from pharmaceutical companies or convenience to the clinician. In addition, the patient should expect and trust that the clinician will act professionally. Edmund Pellegrino nicely summarizes what patients trust in their clinicians: "We trust professionals in realms over which they have expertise. We trust them not to use that expertise to exploit our vulnerability for their own interests. We trust them for accurate information and we trust them to empower and enable us to place their recommendations into the full context of our own hierarchy of values. We also trust them to carry out the procedures in which they are skilled and which we cannot perform for ourselves."[26] We trust clinicians to carry out the expectations we have for them by virtue of their roles as clinicians: to use their expertise to address our sickness and pain and to aid our health and well-being. In addition, we trust clinicians in a testimonial sense: just as clinicians trust us to present ourselves accurately and give reliable testimony of our experience, we trust that clinicians will provide accurate information to the best of their knowledge. When patients have more specific expectations of their clinicians besides general role expectations, they should communicate these with the clinician and have a dialogue about them so the clinician and patient are on the same page, so to speak, as each other.

We have to trust clinicians because of the position of vulnerability that we are in by virtue of being a patient and under a clinician's care. Because clinicians have greater power in the clinician-patient relationship, patients are more vulnerable when placing trust in the clinician than clinicians are when trusting patients. Patients are vulnerable the moment they walk into the clinician office, at least in the context of in-person care. They typically have to wait for an indeterminate amount of time in a waiting room, often surrounded by other patients; many people in the waiting room feel anxious for their appointment, perhaps self-conscious about being observed by others, perhaps worried that they will be recognized by others in the waiting room. When they finally see the clinician, they have to offer up their bodies for probing (in a medical context) or recount details of their psychological state (in a mental health context), either of which can be difficult and embarrassing and be the source of great vulnerability.[27]

In a mental health context, whether in person or through telemedicine, patients are vulnerable when they are asked about symptoms and impairments that are intensely personal, and they are vulnerable when they give an account of their experience and they do not know whether the account will be believed or taken seriously. In such a context, they are vulnerable to being misunderstood, discounted, discredited, ignored, patronized, coerced, and dehumanized, and they often experience anxiety based on that vulnerability. When clinicians type patient responses into a computer while patients are speaking, patients are vulnerable not only in the sense that they are exposed, but also in the sense that they may not be respected. When clinicians or therapists do not make eye contact or exhibit warmth, or when they seem more interested in recording symptoms than listening to patients, patients may feel that their humanity is not being recognized.

When clinicians treat patients as if they are simply a diagnosis, a set of symptoms, they do not feel like they are treated as whole people or as unique individuals. Patients easily feel dehumanized in clinical settings.

While patients are necessarily vulnerable by virtue of their role as a patient, which positions them as being in the care of clinicians, clinicians are never in a position in which they are required to be vulnerable in these ways. Whatever vulnerabilities clinicians show to patients are by choice, not necessity. Clinicians thus have more power in the therapeutic relationship, due not only to their professional expertise and authority, but also to their privilege in not having to be vulnerable to patients in certain ways even as patients have to be vulnerable to them. Patients have more to lose when clinicians violate their trust than when patients violate the trust of clinicians.

Patients are vulnerable to the power of clinicians in many ways, and in some circumstances, this vulnerability can foster distrust. Patients may distrust clinicians when they have had negative experiences in the past, such as being subject to abuse, trauma, or coercive treatment, or when they have been or could be subjected to systemic oppression such as racism or sexism. Negative experiences and vulnerability to oppression can create negative expectations, leading to a disposition of pessimism rather than optimism in working with clinicians, and negatively impact future experiences with clinicians.

When we trust clinicians, however, part of our trust is based on their expertise and authority, or where they are positioned in an epistemic hierarchy of knowledge. This epistemic hierarchy privileges clinicians based on their professional training and experience and necessarily and unavoidably puts patients in a condition of vulnerability by virtue of their role.[28] Clinicians have significant epistemic power based on their professional training and experience, as well as on the epistemic methodologies, techniques, and technologies that are part of their profession. Clinicians have specialized knowledge and skills and access to special resources, and they rely upon practices and techniques that are demonstrably effective within their field. Some forms of epistemic power that clinicians yield based on their professional expertise include the powers of observation,[29] discernment, diagnosis (in the case of psychiatrists), making treatment recommendations, and making resources available to or withholding resources from patients as they see fit. Since clinicians wield significant power over patients in their role, it is vital that clinicians are mindful of this power and take care to respect patients in their vulnerability and empower them where possible.

Clinicians can easily and unconsciously abuse their epistemic power by silencing patients, ignoring or discounting their testimony, interpreting their testimony through preconceived frameworks that ignore other ways of understanding,[30] withholding information from them, discounting their concerns as the product of excessive emotion or imagination, viewing their concerns as symptoms, and dehumanizing patients in the various ways described above.[31] I discuss these abuses of epistemic power more in chapter 6. When clinicians do this, they typically do so unthinkingly, unaware of the effects their action has on their patients. Clinicians can also abuse their power by inflicting violence, coercing patients, or perpetuating systemic oppression such as racism. These kinds of abuses can be unconscious, for example resulting from implicit bias, or conscious and intentional, with various possible motivations.

An ethically minded clinician is mindful of the potential for abusing their power, self-aware and self-monitoring to try to make sure they do not unconsciously fall into such action, and concerned enough to rectify situations in which they unwittingly caused their patients harm. An ethically minded clinician also adopts epistemic humility, acknowledging the limits of their knowledge and power, and being open to learning from patients' perspectives.[32] Because they are entrusted with the care of patients, clinicians have special responsibilities by virtue of their role as clinicians. As Richard M. Zaner says, they must be *"responsive to* each individual within his or her unique circumstances and condition," *"responsible for* whatever is then said or done on behalf of that individual," and *"responsible to and for* the profession itself."[33]

What Clinicians Trust in Their Patients

Clinicians generally trust patients in at least four different ways. First, they trust patients in a moral agency sense, believing that when they treat patients, patients share the same values and goals they have (to promote the patient's health) and act honorably (e.g., they wouldn't generally sue).[34] Second, they trust patients in a testimonial sense, assuming that patients are honest in providing an accurate account of their past history of illness and treatment, of the aspects of their psychosocial context that are relevant (e.g., past history of substance abuse, history of trauma, family status, and socioeconomic conditions), and of their current symptoms.[35] Third, they trust patients in a competence sense, assuming that patients have the epistemic capabilities necessary for hearing and contextualizing information, making accurate and relevant judgments, making reasonable and informed decisions, and collaborating with clinicians about treatment plans.[36] Fourth, they trust patients in a trustworthy sense, expecting that patients will follow through on the agreed upon treatment plan by adhering to prescribed treatment and keeping the clinician informed about how treatment goes and if health conditions are getting worse or better.[37] The forms of trust that are most important for participating actively in recovery are the moral agency, competence, and trustworthy aspects.

Just as it is important for the patient to communicate their expectations to the clinician, so should the clinician communicate their expectations of the patient to the patient. Clinicians should expect patients to carry out their treatment plans to the best of their ability, for example by taking medication as prescribed, participating in advised therapies, and exercising or eating well. Clinicians can also hold expectations around how a patient should participate in devising their own treatment plans and communicate these expectations to the patient. For example, if the clinician wants to give the patient choices in which medication to take, the clinician should make this expectation clear and provide the information needed about the relevant options to make an informed choice. In addition, clinicians should expect and trust that patients will behave in ways that are appropriate to a professional relationship. As long as the expectations are reasonable, it is fair for the clinician to hold the patient to those expectations, and the clinician should be able to trust that the patient will carry out those expectations.

Patients can violate trust in a variety of ways, especially in a mental healthcare context. Patients can betray a clinician's trust when they give dishonest or misleading accounts, when they do not tell the truth about their motives (such as motives to attain opioid medication), or when they share information only selectively and withhold pertinent information. They can also fail to be competent or trustworthy or, for various reasons, not share the same goals as the clinician. Betrayal leads clinicians to feel "burned."[38] This creates negative reactions toward the patient, not only negative emotions, but also causing the clinician to feel less invested in the patient's treatment outcomes and possibly less helpful in their treatment plan. This can also lead to future distrust not only of that particular patient, but of all patients who are relevantly similar. When a patient has a positive therapeutic relationship with their clinician, this can ameliorate some of these concerns, as it is harder for a patient to lie, deceive, or mislead a clinician that they have a relationship with and easier for both to trust the other as they interact with each other over time.[39]

Clinicians generally trust that patients share the same goals that they have: for the patient's condition to improve, and for the patient to regain health and well-being. An implication of this shared goal is the assumption by clinicians that patients will adhere to prescribed treatment in order to try to attain this goal. In other words, clinicians trust that patients will collaborate and participate actively in their treatment. Jessica Miller states:

> Moreover, as preserving or restoring health (not to mention comfort care at the end of life) takes days, weeks, or years, the physician must trust that the patient is committed to the course of care upon which they have mutually decided. The physician invests his or her time and effort in diagnosis and treatment, but, as health is a joint undertaking, little will be accomplished without full patient cooperation. This does not mean, of course, that a patient can never change his mind (say, to opt against participating in an experimental study) without betraying a trust, but it does suggest that the physician deserves consultation on sudden or precipitous changes in care or regimen.[40]

When clinicians know or suspect that a patient is not following treatment recommendations, this may erode trust, and when this happens repeatedly, the clinician may find themselves wondering why they should bother to give treatment advice at all. If the patient does not seem to have the same goal, or the same understanding on how to reach the goal, as the clinician, this undermines the entire clinician-patient relationship. When a patient does not adhere to treatment, they appear to not be invested in their own welfare, as if they do not care whether they are sick or well. Clinicians may find themselves feeling less invested in the patient's welfare as well. This can lead to poorer treatment advice or even negligent treatment. But providing good treatment is an intrinsic element of carrying out the role of a clinician. The challenge for clinicians in this case is to remain invested in a patient's welfare even when the patient themselves does not appear to be so and even when the patient seems to be actively resisting working on improving their health condition.

When clinicians trust patients, they make themselves vulnerable to patients in certain ways. When they trust patients to work on their recovery, they are vulnerable to being disappointed by patients' inaction or to feeling used if the patient deliberately flouts recommendations. They are vulnerable to having their professional expertise disregarded, which can feel like an insult. They are also vulnerable to existential anxieties about what is the purpose of their work; when patients act contrary to clinician recommendations, clinicians may wonder what the point of what they are doing is. In order to continue working with patients with a trusting, optimistic attitude of hoping patients will follow through on recommended treatment, clinicians have to be willing to endure disappointment and not let existential anxieties about the purpose of their work bother them.

Therapeutic Alliance

Collaboration in creating and carrying out treatment goals is an essential aspect of therapeutic alliance. Therapeutic alliance occurs when the clinician and patient are in agreement about what the goals of treatment should be and how these goals should be achieved.[41] In other words, they share an acknowledgment of what the patient's main problems are, ideally agreeing on the appropriate diagnosis and having a similar idea of the nature of the illness; and they agree on what the course of treatment should be. Having a sense of shared meaning is an important component of therapeutic alliance.[42] Collaboration, mutual trust, and support are also beneficial for forming alliance.[43] In addition, empathy is essential for therapeutic alliance: when the clinician empathizes with the patient, this creates a positive relationship between clinician and patient, which contributes to improved treatment outcomes.[44] A positive therapeutic relationship can be characterized as one where there is significant therapeutic alliance.

Patients and clinicians may not always share the same goals, however. In such cases, working together to try to come to a shared understanding is critical for the therapeutic relationship to be productive. There are different ways that patients and clinicians may not be in agreement or have the same understanding about goals. A psychotic patient who feels conflicted about reducing or eliminating their psychosis, or who believes they do not have a psychological problem in need of treatment, will not have any particular goals for treatment because they will regard treatment as unnecessary (at least to some extent). A psychotic patient who seeks treatment to alleviate distress—as I did when I emailed my psychiatrist in the throes of psychosis begging for help—will agree on the need for treatment but may not agree on what the goal of treatment is—for example whether the goal is to reduce or eliminate distress, to reduce or eliminate hallucinations and delusions, to increase organization of thought, to enable functioning in daily life activities, or to enable a person to achieve various life goals. Some of these goals may be desirable to the psychotic person but impossible to achieve (for example, eliminating distress or positive symptoms of psychosis may not be possible); some may be desirable to the clinician and perceived as achievable by the clinician but may not be desirable to the patient (for example, reducing hallucinations and delusions when the patient wants to maintain them) or may appear to be impossible to the patient (for example, functioning in daily life activities). The patient or clinician may desire to eliminate psychosis entirely, but this may not be feasible; a more realistic goal might be to put the psychosis into remission for as long as possible, so the patient has periods of wellness in between periods of illness, or to minimize its effects so a person can function better in their daily life.

When the clinician and the patient disagree about what the goals of treatment should be and how they should be achieved, the clinician must dialogue with the patient to try to come to some form of agreement. The clinician should try to understand the patient's perspective as best as they can, so they can address concerns the patient may have that may be getting in the way of treatment goals and means. Imagining themselves as a guide, the clinician should help the patient perceive what is in their best interests and see what the role of health and well-being is in their conception of a good life, so they can more accurately determine what role treatment should play in their lives. While the clinician should articulate clearly their own views about what the patient's goals and the methods to achieve them should be in the spirit of trying to educate the patient about their situation, they should also be open to revising their ideas, based on the patient's perspective and concerns. Having the most power in the relationship, the clinician should instigate a discussion about the patient's treatment goals and means, guiding the patient to think more clearly about what matters so the patient can articulate their own goals and means to achieve them in a meaningful way.

Incompetence and Coercive Treatment

Sometimes patients who have very different goals from their clinicians are unable to reason about goals and means to achieve them because they are incompetent. As discussed in chapter 2, when a patient is incompetent, they are unable to engage in the rational deliberation required for making autonomous decisions for themselves. Because they cannot make autonomous decisions for themselves, it might be appropriate for someone else to make decisions for them depending on the context. When an incompetent patient is unable to make autonomous decisions about their treatment, they may need someone else to make those decisions for them, because it is important for their welfare that someone make good decisions regarding their treatment. This substituted judgment is a form of paternalism; the need for it may justify coercive treatment.

Coercive treatment involves compelling a patient to accept recommended treatment through persuasion or force and is a form of paternalistic intervention. While paternalistic interference involves interfering with a person's nonautonomous choice for the sake of furthering the patient's best interests, coercive treatment is treatment that "forces" patients to make a certain decision about treatment or to accept certain forms of treatment. In chapter 2, I focused on the justifiability and appropriateness of paternalistic interference with patients' choices, looking at a range of paternalistic interferences, including educating and guiding patients to make better choices; here I am focusing on the justifiability and appropriateness of coercive treatment in particular. When patients are incompetent but in serious need of treatment, clinicians have to decide if coercive treatment is appropriate.

Paternalistic interventions can involve a range of actions, including positive approaches like encouragement, rational persuasion, and incentives and negative approaches like making threats, removing privileges, implementing negative consequences, and physical force.[45] Positive approaches are experienced subjectively as being less coercive or not coercive at all,[46] so I will hereafter not consider them to count as coercion. Negative approaches are experienced subjectively as being more coercive and forceful[47] and constitute what we more readily think of as "coercion." Positive approaches are usually employed before negative approaches are; negative approaches are generally used only as a last resort, when making the patient comply with orders is necessary for patient or staff safety and the clinician feels there are no other options to accomplish this.[48] Hospitalizing a patient against their will, forcing patient to take medication, and making a patient attend group therapy by imposing sanctions on them if they refuse are all examples of coercive treatments used in a mental healthcare context. Coercion commonly occurs in inpatient settings and less commonly in outpatient settings.

Coercive treatment is typically justified in one of three ways: in terms of community safety, beneficence, or restoring competence. In all cases, the treatment under consideration (such as medication use or hospitalization) must be deemed medically necessary and the least restrictive alternative available.[49] The community safety criterion applies when a person is in danger of causing significant harm to others.[50] I believe this is an important criterion employed to protect the community from people who are potentially violent due to mental illness, but I am not going to address this criterion here. Rather, I am going to focus on the two ways of justifying coercive treatment when a person is a danger to themselves due to mental illness.

The principle of beneficence justifies coercion when coercive treatment is seen as necessary to advance the patient's best interests, namely when they are in need of mental health treatment in order to be able to avoid causing danger to themselves, and they are unable to consent to it themselves. This danger can include the risk of suicide, uncontrollable behavior that may harm a person, or inability to get basic needs (such as nutrition) met. Patients may be unable to consent to treatment when they are unable to reason appropriately. Some impediments to reasoning that make them unable to consent include having certain false beliefs, such as a belief that they are not ill or a belief that mental health professionals are trying to control them; lacking certain information, such as information about the ways that mental health treatment will help them, which they may lack because they are unable to process information that is given to them in meaningful ways; being unable to form desires that advance their interests, for example by forming instead desires that are self-defeating; or being unable to act on their desires, such as by being unable to control impulsive actions that thwart their interests. Situations where beneficence justifies coercion are cases where paternalistic interference is justified to promote a patient's welfare.

Clinicians can determine the patient's best interests in at least three ways. In some cases, they can ascertain what patients wanted before they became incompetent, such as when patients create advance directives that specify their treatment choices.[51] Often, patients have not clearly expressed their wishes, however, so clinicians must rely on substituted judgment or the patient's best interests objectively determined. In the substituted judgment standard, they can try to figure out what the patient would choose if the patient were competent (what we might think of as the hypothetical desires of a more rational and sane version of the person[52]) and treat the patient's own (hypothetical) desires as their best interests.[53] In the best interests standard, clinicians can simply determine what is in the patient's best interests in an objective way, irrespective of the patient's desires.[54] Determining what someone would hypothetically want can be highly problematic and can lead to results that are difficult to justify or that are even bad;[55] determining what someone *should* want is easier to do, and the results are easier to justify. What is in a patient's best interests is the improvement of functioning in various areas of life so that the patient can avoid harming themselves and others and live a flourishing life. Coercive action undertaken to advance a patient's best interests can be redescribed from a care perspective as "compassionate interference," where the patient's best interests are promoted through actions taken on their behalf.[56]

The other way that coercion is typically justified is according to a competence criterion, in which people who are too incompetent to make rational decisions on their own are medically treated in order to restore their competence so they can make rational decisions in the future.[57] This is analogous to the argument, discussed in chapter 2, that paternalistic intervention is justified for patients who are unable to make autonomous choices in order to restore or increase their autonomy so they can make such choices. In the competence criterion view, coercion is justified not simply by the fact that the patient is incompetent, or that they need treatment (though these are both necessary elements of this criterion), but rather by the idea that actions should be taken that would restore a person's competence by making them capable of making meaningful decisions about their situation. The relevant issue for this model, therefore, is not the patient's need—which is what is central to the beneficence model—but rather the loss of the patient's decision-making capacity.[58] Mental incompetence justifies coercive treatment insofar as the treatment will help the patient to regain their decision-making capacity.

The competence criterion and the beneficence principle often collapse into each other. The competence criterion falls under the beneficence principle in the sense that regaining one's decision-making capacity can be regarded as what is in the patient's best interests; the loss of the patient's decision-making capacity justifies paternalistic action that advances the patient's interests, namely the restoration of this capacity. The competence criterion can thus be seen as one form that the beneficence principle may take. At the same time, the beneficence principle often falls under the competence criterion. In the vast majority of cases, when a patient who is in dire need of treatment to prevent a significant harm that would occur without treatment, they are too incompetent to make the decision to receive treatment autonomously. When they refuse treatment in such circumstances, such a decision reflects nonautonomous desires that should not be respected. In such a case, treatment should be administered so the patient can regain their ability to make rational decisions for themselves. Most of the time when the beneficence principle applies, the competence criterion applies as well. In most cases where either criterion can be used to justify coercive treatment, therefore, the other can be used as well. For the sake of argument here, however, I will focus on the competence criterion. As I argued in chapter 2, one of the patient's primary interests is to be able to make autonomous choices for themselves. Given this, it is in their best interests to have the competence to be able to make autonomous decisions.

Clinicians rightly want to avoid coercion as much as possible, because they would rather have patients decide for themselves that they need to accept treatment. They want to encourage patients to act as autonomously as possible, but within the constraints entailed by the need for treatment. Coercion can cause negative treatment outcomes, resulting in alienation, disaffection, nonadherence, and fear of seeking out treatment voluntarily; it reinforces feelings of incompetence and hopelessness while diminishing internal motivation to get better and self-efficacy; it can even promote psychological dysfunction and induce learned helplessness.[59] In addition, it can create trauma and induce posttraumatic stress disorder.[60] When patients make choices about their own treatment, on the other hand, this increases competence, internal motivation, self-efficacy, adherence, and willingness to ask for help.[61] The ability to avoid coercion is a matter of trust: patients can learn to make good choices about their treatment when they have positive therapeutic relationships where they trust their clinician and can work productively with their clinician to determine treatment goals and means to achieve these goals together, and where their clinician trusts them to make reasonable decisions.[62]

While clinicians try to avoid coercion, sometimes coercive treatment is necessary. When education, guidance, and encouragement are ineffective, and a patient in dire need of treatment refuses to accept it, coercive treatment may be warranted, though it should be used sparingly. Usually these are cases in which a patient needs hospitalization to avoid causing harm to themselves or others, and the patient refuses to hospitalize themselves, so a clinician or first responder must determine whether the patient should be committed to a hospital for a short time for their own safety until they can recognize their need for treatment and consent to it themselves. Patient choices to refuse treatment in such cases, when their need for treatment is evident to all but possibly themselves, should not be respected and should be overridden by paternalistic interference, namely coercive treatment.

My choices to not be hospitalized all of those times my clinicians asked me about it were low-voluntary choices: they reflected some first-order desire I had—I did not want to be hospitalized—but they did not reflect my valuation system—I knew in some of those cases that I needed hospitalization. The first-order desire that I had came partly from myself—hospitalization is simply undesirable—and partly from my psychosis—my psychosis wanted me to not receive more intensive treatment so it could stay present and alive. My choice to not be hospitalized was nonautonomous and low voluntary, but it had significant potential negative consequences. Not allowing myself to be hospitalized again—and to receive appropriately intensive treatment— kept me stuck in a perpetual state of crisis that I never really dealt with, to the point that, for many months, almost every time I saw my psychiatrist or therapist, they asked me if I thought I should be hospitalized.

I know from my own experience that patients in the throes of illness can make decisions based on what the illness "wants" and not be able to assert what they in fact need. I could never agree to hospitalization after the one time I sought it out voluntarily because I felt like my illness was dictating what I should do, allowing it to perpetuate itself. In fact, when my clinicians refused to hospitalize me themselves, I actually got mad at them for not being able to see past my illness. It seemed to me that they saw my refusal to be hospitalized as a choice that emanated from my will and ought to be respected, whereas I saw it as a choice that came from my psychosis, as it wanted me to stay sick so it could perpetuate itself. The fact that my clinicians could not see that angered me because I felt like they were letting my illness stay in control instead of helping me to fight it. Shaped by my psychosis, my choice to refuse hospitalization was not autonomous. In such a case, it would have been quite justified if my clinicians had determined that I needed coercive treatment and part of me wanted them to make this determination because I knew, deep down, that I needed it.

What my clinicians knew, and what I did not understand until much later, was that treating me as if I were autonomous actually helped me become more autonomous. It is important to treat the desires of someone who is incompetent seriously and to respond to the reasoning behind them as if it is rational. When people who are in dire need of treatment refuse treatment, they are usually incompetent in that their rationale for refusing treatment is often based on poor reasons motivated by their illness. Because they are usually incompetent, the competence criterion often applies, justifying treatment to restore their autonomy; when not obtaining treatment will threaten their life or basic flourishing, the best interests standard may apply as well.

At the same time, it is always best to use the least restrictive means of paternalistic interference so as to encourage patients to take responsibility for their own recovery. When my clinicians tried to guide me to make choices in my best interests, they were trying to get me to take responsibility for my own recovery. When I refused hospitalization, they gave me other options to try to stay safe and work toward getting better, such as participating in IOP and trying new medication changes. Giving me options was a way of guiding me to make good choices. I was more amenable to these suggestions as they restricted my freedom much less. Although I struggled to make choices to work on my recovery consistently, sometimes I had success making these choices, and this success was due in part to the optimism and trust my clinicians held for me and the ways that they tried to guide me to make positive choices. They would have been justified if they had determined I needed coercive treatment, but by giving me options and guiding me to make good choices instead, they allowed me greater freedom, which allowed me to practice making voluntary choices so I could learn to make truly autonomous choices. In doing this, I could take responsibility for my recovery and learn to work toward it more consistently, choosing over and over again to participate in treatment rather than resisting.

Encouragement to Trust

Trusting a patient takes courage, because the outcome of putting trust in someone to act well, especially when evidence suggests that the person may choose *not* to act well, is uncertain and carries with it risks. In nonacute situations in which the patient's life is not on the line, and the patient is not causing significant harm to themselves or others, clinicians should do their best to trust their patients and to develop the kind of therapeutic relationship with their patients that enables the patient to trust them, because this is how a patient learns to act well. In a positive therapeutic relationship, clinicians and patients can dialogue with each other with honesty, compassion, empathy, and humility about the merits of following treatment recommendations. In such a relationship, patients can try to explain why they do not want to adhere to treatment (to the best of their ability), and clinicians can listen with empathy. Clinicians can try to respond to patient concerns in ways that assuage the patient and make it easier for the patient to heed their clinician's recommendations, for example by prescribing medication in ways that minimize side effects or otherwise make it easier to take. Through dialogue with their clinicians, patients can learn to make positive choices to take care of themselves by following treatment recommendations.

Karen Jones notes that sometimes our desire to trust someone is not based on evidence of trustworthiness, or evidence that would support a belief that they will fulfill our expectations of them, but rather a desire to inculcate the trustworthiness that they do not already possess. She says, "Sometimes we set about cultivating trust because we think that by trusting, and displaying our trust, we will be able to elicit trustworthy behavior from the other. When we do this our hope is that by trusting we will be able to bring about the very conditions that would justify our trust."[63] In such a case, we do not actually trust the person—because they do not appear to be trustworthy—but we nonetheless act *as if* we trusted them, in order to try to encourage them to become trustworthy, to live up to our expectations of them. She argues, however, that this is a "pointless strategy," and that acting as if we trust someone does not lead to the same results that actually trusting someone does.[64] She says, "Our attempts at giving positive reinterpretations of those aspects of a person that might otherwise have tended to support the hypothesis that she is untrustworthy have the feel of fantasy and wish fulfillment. They do not ring true."[65] And, she argues, they are unlikely to lead to the desired result of developing or proving trustworthiness.

I disagree with Jones's assessment of this practice as a pointless strategy. Even if it does not lead to the desired outcome—in this case, of the patient participating actively in their treatment—it does do something fruitful: it helps create the conditions that enable change to occur. People are able to make different decisions and act differently than they have in the past when they have genuine options as well as encouragement to do so. People do not always respond to our confidence in them, but they do sometimes respond, and only when we do have this confidence in them do they have that opportunity to respond to it. To deny them that confidence is to close off the option that they might respond to that confidence. Denying them one's confidence in them does not foreclose the option of acting differently—a person still has the option to choose to respond to expectations of them by living up to them and fulfilling their commitments. But they do not in this case have the *encouragement* that could provide an additional boost in favor of such a decision.

Jones characterizes our trust in people in such conditions as "fantasy" and "wish fulfillment." But this assumes a certain kind of response we may have if people fail to fulfill our expectations of them: that we will be disappointed in them and perhaps hold reactive attitudes like blame or resentment toward them. In fact, we do not have to respond to people who do not fulfill our expectations of them in this way. We can hold asymmetrical attitudes of trusting that they will follow through on what we expect them to do while refraining from blaming them if they fail to follow through.

We can choose to not be personally affected by whatever choice they make, even as we maintain a trusting attitude toward them. In doing so, we create a small distance between ourselves and their act, being connected to it in the sense that we want people to choose what we think is in their best interests but remaining distant from it in that whatever actually happens does not affect how we feel about the person or the situation.[66] Hanna Pickard describes this attitude of holding a person responsible for their behavior while not being personally affected by it as "detached blame." In this way, a clinician can hold a trusting attitude, by being optimistic toward their patient that the patient will participate actively in their treatment, and be ready to praise the patient if they follow through, yet not feel disappointed, hold reactive attitudes like blame, or be otherwise personally affected by whatever the patient chooses to do.

Some philosophers object to this view as an impersonal attitude that treats the person more like an object than an agent, assuming that treating people as agents necessarily entails being personally affected by what they do.[67] But it is unclear to me why we must always be affected by what others do in order to treat them as agents. It seems perfectly compatible to me to regard someone as an agent who can make sufficiently free and rational choices in the relevant domain while not being affected by what they choose to do.

Trusting in circumstances such as those I describe here takes courage. It is an act of bravery to trust someone to meet a commitment, especially when there may be good reasons not to trust, whether that be a lack of trustworthiness on the part of the patient or patient incompetence that threatens to prevent a patient from having the capacity to carry out commitments. Some may argue that trusting under these conditions is an act of foolhardiness, but it all depends on how we look at it. If we feel like a lot is personally at stake in trusting someone, it can feel foolhardy to trust when there are reasons not to trust. But if we feel like little is at stake personally, it can be worthwhile and even noble to trust someone even where are reasons not to trust. Whatever is lost in being let down by a patient's action or inaction is small compared to what is gained in trusting a patient to do the right thing. Even if the patient does the wrong thing, they gain by being put in a position where they can make a meaningful choice. In this way, they exercise their agency and develop their autonomy. When the consequences of a patient not meeting their commitment to participate in treatment are graver, clinicians may need to employ coercion to get patients to comply with treatment. In most normal cases, however, patients ought to be allowed to choose how they participate in treatment in order to feel invested in their recovery and make good decisions regarding their treatment.

Conclusion

During my psychotic period, I experienced coercive treatment a few times. Some of these occurred when I was hospitalized. Both the process of becoming hospitalized and the experiences I had while in the hospital were coercive. Although I went to the crisis center voluntarily, I was placed under a seventy-two-hour mental health hold so I was hospitalized involuntarily, meaning that I could not leave if I wanted to do so. This coercion did not bother me, as I thought it was appropriate given my circumstances. While in the hospital, I was given certain choices that had only one live option, making the choice seem coercive. Taking medication and attending group activities was one type of coerced choice: I had no real option of refusal, as I had to take medication and attend group activities if I wanted eventually to be discharged. This coercion also did not bother me, as I thought it was reasonable that one had to adhere to treatment in order to be discharged, as long as treatment was generally reasonable. Being coerced to act in ways that are generally reasonable, for reasons that make sense, is justifiable.

Remaining in the hospital after the seventy-two-hour hold was up constituted another type of coerced choice: again, I had no real option of refusal, for if I did not voluntarily sign myself into the hospital, the doctor would apply for a court order to keep me in the hospital involuntarily. Bruce Winick notes that many patients who are voluntarily admitted to a hospital feel that their decision was coerced because they felt pressure or experienced threats resulting in this choice (for example, the threat of being involuntarily admitted if one does not choose to admit oneself voluntarily).[68] This coercion bothered me because it was presented as a choice but in fact was not a choice at all. I would have felt more comfortable had the need to sign myself in voluntarily been presented in a different way, and not couched falsely as a "choice." Coercion presented straightforwardly as coercion is transparent and as a result easier to accept, but coercion couched falsely as a choice is confusing, manipulative, and deceitful and thus harder to accept.

Very rarely was I coerced while in outpatient treatment. The only times my therapist coerced me were when I had bought over-the-counter pills "just in case" I needed to overdose. When I admitted that I had bought them and that they were hidden in my car, he made me bring them to him; if I didn't, he said he would need to hospitalize me because I had the means and intention to kill myself. So I had a choice, but it was a coerced choice. I brought him the pills. The whole thing seemed really silly because I could just go out and buy more pills, which I did; we replayed this scene a few times in successive therapy sessions. Each time, he had to make sure that I did not in that moment have the (intended) means to kill myself. In retrospect, this act of coercion seems justified in order to prevent me from having the means to cause imminent harm to myself. As my inclination toward suicide was not autonomous, the principle of beneficence heavily outweighed my low-voluntary choice to have the means of suicide at my disposal.

Outside of the hospital, I was never coerced into receiving treatment and only rarely (as with the pills) was I coerced while in treatment. Sometimes I felt as if I had no other options, but in fact I always did. My clinicians knew that forcing me into treatment would cause me to feel passive, detached, and uncaring about my recovery. They knew that the long-term solution required me to be invested in my recovery. To be invested, I had to make choices on my own to participate in treatment. While guiding me to make choices in my best interests, my clinicians ultimately had to trust me to make the choices on my own. When they put this faith in me and helped give me the tools to make choices successfully, I was able to develop the ability to do so.

Trust is a crucial component of the therapeutic relationship and is often critical for recovery. When patients trust clinicians, they are more likely to share the same treatment goals and agree on means to reach those goals, which encourages patients to make good decisions regarding their treatment. And when clinicians trust patients to make their own decisions about treatment, patients feel encouraged to take responsibility for themselves and to act on their own will whileparticipating in their recovery. Building trust on both sides of the therapeutic relationship helps patients to participate more actively in their recovery, which increases their agency and autonomy and improves their treatment outcomes. In the next chapter, I examine another crucial component of the therapeutic relationship: empathy.

5 Empathy

Introduction

Shortly before I was hospitalized, I started seeing a new therapist. The last time I had seen a therapist was a few years prior to that. I had liked that therapist a lot, but she left the practice. When she left, I tried a new therapist, but this one did not seem to understand me, so I stopped seeing her after three sessions and went therapist-free for several years. During this time, I met with my psychiatrist annually. Since my symptoms during this time period were under control, I did not feel the need to see clinicians more frequently and was pessimistic about my ability to find a therapist with whom I could really connect.

When I met with my psychiatrist in the spring of 2018, psychotic and suicidal, he strongly recommended that I start seeing a therapist again. He gave me the names of a couple of people with whom he was familiar and recommended. I was able to get in to see one of these people, but I never clicked with her. She thought I had too much insight for the problems I had and did not believe me when I told her I heard a voice telling me to kill myself. I left every session feeling worse than I did when I went into it. With the person who is supposed to be helping me not taking me seriously, I felt extremely isolated. While I needed her to be on my side and help me understand and fight my mental illness, instead I felt like she was laughing at me.

After seeing her three times, I realized the relationship was not going to improve and I opted to end it. My suicidal ideation grew worse over the course of seeing her that spring, and after the third time, I became unhinged. I called the crisis hotline several times that weekend because I was so suicidal that I felt like I was running out of options. The first time I called was later that day after my appointment; I told the nurse on the phone that I needed to see a different therapist because the one I was seeing wasn't working. She was able to get me in to see the other person who my psychiatrist had recommended the following week when he must have had a cancellation.

Seeing this therapist was an entirely different experience. The first thing he did at our initial session was to lean in toward me and ask me what was going on. His body language indicated that he was deeply interested and fully engaged. He never looked at his computer during the session. After I spoke, he rephrased what I said in a way that made me know that he understood what I was saying. He validated my suffering and noted that I was barely holding on. He took my psychotic symptoms seriously and helped me identify them as psychotic. His ability to read me so well made me trust him inherently. At the end of the session, he suggested I think about hospitalization since I was having such a difficult time keeping myself safe. Although I did not really want to be hospitalized, I trusted him enough to take his suggestion seriously. The seed was planted. Two days later I went to the crisis center and turned myself in to be hospitalized (or so it felt, since I had felt like I had been running on the lam for months). I only had the courage to reach out to the crisis center because of his suggestion and because I inherently trusted him, even though I had just met him. I trusted him because I felt that he understood me in a way that few people did.

Having a good working relationship with clinicians is vital for recovery from mental illness. In a medical model of psychiatric disability where medication and therapy are seen as essential to addressing a patient's illness, the quality of the therapeutic relationship is critical. In chapter 4, I explained the crucial role that trust plays in the therapeutic relationship. Here I explain the role that empathy plays.

Some of the greatest needs that patients have in the therapeutic relationship are to be understood and to be given compassion and care based on that understanding. When clinicians empathize with their patients, they can appreciate the patient's perspective on their illness and work more effectively with the patient to develop shared goals and shared ideas about how to achieve those goals. Empathy is thus crucial for therapeutic alliance and the creation of a positive therapeutic relationship. Patients have a great need to be treated with respect, empathy, and compassion, particularly within the therapeutic relationship, and to be taken seriously at all times; clinicians can foster a healthy and productive therapeutic relationship that meets these needs by interacting with patients empathetically.

Empathizing with Psychotic Patients

Empathy toward people who exhibit psychotic symptoms is more difficult than empathy toward people showing other symptoms, even other mental health symptoms. This is because psychosis is harder to understand, so the knowledge condition of empathic understanding is not satisfied as easily. As one study on voice hearing simulations notes, "While the helping professional can acknowledge and appreciate that such symptoms produce problems, it is unlikely that she or he will have personally experienced such symptoms."[1] Psychotic patients engage in behaviors and entertain ideas that seem foreign and mystifying. In part this is because psychotic patients operate from a different context than people who do not experience psychosis. They experience the world very differently from others, and this different experience of the world colors what they think, feel, believe, desire, do, and say. Without sharing this context, people who do not experience psychosis find psychotic thought and behavior to be strange and confusing. Clinicians often have to make a special effort to learn how to empathize with patients who experience psychosis.

One element of psychosis that is difficult to understand is why many psychotic patients do not seem to work hard on getting better. Many patients who experience psychosis seem uninterested in improving their health and well-being, unmotivated to make changes in their life that would decrease their symptoms and increase their functioning, and/or unable to make such changes. These involve both lifestyle changes and actions that address their illness. Such patients do not take the steps required for well-being, such as eating healthier, sleeping on a regular cycle, or exercising. Oftentimes they do not take their medication as prescribed. Sometimes they do not attend or participate in recommended therapy sessions. This lack of interest, motivation, and ability to change can be very frustrating for clinicians who want to see their patients get better.

From the clinician's point of view, it would seem obvious that a person experiencing psychosis would want to get better. Being out of touch with reality and experiencing hallucinations, delusions, and paranoia sounds scary. Hearing voices that are usually negative in nature would be distressing. Having confused thoughts and illogical ideas seems like it would be terrifying. Being unable to interact with others in socially appropriate ways and unable to maintain meaningful relationships seems tragic. From this vantage point, why wouldn't someone want to work hard to alleviate their psychosis?

The fact that many psychotic patients do not appear to work hard at getting better is usually a function of their illness. Sometimes the problem stems from negative symptoms of psychosis. Apathy, disinterest, lack of motivation, lethargy, social withdrawal, and difficulty completing tasks can make it so a patient does not care about getting better, or so they do not have the motivation and energy required to make changes, or so they simply are unable to translate their will into action. Sometimes the problem results from cognitive symptoms of disorganization, cognitive dulling, and memory loss. It can be too difficult for a person to comprehend what changes they need to make, or to organize themselves enough to commit to make changes and follow through on this commitment. In addition, positive symptoms can play a role, as hallucinations and delusions can provide contrary motivation that make a person resistant to making changes.

Clinicians often do not realize the influence hallucinations and delusions have on making a patient not want to get better. This is often because they have mistaken stereotypical views about what hallucinations are like that lead them to think that hallucinations are so debilitating and distressing that patients should want to be relieved of them. These stereotyped views are reinforced by auditory hallucination simulations, which are commonly used in nursing education. Clinicians who adopt stereotyped views of psychosis often don't realize that hallucinations and delusions can exert a pull over a person that make the person want to pursue them rather than eradicate them.

Staying committed to working on recovery was something I struggled with quite a bit, as I often went back and forth between begging my clinicians to help me deal with my distress and resisting their recommendations, because, in my psychosis, I wanted to stay psychotic. Here I want to shed some light on why a psychotic person might not want to let go of their psychosis by focusing on the role that hallucinations can play in a person's life. This can help us to comprehend psychotic patients' motivation in resisting their clinicians' attempts to treat their hallucinations.

Let us look at some of the assumptions that people commonly have about hallucinations to see how psychotic patients' experiences sometimes differ from these assumptions so we can better understand why a person might want to hold onto their hallucinations.

What Hallucinations Can Sometimes Be Like

One assumption that is commonly made is that hallucinations are unequivocally distressing. When people who do not hallucinate imagine what it is like to hear voices telling a person what to do, they imagine that this would be a difficult and terrifying experience.

Auditory hallucinations *can* be distressing, of course. Factors that contribute to distress include the belief that voices are omniscient and omnipotent, the belief that voices have malevolent intent, and the belief that voices are uncontrollable.[2] Auditory hallucinations are not always distressing, however. Many people have voices that are benign or even positive,[3] and most people hear both positive and negative voices (voices that are disparaging).[4] Positive voices give advice, encouragement, and information, and they provide reassurance, comfort, and companionship; sometimes they help patients deal with negative voices. Whether the voices are experienced as distressing or not, many people like their voices because the voices keep them company, are comforting, or confer a sense of specialness.[5] People frequently form complicated relationships with their voices.[6] Voices can keep loneliness at bay, provide motivation, shape identity, and exact a pull over a person that dictates their action and way of being in the world (particularly command hallucinations). As a result, people often hold complicated feelings toward their voices even when their voices are predominantly negative.

For example, even though the voice I heard frequently told me to kill myself, I welcomed the voice as a companion. One afternoon after my depression had finally receded in spring 2019, I was sitting in my office waiting for the hours to pass until it was time to attend a late afternoon meeting and feeling desperately lonely and empty. Suddenly the voice appeared and told me that if I let it out of its cage, it would keep me company at all times; I would never have to feel lonely again. That night I started reducing my antipsychotic medication so the voice would stay with me, and I continued to struggle with taking my medication for much of that spring. While the resulting increased psychosis caused me distress, I no longer ever felt lonely. For me, the voice solved a problem. Clinicians wanting to understand why I struggled to take my medication as prescribed would have to understand what roles the voice played for me.

Voices can also provide meaning. Hallucinatory experiences often involve heightened sensory awareness and can feel momentous and significant. Hallucinations can be imbued with meaning that is only accessible to the person experiencing them. One of the features of auditory verbal hallucinations is the way their meaning supersedes whatever linguistic meaning the words heard convey. In other words, a person may hear a simple message—for example, "Act natural"—but the meaning of this message to the voice-hearer may involve persecutory delusions and beliefs about what it is to be "natural" that go beyond what the words by themselves suggest. Voice-hearers may not be able to articulate verbally the meaning that is conveyed in a message, perceiving that the message opens up a layer of reality that was previously inaccessible, and that is apparent to no one but the perceiver. There is a richness of meaning that hallucinations may convey; hallucinations can be experienced as sources of awe and wonder. Even when they are distressed by their voices, people often find meaning in the voices that they are hesitant to eliminate.

It is important to note that, while many people who hear voices do suffer from the experience, they tend to be harmed more by other connected aspects of psychosis than by auditory hallucinations themselves. Delusions can impede a person's ability to have knowledge about the world and self-understanding and insight, leading to losses of epistemic and moral agency. Delusions also can impact the way a person engages with other people and with the world much more than hallucinations do; feeling a gap between the world inside one's mind and the external world can make interacting with the external world very difficult, awkward, and distressing. Moreover, cognitive dulling, memory loss, detachment, social withdrawal, and other negative symptoms related to psychosis can create more problems with functioning than hallucinations do. In my experience, feeling like I had dementia was by far the most debilitating aspect of psychosis because it made it so that I could not understand the world around me even when I tried to. By creating massive confusion and misunderstanding and by severing the connection a person has to the world around them, cognitive dulling can decrease epistemic agency in a significant way. Furthermore, memory loss can separate a person from their past; by erasing their connection to the past, memory loss erases self-identity. Social withdrawal can isolate a person, leading to many losses, while apathy and lethargy can make a person unable to make choices and take action. We often treat hallucinations as if they are the chief problem of psychosis, but delusions, cognitive dulling, memory loss, lethargy, and apathy can be just as debilitating.

Another assumption that is sometimes made is the idea that auditory hallucinations are an isolatable symptom that can be experienced apart from other symptoms. For people who experience auditory hallucinations due to neurological disorders, or for people in the general population who experience them, this impression may be true: auditory hallucinations may stand alone, isolatable from other aspects of experience. For people who are psychotic and experiencing auditory hallucinations, however, this is often not true. Hallucinations are usually connected to other aspects of psychosis, including delusions, paranoia, a sense that the world is less real or has a changed reality, a feeling of alienness that affects one's interaction with other people, and disorganized thinking that sees connections where there are none and that reasons in illogical ways. Hallucinations are typically tied to delusions about the source of the hallucination (for example, coming from an object or entity) or the nature of the hallucination (for instance, a command from God, a message aimed directly and solely at the person having the hallucination, or secret messages hidden in the universe needing to be decoded). Hallucinations are often part of the person's overall distorted sense of reality, affecting how the person interacts with others and with the world, and are in some cases connected to paranoia.

A third assumption that is commonly made about hallucinations is that what is frightening about hallucinations is the incorrectness of the perception, the way that it does not match reality. Hallucinations are often not experienced as being out of sync with an otherwise correct world, however. Instead, they tend to be part of an overall change in one's experience that affects one's way of being in the world. A common misconception about hallucinations is the assumption that people who hallucinate cannot tell the difference between their hallucination and the shared reality that everyone experiences. For example, authors of a study on voice hearing simulations claimed that "a person who does experience auditory hallucinations will not know whether other people can hear the voices or noises that they can."[7] In fact, most people who hear voices know that they are having hallucinations and can tell the difference between what they experience and the shared reality that others experience.[8] What is significant is that this knowledge does not negate the knowledge and insight they gain from the experience of having the hallucination; in other words, knowing that others do not hear their voices does not take away from the way the voices are experienced as subjectively real to them.[9] The fact that the experience of hearing voices does not match shared reality is not the basis of fear or distress for people who actually hear voices; psychotic individuals accept that their experience does not fit with the reality that others experience.

What is sometimes frightening about hallucinations is not that they involve incorrect perception, but that they shift a person's attention away from shared to reality to an idiosyncratic experience of reality that only they experience. Psychotic patients often know that the voices they hear are not part of the reality that everyone else experiences, but they have the sense that the voices are part of a reality that only they can experience, which makes their experience special and significant. This added layer of meaning can be frightening when a person recognizes that it removes them from the reality that everyone experiences, but it can also be thrilling because it provides purpose, meaning, joy, and pleasure. Typically, hallucinations are not experienced by psychotic patients as being wrong or in error, the way some people might suppose; they are experienced as being absolutely correct. Thus, the problem for people who actually experience auditory hallucinations often is not that they perceive a wrong reality, but that the reality they perceive removes them from the reality they share with others. This retreat into their own private mental world has significant effects on functioning and well-being, and it can lead to dysfunctions in work and home life, changes in attention, sleep, and appetite, social withdrawal and avoidance, and neglect of personal hygiene.

The authority of command hallucinations is particularly hard to understand. A person who has not experienced command hallucinations may suppose that hearing a voice issuing a directive is like hearing someone else telling a person what to do, where the person has the freedom to obey or not and can articulate, if they so choose, reasons why they should or should not obey. For a person who actually hears voices, on the other hand, hearing a voice issuing a directive can be like having a family member telling them what to do. A person who hears voices may have been hearing them for some time and may have developed a relationship with them. Within the context of that relationship, a command holds special meaning and has special force. Disobeying a command can be more like disobeying one's parent, something many of us are not comfortable doing. The agony that a person who actually hears voices may experience when they hear commands telling them what to do, when they do not want to follow through, is not only the annoyance of being told to do something contrary to one's will. In some cases, the agony comes from the persistence of the command, the way it will not go away no matter how much a person tries to resist it and distract themselves from it. But in many other cases the agony comes from the existential struggle involved with wanting to resist something that has special hold over the person. Again, it is like the agony many of us would experience if we tried to resist doing what our parent requested of us. It can make us question our identity (whether we are still good children to our parent) and second-guess ourselves ("Am I doing what is right by trying to resist?"). Resisting a voice that a person has a relationship with can feel like committing a betrayal, and it is not something a person can do lightly, if at all.

Another assumption that people commonly have is that hallucinations and delusions are globally debilitating, that they can make it impossible for a person to function. When people believe this, they endorse the stereotype that people with severe mental illness are incompetent and unable to succeed in life. This assumption was probably underlying the reaction of the first therapist I saw when I was psychotic: she couldn't see how someone as functional as I generally am could be as sick as I claimed to be. But a person can sometimes function reasonably well while psychotic because they can compartmentalize their psychotic experience and separate it from other aspects of their life. Knowing that others would not approve, sometimes a person can become good at hiding their psychosis from others.

Moreover, a person who gets sick episodically, like myself, can function very well when their illness is in remission but then function very poorly when the illness blossoms. If a person has a job with a lot of flexibility, and supportive family and friends (as I do), they can manage to get by through their less functional periods without necessarily causing great and lasting harm to their lives. I am successful because I have periods of my life when I am well, and I have a job with a lot of flexibility, which makes it easier to get by when I can't function well. When I am doing poorly, this does impair my work and family life and threaten my job and family stability.

A good therapist can recognize that a person can appear to function well despite severe illness, but also needs to recognize that illness can threaten the building blocks of a successful life.

When clinicians believe that hallucinations are intrinsically distressing, they may have no appreciation for the role that hallucinations can play in a psychotic person's inner life: the way they can affect a person's meaning structure, orientation to the world, and even identity and agency. When clinicians believe that psychosis is globally debilitating, they may fail to recognize when patients who appear to be functioning reasonably well are sick. Even when psychosis is on the balance impairing and distressing, it can still hold value to a person that must be acknowledged and accounted for. Without an appreciation of this value, clinicians may not understand how a person who experiences auditory hallucinations can become attached to their hallucinations. When a person sees their voices as disclosing secret meaning, when the voices color experience as momentous and significant, and when the voices confer a status of specialness to both the experience and the person experiencing it, the voices are something to be welcomed and even sought after rather than something to avoid. For this reason, people who experience auditory hallucinations may not want to take prescribed antipsychotic medicine: they may like the connection they have to a special and unique reality that psychosis offers them. Clinicians who do not understand how attached someone can get to their voices lack an understanding of one of the sources of nonadherence to treatment and will be frustrated when patients refuse to take their medicine or otherwise participate in their treatment.

Psychotic patients often want to hold onto their hallucinations for many reasons, including to experience the special meaning they convey, to see the world as extraordinary, and to obey the voices that tell them to do so. All of these factors played a role in my struggle to participate in recovery. In order to be more committed to my recovery, I needed to work with clinicians who understood these aspects of psychosis so they could help me address them. I needed my clinicians to have empathetic understanding of what my psychosis was doing to me.

Empathy

In order to understand why a patient might not want to eradicate their hallucinations with treatment, clinicians need to try to empathize with the patient so as to understand the patient's experience from their own point of view. Empathizing with patients is necessary for clinicians to move beyond their own assumptions about patient experience to understand what it is really like for the patient in experiencing their situation. Empathy provides more accurate understanding, and thus enables more effective treatment, than mere clinical observation and reasoning.

Empathy is understood in myriad ways,[10] suggesting that there is a lot of conceptual confusion around the term.[11] Most accounts of empathy identify both an affective component, in which a person feels what another person feels or at least is emotionally affected by the emotions and experiences of someone else, and a cognitive component, in which a person takes on the perspective of another person.[12] Sometimes the affective component is connected to compassion or care for a person based on an understanding of what they are going through.[13] The affective component is commonly understood to involve an intuitive, pre-reflective grasping of another person's feelings, while the cognitive component is typically seen as an imaginative and reflective reconstruction of trying to understand another person's perspective.[14] This requires recognizing and acknowledging someone else's psychological state and drawing on one's familiarity with similar states (whether through imagination or past personal experience) to understand—either cognitively or affectively—what the person is experiencing.[15] In some accounts of empathy, by imaginatively reconstructing someone else's experience, we also develop similar emotional states as the person whose experience we are imagining, which we may understand as emotional "matching."[16] As a form of perspective-taking, empathy is a skill or capacity that we can develop through practice.[17]

I endorse Jodi Halpern's definition of clinical empathy as the ability to understand a patient's emotional point of view.[18] Empathy is best understood as a cognitive trait of imaginatively reconstructing another person's experience in order to have an understanding of that person's situation from their own perspective.[19] In a clinical context, the third-person point of view of detached observation of a patient's emotional states is insufficient; the first-person perspective of experiential knowledge is necessary. As Halpern says, "Empathy requires imagining, and not just logically understanding, a patient's world."[20] Through this, a clinician can gain greater knowledge of the patient's perspective. By imagining the patient's emotional perspective, a clinician can pay more attention to what is relevant and meaningful to the patient and thus better understand the motivations and intentions underlying the patient's actions.[21] This deeper understanding is useful clinically as it helps the clinician determine what is the best response to a patient's situation as well as determine how to interact and communicate with the patient more effectively. Empathy is especially important in the context of trying to understand a psychotic patient, because what is salient to a psychotic person is often not what is apparent or salient to others; understanding a psychotic person's reasoning and perspective requires imagining the psychotic patient's world and emotional experience from their own point of view.

In a clinical context, the most valuable form of empathy is imaginative reconstruction of a patient's experience. Emotional matching or contagion is not a helpful trait in a clinical context, as emotions can impede the kind of rational judgment that clinicians have to make in the course of their work. When clinicians adopt the feelings of their patient, they risk experiencing emotional upheaval that may interfere with their ability to reason about the patient's situation appropriately; they also risk emotional burnout and the possibility of overrelating to patients in an unprofessional way.[22] When clinicians *understand* what a patient feels, on the other hand, they have valuable information that they are able to use to help them reason more accurately and thoroughly in determining what should be done for the patient; they can thus make better treatment decisions and relate to patients in more productive ways. In trying to understand the patient as best as possible, the clinician is able to treat the patient as a whole person.[23]

Developing an understanding of what another person experiences can occur in at least two general ways. We can adopt self-oriented perspective-taking, in which we imagine what it is like to be ourselves in someone else's situation, or we can adopt other-oriented perspective-taking, in which we imagine what it is like to be someone else in their own situation. Peter Goldie claims that other-oriented perspective-taking is impossible, as we cannot literally get inside someone else's mind and see the world from their point of view.[24] We have not had the range of experiences they have had in order to develop the perspectives they develop; we do not have the same resources to draw upon in feeling, thinking, and responding to the world and so cannot know or act the way they would. Because we cannot actually get inside other people's minds to understand their situation and motivations exactly, when we adopt other-oriented perspective-taking, we can easily be wrong in our understanding and may ascribe reactions, feelings, and motivations to people that they do not actually have.

For this reason, Goldie rejects other-oriented perspective-taking, which he calls "in-his-shoes imagining," in favor of self-oriented perspective-taking, in which a person imagines what it is like to be themselves in another person's situation.[25] Goldie describes empathy as "a process or procedure by which a person *centrally imagines the narrative* (the thoughts, feelings, and emotions) of another person" by placing themselves at the center of the narrative.[26] Such narrative reconstruction is important to understand someone else's situation, but Goldie is wrong to think we must put ourselves in the narrative; rather, we must understand a person's narrative from their own perspective.

This is because self-oriented perspective-taking is highly problematic. When we imagine what it is like for us to be in someone else's situation, we focus on what is salient to *us*, such as what excites or distresses us, and we easily ignore what may be salient to the other person. We may get so caught up in our own distress or excitement that we do not notice that other people's reactions to their situation may be very different than our own responses to their situation. This can cloud our judgment and create epistemic inaccuracies in our understanding. For example, clinicians who focus on how debilitating and distressing hallucinations would be to them may not realize what value hallucinations can hold to psychotic patients. In addition, self-oriented perspective-taking can deter us from feeling care and compassion toward others, impeding our moral motivation to help others. When we imagine ourselves in a distressing situation, we may become self-absorbed, interested in alleviating our own distress rather than that of others. We may try to escape distress by avoiding the situation that causes it or by avoiding the people who actually experience what we are imagining.[27] In a clinical setting, this can contribute to clinicians distancing themselves from their patients as they try to avoid feeling their patients' suffering, resulting in aloof or fearful pity rather than compassion.[28]

Clinicians who adopt self-oriented perspective-taking and try to put themselves in the shoes of their patients, so to speak, can sometimes learn new perspectives that can be useful, but it can also be harmful. When clinicians imagine themselves as patients, they may downplay the amount and kind of pain and distress they feel and wonder why actual patients make such a big deal of it. They may feel comfortably compliant in the hands of clinicians they trust, or they may retain their sense of authority and speak to clinicians as peers; in either case, they fail to understand what it is like for patients who are not comfortably compliant, who do not uniformly trust their clinicians, or who feel like they have little authority and struggle to make their voice heard. When clinicians imagine themselves as patients, what they can learn about the patient experience is very limited, based on their own experiences and not on the actual experiences of someone else. Moreover, when clinicians try to understand patients' experiences by imagining what it is like to have certain symptoms, they can misrepresent what the experience of actual patients is like, for example misconstruing the experience of psychosis as uniformly debilitating and distressing. While the self-oriented approach may help clinicians gain some epistemically useful knowledge, therefore, it is at the same time very limited knowledge and not as useful as actually understanding a patient's perspective of their own experience.

Clinicians who adopt other-oriented perspective-taking and try to understand what patients experience from the patient's own point of view, on the other hand, can develop a greater scope of knowledge of what it is like to be a patient. In order to gain this knowledge, they must try to understand the patient's situation as broadly as possible, including understanding relevant aspects of the patient's history, relationships, beliefs, and worldview. They must try to develop a third-person perspective of the patient's situation as a whole in order to understand what the patient feels and thinks and why. They cannot simply imagine what it must be like for the patient; imagination can be helpful, but it can also lead us astray. Rather, clinicians must engage in dialogue with patients in order to ascertain what they feel and think and try to gain a larger understanding of the patient's situation.[29] This way they can learn the patient's motives and interests—why the patient believes, thinks, feels, and acts the way they do—in order to develop a greater understanding of what it is like for the patient to be themselves in their situation.

Understanding another's experience from their own point of view involves, in part, listening attentively to their testimony, to the stories they tell about their experience. Thus, one set of skills that facilitates empathizing with patients is narrative competence, "the competence that human beings use to absorb, interpret, and respond to stories."[30] Narrative competence is important for both developing other-oriented perspective-taking and for creating the conditions that enable epistemic justice, which I discuss in chapter 6. Rita Charon regards narrative competence to be essential to medicine, and I would argue that it is essential to therapy as well.

Although other-oriented perspective-taking may be impossible to achieve fully, we must try to develop it to the extent that we can in order to develop true empathy. Other-oriented perspective-taking can increase our epistemic resources by helping us to see how a person perceives their own situation and what their motives are from their own perspective. Other-oriented perspective-taking can also enable us to see the broader psycho-social context in which they make their decisions about how to act. This third-person perspective of trying to understand other people's actions, motives, and intentions from their point of view rather than our own can be understood as what Ann Arber and Anne Gallagher calls "empathic maturity,"[31] what Jean Harvey and Barrett Emerick identify as "empathetic understanding,"[32] and what Larry Davidson describes as "building empathic bridges."[33] In a clinical context, other-oriented perspective-taking provides valuable clinical knowledge by enabling clinicians to understand their patients' motives and experiences and to see the psycho-social context that informs how patients act.

In order to attain more accurate and useful information about other people's experiences, other-oriented perspective-taking must be dialogic rather than monologic.[34] Engaging in dialogue with a person can help us to avoid the problems involved with trying to imagine someone else's experience in our own minds and helps us to acquire more accurate information about their experience. Ideally, this involves active communication with someone through interpersonal dialogue; when this is impossible, however, more passive or one-way communication can provide at least some of the benefit of dialogic engagement. Reading memoirs, vignettes, or case studies, or hearing speakers tell their personal stories, can give us firsthand perspectives of other people's experience. Even if we do not have the ability to communicate back and forth with the person telling their story, we can learn what their experience is like through their own eyes to the extent that they can share it in a story. Sometimes we are unable to reconstruct another person's experience imaginatively because it is so different from our own; in such cases, we must trust people's narratives of their own experience so that we may still learn from them.[35]

Empathizing well with someone requires us to understand their experience in their own way and as their own experience. When we empathize with people, we have a tendency to assume that they are like ourselves in a variety of ways and a tendency to ascribe to them the same feelings, desires, beliefs, attitudes, and judgments that we have ourselves.[36] But empathizing well with someone requires that we recognize and respect the alterity of people's experience as their own and not try to put our own interpretation on it or see it through our own lens.[37] This involves, in part, recognizing the ways that someone else's experience is different from our own. As Jake Jackson notes, "Empathy does not attempt to feel the same way as the other, but rather to understand the difference between the experience of oneself and the other. Although there are similarities between myself and the other, our differences matter considerably."[38]

Matthew Ratcliffe recommends that we adopt what he calls "radical" empathy, which emphasizes the otherness of another person's experience, or a recognition of their alterity;[39] it is an openness to another person's perspective as their own.[40] Radical empathy requires putting aside the assumption (which we normally take for granted) that we share experiences and perspectives with others, and instead open ourselves up to another person and their "modes of existence" or ways of being in the world and ways of seeing the world.[41] One way that we come to understand someone's modes of existence is through dialogue with them, asking them about their experience and perspective and trying to make sense of it as best as we can. When a person has diminished capacity to participate meaningfully in dialogue or to relay a trustworthy and meaningful story, however, such as when delusions make it difficult to communicate effectively, we may have to reconstruct the other person's experience through a narrative that we construct of their experience based on what information we are able to ascertain about them.[42]

Empathetic understanding thus requires us to be open minded, open to seeing and being in the world in ways other than our own, and it requires the curiosity to learn about these different ways of seeing and being. Jodi Halpern in fact defines clinical empathy in terms of curiosity, calling it "affectively informed engaged curiosity."[43] She specifies that the goal of clinical empathy is for a clinician to understand the patient's experience in a way that allows the clinician to treat the patient's illness effectively. Clinical empathy requires communication practices that successfully build therapeutic alliance.[44] Part of this involves repeating patients' exact words as a way of validating their experience, rather than smuggling in an interpretation of one's own that could get it wrong.[45] Halpern notes that what matters to successful clinical empathy is not that the clinician gets it right the first time they try to understand the patient, but rather that they keep on trying continuously to seek better understanding. Thus, the clinician should adopt an attitude of curiosity, of always trying to gain better and fuller understanding, rather than seeking an end point in which one has fulfilled some criterion of understanding. She notes that observational studies show that patients who perceive their doctors as empathetic "give fuller histories, adhere to treatment, and take steps to treat their diseases."[46] When clinicians empathize with psychotic patients, trying to understand the experience and perspective of the psychotic patient as best as possible, this improves communication and interaction, increasing patients' receptivity to proposed treatment and enhancing treatment adherence.

The Role of Empathy in Developing Autonomy

Having empathy for patients is important for helping patients to develop autonomy. Recall Jodi Halpern's definition of autonomy as "a psychological capacity to make decisions that reflect one's own goals and an ethical ideal of individual self-determination."[47] Autonomy is a capacity to use reason to deliberate about ends, determining what is valuable and what is worth doing. This capacity requires that a person can see that the future is not wholly determined and perceive that their agency has an effect on the world. Autonomy also requires imaginative capacities, in which a person can imagine goals for the future and can imagine acting in ways to try to achieve their goals. To have these imaginative capacities, a person must be able to perceive that they have a future (that they exist in the future) and that their own immediate future is tolerable. Suffering often impairs both of these making it so that a person is unable to think through life goals, unable to exert control over their actions so as to implement their goals, and sometimes unable to conceptualize themselves in the future at all.[48] As we saw in chapter 2, psychosis can also impair these abilities to a significant degree.

Through empathy, clinicians can understand the patient's own perspective on their situation and better understand the nuance of their particular suffering. This enables the clinician to communicate and interact with the patient more effectively. Respecting a person as someone who can determine their own ends requires understanding their particular state of mind[49] so the clinician can better understand their reasoning about their values and goals. This deeper understanding allows clinicians to dialogue with patients more effectively about what goals are important and how they can best be achieved. Through this dialogue, clinicians can help patients see their situation in different ways, allowing them to consider possibilities for the future that they couldn't envision on their own.

In order to act autonomously, a patient must be able to form treatment goals that reflect their values.[50] Halpern notes that, most of the time, values are not reducible to a single scale of well-being but rather involve tradeoffs of losses and benefits set against the person's conception of a worthwhile life; individuals will calculate these tradeoffs differently depending on their overall scheme of value.[51] Patients struggle with setting treatment goals when their suffering interferes with their ability to see themselves in the future and their ability to see their action as having effects in the world. When patients' suffering interferes with their ability to imagine goals for the future, they need assistance from clinicians to help them develop the capacity to set future goals.[52] When clinicians empathize with patients, they are able to work with patients more effectively to help patients set goals for themselves and figure out the means to achieve them.

For some patients, and especially for psychotic patients who lack a strong sense of self, this requires developing a sense of oneself as a center of motivation and efficacy.[53] Finding ways for patients to increase and exercise their agency in the process of their recovery is important to help patients develop this sense of agency. Giving patients opportunities to participate actively in their treatment, such as by giving testimony that is taken up appropriately, making sense of their experiences in the context of a larger framework of meaning, and making treatment decisions are all important aspects of this. Alleviating suffering is also paramount, so patients find it tolerable to go on living and can start to imagine themselves as having a future.[54] In addition, addressing cognitive symptoms of psychosis through antipsychotic medication is important so patients have increased epistemic and moral capacities and thus can develop and exercise agency and autonomy.

The Role of Empathy in Clinical Care

Empathy does important epistemic and moral work that helps people be better knowers and better moral agents, and it is best employed in balance with epistemic humility. Empathy is epistemically efficacious because it enables people to have knowledge that they might not be able to gain through other means.[55] In taking on someone else's perspective, a person can gain knowledge of the other person's mental states that they would not be able to have otherwise.[56] Empathy plays a distinctive epistemic role in allowing people to know how other people feel.[57] Having this knowledge can help people to identify morally correct action to take in a given circumstance,[58] in part because it can help people to figure out what moral weight to assign to factors related to the person's experience.[59] Empathy may also play an important role in certain speech acts. For example, empathy can enhance the processes of questioning and asserting, allowing speakers and listeners to engage with each other more closely.[60]

Arthur Frank notes that empathy should not be understood as an asymmetrical relationship where one is the giver (the empathizer) and one is the taker (the object of empathy). Rather, empathy should be seen as a reciprocal relationship with mutual benefit, where the person who suffers can teach the person who empathizes about their suffering. The empathizer receives the benefit of learning about suffering from the person with whom they empathize.[61] A clinician working with psychotic patients does not just bestow compassion to their patients; they also learn from their patients what the patients' suffering is like and how to deal with it. This helps clinicians perform their jobs better by interacting more effectively with patients.

In a clinical context, empathy is important in enhancing *phronesis*, or practical wisdom, which is the kind of knowledge and reasoning used when making moral decisions. In helping people to be attuned to others, especially when others are in distress, empathy helps a person to identify what is morally salient in a situation, so they pay attention to the right sorts of things in their moral reasoning. Clinicians use practical wisdom in the decision making they do as part of their jobs. When clinicians have empathy, they are attuned to how a patient is feeling and what a patient is experiencing, and they can discern the patient's needs and interests more intuitively. This helps them pay attention to the salient aspects of their patient's situation when they make decisions that affect the patient's well-being. Empathy also helps clinicians avoid the fundamental attribution error of ascribing intentionality to other people's actions in an unfair way, assuming they have more free will and control over their actions than they in fact do. The third-person perspective of other-oriented perspective-taking helps clinicians to understand the broader psycho-social factors that underlie a patient's action, allowing them to see the way that patients' actions are mitigated by factors beyond their control, or the way that patients' actions make sense to them given their circumstances even if they do not seem to make sense to others. Clinicians who adopt this third-person perspective can be more understanding and compassionate toward their patients. In addition, when clinicians have empathy, they can also more effectively and calmly de-escalate crises or help patients avoid crises. Understanding a patient's experience from their own perspective enables clinicians to interact with patients in more genuine and productive ways.

At the same time, clinicians should not believe they understand patients more than they in fact do. It would be hubristic for a clinician to claim that, because they can imagine what it is like to be a patient, they can fully understand the patient's experience and perspective. Patients want clinicians to understand them as much as possible, but they also need clinicians to acknowledge the limits of that understanding. Clinicians need to recognize that there is a lot that they can never understand, simply because they are not the patient and there is no amount of imaginative reconstructing that can replicate what the patient experiences and how the patient sees the world. In other words, clinicians should have epistemic humility, recognizing the limits of their knowledge while being interested in trying to broaden that knowledge as much as possible. Empathetic understanding must be coupled with epistemic humility in order to serve patients well.

Epistemic humility goes hand in hand with the curiosity involved with clinical empathy: epistemic humility is the recognition of one's limits of knowledge while curiosity is the continuous desire to seek greater understanding, to expand one's knowledge as much as possible. Patients want their clinicians to recognize that the clinicians cannot truly, fully understand what it is like to be the patient, but patients want them to *try* to understand, to make the effort, to ask patients what they should know about patients instead of presuming to know. As Jodi Halpern notes, clinicians should engage with patients by asking, "What am I missing?," rather than by asserting, "I understand what you're feeling."[62] What patients really want their clinicians to do, therefore, is to make the effort in *trying* to understand them, always acknowledging the limitations of that understanding.

Empathy and Compassion

Clinical empathy is inextricably linked with compassion and care. Some philosophers argue that empathy is necessary for sympathy (feeling with another person) or compassion, as understanding what someone else is feeling enables us to feel with them and to care about their welfare.[63] Some philosophers also argue the opposite, that sympathy is at least as morally important as empathy in a healthcare context and that sympathy is necessary for empathy to be of any use.[64] Clinicians who understand what their patients are feeling and experiencing are in a better position to provide the care that is necessary for good treatment; clinicians who care about their patients are better able to empathize with them and understand what they are going through.

Compassion can be understood as care or concern for another person, often based on an understanding of what that person is going through. In a healthcare context, Petra Gelhaus views compassion as an attitude of helpfulness, or a benevolent response to suffering.[65] Emphasizing the affective dimension of compassion and downplaying the cognitive aspect, Roger Crisp defines compassion as feeling pain or distress at the pain or distress of someone else.[66] Noting that compassion often has an action component to it, Brian Carr understands compassion as appreciating the suffering of another and being motivated to respond to it.[67] In a clinical setting, it is most useful not to regard compassion as feeling distress at someone else's distress, for the same reasons that it is not useful to feel what the patient feels, but rather to understand it as recognizing the patient's suffering and being moved to try to alleviate it. Compassion thus motivates good clinical work.

Compassion can be problematic for clinicians when it is assumed to be a spontaneous response of warmth and emotional closeness toward a person. This form of compassion potentially can lead to excessive demands put on the clinician, emotional burnout, justice, and fairness concerns (when compassion is not distributed equally or fairly among patients), and possible threats to patients' dignity and autonomy.[68] In the context of healthcare, therefore, compassion should be understood not as emotional closeness, but as a professional attitude of helpfulness combined with empathetic understanding of the patient. Compassionate clinicians "will be personally engaged and willing to help one, understand that one is not well, and they will not expect something from the patient in return."[69] To be most effective in clinical work, compassion should be combined with empathy and care.[70]

Compassion can lead to either emotional overload or emotional distancing if it is not tempered with an attitude of equanimity.[71] Equanimity is an attitude of calmness and acceptance of suffering; it helps a person avoid both emotional overload, by decreasing the strain that being exposed to so much suffering can bring, and emotional distancing, by removing whatever fear a person may have in relation to suffering. Equanimity can also help a person to deal with the potential emotional overload that can occur when empathizing with someone else, when understanding someone else's experiences (especially experiences of suffering) creates an emotional reaction. Self-regulation of one's emotions is thus important for dealing with the emotional effects of empathy.[72] Equanimity allows a person to empathize more fully by providing just enough distance from the other person's suffering to enable the empathizer to experience the other person's experiences *as* the other person's rather than as their own.

By engaging in dialogue with the patient, listening without imposing their own meaning structure to the patient's experience, having both empathetic understanding and the epistemic humility to acknowledge the limitations of that understanding, and having compassion toward the patient, a therapist can help the patient value their own life and health and set appropriate life- and health-affirming goals for themselves, as well as develop the pathway to reach these goals. The therapist can help the patient clarify their conception of what a meaningful life consists of, as well as the steps needed to achieve this conception of a good life, and help the patient recognize the objective aspects of leading a meaningful life, namely the health-conducive steps necessary to achieve a good life.

When a clinician exhibits empathy and compassion toward a psychotic patient, this counters the power that psychosis may have over the patient. Psychosis can act as a mirror image of the therapist, appearing to the patient to be trustworthy, understanding, and helpful in aiding the patient to determine what is of value and how to achieve one's goals.[73] The therapist must recognize the power of psychosis to act in this way and counteract and thwart the psychosis by being a more empathetic, helpful, and compassionate agent than the psychosis can be, so the therapist appears more trustworthy than the psychosis and the patient is more willing to listen to the guidance of the therapist than that of the psychosis. Psychosis can mimic many of the activities of the therapist, trying to supplant the work of the therapist in the patient's mind, but it cannot be truly compassionate and caring because it often acts as a dictator. The therapist can overcome the power of the psychosis by being deeply compassionate, forgiving, kind, warm, and caring toward the patient.

Empathy and Compassion of the Patient

While empathy of the therapist toward the patient is necessary for therapy to be effective, empathy of the patient toward themselves, and perhaps even toward the therapist, is also necessary. As the patient experiences the empathetic understanding of the therapist, they can learn to see themselves through the therapist's eyes and develop empathetic understanding toward themselves. Seeing themselves through the eyes of another can broaden their perspective of their situation and increase self-knowledge and self-understanding. By understanding their own experiences and perspective more deeply, they can develop compassion toward themselves and treat themselves with more patience, kindness, and care than they otherwise would.

As their self-understanding increases, a patient might also learn to see others through empathetic eyes and adopt empathetic understanding toward other people in their life, including their therapist. This greater understanding can lead to better interactions with other people, improving the patient's interpersonal relationships, as well as enhanced therapeutic alliance, leading to a more constructive therapeutic relationship and more effective collaboration on treatment goals and the means to achieve those goals. Greater empathy toward others can lead to greater compassion for others, which can be transformative to the patient.

Conclusion

The therapist I started seeing right before I was hospitalized demonstrated empathy with me by being curious about my condition and my state of mind. He asked me questions to try to understand what I was going through, he listened intently to what I said, and he repeated back to me what he heard me saying so as to be sure that he comprehended me correctly. He both understood me and acknowledged the limitations of his understanding. His special understanding of what I was experiencing came at least partly from having many years of experience working with psychotic patients in a psychiatric hospital before he became a clinical therapist. Because of this experience, he was very familiar with psychosis, which my other clinicians lacked.

Some of the clinicians I have seen as an outpatient have treated few patients who struggled with psychosis, and so are not very familiar with it; this therapist's experience, however, allowed him to help me identify what I was experiencing as psychosis and help give me conceptual tools to understand my experience. When I talked about having incessant noise in my head and feeling pulled by the psychosis into an inner world, he understood what I meant as well as anyone who has not experienced this could understand. Feeling like I was understood aided me tremendously, as it helped me feel less alone in the world and less isolated inside my own head. Feeling like he understood me made it easier to talk about what I was experiencing, to be honest with both him and myself, and to explore some of the issues raised by my psychosis. I was able to go deeper in my therapy sessions with him than I would have had I not felt so well understood.

At the same time, he acknowledged that he did not fully understand the particular details of what I was experiencing but was committed to trying to do so. He expressed curiosity in the details of my experience and gave me the space to explain not only what I was feeling, but also why I thought I was going through this; in other words, he was open both to my testimony and to my interpretation of my experience. This allowed me to express myself and have some say over what my experiences meant, which was empowering.

Through empathetic understanding, my therapist helped me to understand what meaning my inner world held to me and what roles my psychosis played for me, and he helped me to try to find greater meaning in the external world, the world outside my mind. By understanding the dichotomy I experienced with the inner and outer worlds, he was able to help me to distinguish these so I could identify them more clearly and exert some control over the way I related to them. Comprehending the way that the inner world held vast meaning for me, he helped me see that the external world had meaning, too, and helped me to pay more attention to this meaning. Where normally the psychosis drowned out the meaning in the external world, he helped me pay attention to it. In understanding the pull that psychosis had over me, he recommended strategies to try to ignore the noise in my head and the strange sensations I experienced so they would have less sway over me. He helped me problem solve so I could deal with problems such as loneliness in more productive ways that did not include retreating into psychosis. He gave me tools and motivation to resist the voice that often told me what to do. Fighting the suicidal ideation, he helped me to see that my life had meaning and value outside of my subjective experience and to see that I was able to make effective changes in how I related to the world.

Moreover, with his empathetic understanding, he was able to be an effective guide in helping me to improve my ability to value appropriately and make autonomous choices. Through open-minded dialogue, he was able to meet me where I was and help me recognize from there what is of value and what makes a worthwhile life. He helped me recognize more firmly how much I cared about my family and helped me to make this a motivation for my actions. For example, he encouraged me to take actions to show my appreciation and love for them such as by giving them more hugs. This might sound like a small thing, but it was huge at the time, for when I was in the emotionless, zombie-like state of psychosis, I found human contact to be nearly unbearable. Making the effort to give my family members more hugs was difficult, but it connected me to them in many important ways. In helping me to recognize what was of value, my therapist also helped me to care about myself and my future, making it possible for me to make decisions that were in my best interests. He enabled me to be motivated by the prospect of health and well-being. Only through his empathetic understanding of the effects that psychosis had on me was this possible.

In addition to helping me to perceive the meaning and value in the external world and to resist the pull the psychosis had over me, my therapist also helped me wade through practical problems that I was having trouble navigating. For example, at the time, I was having difficulty interacting with my psychiatrist in a productive way. My therapist helped me to recognize the power dynamic that underlay our relationship and that led me to want to resist his recommendations. Recognizing this power dynamic helped me to change my role in it.

My therapist's empathetic understanding of my situation was critical in my ability to trust him and to feel like he could offer effective help. I would not have shared so much with him if he was not so open minded and curious. Because of his special understanding of psychosis due to his experience working with psychotic patients in a psychiatric hospital, I was able to explore the contours and meaning of my psychosis in a way that would have been impossible with another therapist. He understood me like few other people have, but in a way that was epistemically humble rather than presumptive, and this helped me to address my problems more effectively.

In helping to deepen my self-understanding and helping me to address some of my problems directly, instead of trying to avoid them, he helped me to feel more connected to the world and to other people. As a result, this improved my ability to see myself as an agent, as a source of ideas and action who could make changes that would have an effect. It also helped to address the despondency I tended to feel when I believed that I was unable to do anything to improve my plight and believed that I would be sick for the rest of my life. He helped me to see that I could make effective changes if I chose to do so. Through an empathizing and epistemically humble approach, he helped give me tools to increase my sense of agency as well as my capacity for autonomy.

Helping patients increase their agency and autonomy is one of the crucial roles that clinicians can play in a patient's recovery. In the next three chapters I explore three places where patients should be encouraged to exercise their agency: in providing testimony, in making meaning of their experience, and in making choices regarding their treatment.

6 Testimony

Introduction

When I was hospitalized for psychotic depression, I was first placed in an intensive treatment unit for the most severely ill patients, who tended to be psychotic and/or suicidal. In many ways it fit a stereotype of a mental hospital. Nurses and mental health technicians worked behind a long desk from which they could see the common room and corridors to the bedrooms. Patients milled about the common room, reading, playing games, watching television at designated hours, or talking to themselves, except when they were in supervised group activities. Some patients were reasonably intelligible to others while others were less so. While those who were coherent tended to be social, talking and playing games with fellow patients, other patients were more solitary. Some patients spoke to their voices and were ignored by others. Some patients moaned, screamed, or made other incoherent noises.

Nursing students from area colleges came through the unit daily to observe us. Mostly they stood against a wall and watched us, looking extremely uncomfortable; some sat in the common area with patients but just stared at the television. Only a few students made the effort to communicate with patients.

One day, a nursing student struck up a conversation with me and asked me what my life was like outside the hospital. When I told her that I was a professor at Regis University, I could tell immediately that she was not sure whether to believe me. After all, I was on a unit where many patients were delusional; how could she tell whether I was stating the truth or a delusion? It was not until I described my experiences teaching at Regis that I could see her relax; in that moment I saw her skepticism fade as she realized I was not delusional. She had a friend who went to Regis and was familiar enough with the school to see that I was telling the truth. We had a really nice conversation until I had to leave for an activity.

I am grateful to her for being brave enough to strike up a conversation with a mental patient, and I had a really nice time talking with her. But the experience of her initial skepticism was surreal. She was the same age as my students; I teach nursing students in my introductory philosophy and first-year writing courses at Regis and could have easily been her professor. (I was relieved that Regis students did not make their rounds on the unit while I was there.) I was used to being in a position where I had credibility and authority, where students and colleagues alike treated me with respect. Now I was in a position where my credibility was questioned, where not only was my authority as a professional and an academic irrelevant, but where my claims were met with skepticism. There was nothing surprising to me about the shift in power that this conversation evoked, as I saw how my social position had changed since being in the hospital. But it was nonetheless surreal; it somehow went beyond my understanding. In that interchange, the nursing student possessed the unquestioned credibility, professional power, and credibility that I now lacked. My position of credibility and authority had diminished dramatically; the nursing student, aligned with the nurses and mental health technicians who worked behind the desk, now held all the relevant social power.

My diminished epistemic power was all the more apparent when I tried and failed to make myself understood while going through withdrawal of my antipsychotic medication. At my initial intake session with the psychiatrist, the psychiatrist decided to replace my current antipsychotic medication (ziprasidone, brand name Geodon) with a different one (lurasidone, brand name Latuda). I believe that he assumed I wound up in the hospital because my medication wasn't working and thought I should see if a different one would work better. The ziprasidone seemed to work just fine, however: it seemed to be effective at reducing my psychotic symptoms when I took an adequate dose; the problem was that I had decreased my dose, allowing the psychosis to bloom. If he had just kept me on ziprasidone and increased the dose, I believed it would have taken care of the psychosis. However, he seemed to be putting everyone on lurasidone—all the patients I had talked to about it were on it—me included.

For some reason he thought it would be a good idea to take me off ziprasidone all at once, rather than withdrawing from it slowly, and simply replace it with lurasidone. I had gone down on my medication dose enough times that spring to know exactly how it would make me feel: physically and mentally agitated, creating loud noise in my head, inducing music refrains to repeat intensely and incessantly and burn tracks in my brain, and reawakening the voice I sometimes heard from its slumber. The night I stopped taking ziprasidone, I could not sleep and felt like nightmares were coming alive and engulfing me. I went into the common room at 2 a.m. and said I was going through withdrawal and begged to be put back on ziprasidone. The mental health technicians who were working the night shift suggested I was having anxiety about the idea of stopping the medication. No, I was not anxious about the change; I really was going through withdrawal, and I knew this from previous experience.

Nothing I said could convince them of this. They gave me an additional dose of hydroxyzine to help calm me down and gave me Sudoku puzzles to occupy my mind. Shaking like crazy, I did Sudoku puzzles in the common room until the hydroxyzine did calm me down and I was able to go back to bed. I slept for about three hours and woke up as usual at 5:30. I was still agitated and felt truly like I was going out of my mind. I begged the staff again to put me back on ziprasidone, and they said I could talk to the psychiatrist about it later in the day.

When I had my opportunity to talk with him, I explained that I was going through withdrawal and desperately wanted to get back on the ziprasidone. I explained that it truly was effective (or so I thought at the time); the problem that got me into the hospital had been that I had stopped taking my prescribed dose. I managed to convince him, and he put me back on the ziprasidone. I even negotiated a schedule to help me take it in a way that wouldn't sedate me too excessively, taking 20 mg with breakfast, 20 mg with lunch, and 40 mg with dinner. Upon taking the first dose I felt better immediately.

In this situation, I had a lot of self-knowledge. I knew what was wrong with me, what my needs were, what was good for me, and what I needed in order to get my needs met. It was very difficult to make myself heard, understood, and taken seriously, however.

Was I viewed as an unreliable reporter because I was a mental patient struggling with psychosis? Was I assumed not to have accurate insight into my situation? Was my account discreditable because of how I was situated? Such downgrading seemed automatic; staff members were sure I was wrong and did not even entertain my ideas. My ideas were discounted because I had a mental illness and because I was a patient in a psychiatric hospital receiving care from mental health professionals. Staff members may have had certain negative stereotypes that people who were mentally sick were unreliable reporters, that our testimony and ideas could not be trusted, that we lacked the epistemic capacities to engage in meaningful epistemic discourse, that we lacked the capacity to contribute anything salient, that above all we were too incompetent to be credible. They apparently had certain beliefs about the way medications work that led them to assume I couldn't be going through withdrawal. Perhaps they trusted the epistemic authority of the prescribing psychiatrist too much and figured that he would not have taken me completely off ziprasidone if he did not think it was a good idea (perhaps he thought I would not go through withdrawal or perhaps he saw the withdrawal as insignificant). Whatever the reason, staff members ultimately discounted my ideas because of how I was situated as a mental patient.

Giving testimony is an integral aspect of epistemic agency that is crucial to recovery yet sometimes denied to mental patients, especially in hospitals where patients are disempowered by the way they are situated within the hospital setting. Giving testimony increases a person's sense of self and agency and thus can increase voluntariness, leading to greater autonomy. Sharing information about oneself is a way for a person to own their experiences by claiming the experience as their own and interpreting the experience through their own lens of understanding. This helps address the detachment that psychotic patients often feel with respect to their experiences, actions, and mental states. Through this ownership of experience, a person can come to view their beliefs, desires, thoughts, experiences, and actions as coming from themselves in a meaningful way instead of feeling as if these are imposed on oneself from the outside. In addition, by giving testimony about their experience, patients engage in processes of knowledge production and meaning making as they impose order on and interpret their experience through their act of sharing. Giving order to their experience and interpreting their experience are important activities in recovery, where part of participating actively in recovery involves processing one's experiences. By making sense of their experiences, a person can exert some control over the experiences and their impact on the person; this control contributes to a person's development and exercise of agency and autonomy.

In order to be a meaningful activity, giving testimony requires not only a speaker, or a testifier, but also a listener who receives the testimony. Appropriate uptake is necessary for giving testimony to be an effective exercise of epistemic agency. Giving testimony involves action not only of the testifier, who constructs and conveys the information, therefore, but also of the listener, who is responsible for uptake. When patient testimony is deemed credible and taken up appropriately, it is taken seriously, regarded as valuable information that adds to overall knowledge, and used in making decisions on behalf of the patient. When patient testimony is seen as discreditable, on the other hand, it is ignored and discounted, viewed as false, misleading, or irrelevant, and not factored into decision making. Whether patient testimony is taken up appropriately depends on how credible the patient is viewed as and how relevant their testimony is regarded. Sharing testimony can play a huge role in a patient's process of recovery, but only when it is taken seriously and taken up appropriately.

Patient Testimony

Epistemic agency involves the disposition to act in one's capacity as a knower. Giving testimony is an important aspect of epistemic agency because sharing information is one of the central activities we do as knowers. We share information in a variety of ways and contexts. Patients are epistemic agents in various ways; one way is through the practice of giving testimony about their experience.

Patients and clinicians both share testimony in their interactions with each other, but the type of testimony they share is different based on their respective roles. Clinicians give testimony about diagnosis and treatment, sharing their professional knowledge about how to understand the patient's experience and what treatment options are available; sharing professional knowledge is a crucial aspect of the clinician's responsibilities toward the patient. Clinician testimony is important for patients to better understand their condition and available treatment options. While patient uptake of clinician testimony is important, this chapter focuses on patient testimony as an epistemic activity crucial for recovery and the way that clinicians' uptake of testimony affects the quality of patients' participation in such epistemic activity, so I will not address clinician testimony further here. I discuss the epistemic trust involved with receiving clinician testimony in chapter 7.

Patients give testimony about their experience; in the context of recovery, giving testimony typically involves sharing information about what one is going through and about one's mental states. Sharing information in this way is important to let others know about one's situation; sharing about experiences and mental states is important because only the person who has these experiences and mental states has first-person access to them, so only that person has immediate knowledge of these and is in a position to convey this knowledge to others. Patients' first-person access to their own experiences and mental states allows them to know these experiences and mental states in a way that no one else can know these states and experiences and thus enables first-person authority over these. In this way, they have testimony that is worth sharing with others. Both patients and clinicians thus have specialized knowledge to share with each other: while clinicians have expert knowledge to share by virtue of their role, patients have first-person knowledge of their experiences and mental states.

Clinicians need patients' testimonial knowledge to help them make decisions on behalf of patients. Clinicians need to understand a patient's experiences, mental states, and behavior to the best of their ability in order to make the best decisions they can based on this knowledge. A good deal of their knowledge of a patient's experiences, mental states, and behavior is based on their observation of patients. But clinicians are limited in what they can know through observation, especially since they see patients for only limited amounts of time and only in therapeutic contexts (not in the patient's daily life). So, they must also rely on patient testimony of their experience to have a broader understanding of what a patient is going through.

In certain settings, patient testimony is deliberately ascertained and taken at face value, or, if it is critically engaged, it is done so along with the patient (as in therapy, where the therapist and patient together try to interpret the patient's experience). In intake sessions, patients are asked to recount their story of mental suffering and history of diagnosis and treatment with psychiatrists, therapists, or other mental health professionals.

Their story is usually accepted as is, though questions may be asked to add further detail or to illuminate aspects of the story. In therapy or psychiatry sessions, patients are asked about their recent experience and their own interpretation of their behavior, and this too is generally accepted as fact and questioned only to add deeper understanding.

In some other settings, however, patient testimony is not sought out, and, when it is given, it is disregarded. In settings where a patient has minimal power and others have power over them, such as in psychiatric hospitals, patients are regarded as having little credibility and thus granted little power to express testimony; when they do express it, it is not taken up appropriately and is instead ignored and discounted. In such settings, even patients' firsthand account of their experience is regarded as discreditable; patients are not even seen as a source of knowledge, never mind as collaborators in interpretation.

Yet it is very important for patients to share testimony about their experience and to offer their own interpretations of it because sharing testimony is a way of taking ownership of their experience. The act of recounting a story requires a patient to select what is salient to the story and put order on events through how the story is told (for example, chronologically). Telling a story of one's experience is a way of cognitively engaging with the raw materials of experience and making sense of it by making it intelligible, at least to oneself, and ideally to others. By telling a story of one's experience, a person can claim the experience as their own and put their own interpretative lens on it, thereby making meaning of it. This is especially important for psychotic patients who struggle with recognizing their experiences and actions as their own. When others try to tell a person's story through their own interpretive lens, this can be alienating if it does not reflect the person's own interpretation and so does not resonate in a meaningful way. A person needs to be able to impose their own order on their experience and make sense of it on their own terms in order to be able to recognize and claim it as their own.

Having a listener who takes up testimony appropriately is an important dimension of giving testimony effectively. Uptake is "a dialogical responsiveness and openness"[1] to testimony, involving respecting the testifier, attending to the testifier, and empathizing with the testifier. As Nancy Nyquist Potter says, "Giving uptake well is a disposition to attend carefully, actively, and openly to the communication of another."[2] As a virtue, uptake is a middle state between requiring certainty in accepting someone's testimony as true or reasonable and dismissing, discrediting, or ignoring the testimony; it involves accepting and tending to a person's testimony while being open to learning more that might support or undermine it.[3] Uptake involves taking seriously the reason a person gives for their actions and beliefs, treating the patient as a conversational partner, a moral equal, whose participation is necessary for understanding and managing their illness.[4] Epistemic features of uptake include understanding (comprehending both the causal history and the social context of the testimony), grasping (involving a deeper level of understanding), openness (both to the testifier's credibility and to the possibility that the testimony is true), and nondefensiveness. Taking up testimony appropriately fosters trust between the testifier and listener and indicates trustworthiness. As a stance of openness to the possibility of the truth of the testifier's perspective, uptake is related to but distinguishable from validation, which involves complete and active acceptance.[5]

There is a moral imperative for being attentive to testimony and taking it seriously. Arthur Frank argues that uptake of testimony involves empathizing with the testifier. Sharing testimony calls on people to receive the testimony as communicative bodies who are responsive to the speaker's story. As he says, "The only mode for receiving testimony [of suffering] is *being with*."[6] Clinicians take up the testimony of patients appropriately when they empathize with patients in their suffering.

In addition to paying attention to what is said, part of listening involves paying attention to what is *not* said by being aware of the power differential between clinician and patient and by being aware of how each is socially situated in relation to the other. Being open to the patient's perspective, through both what is said and what is unsaid, helps the clinician avoid subjecting the patient to structural violence and oppression. Clinicians can reproduce structural violence and oppression when they do not take clients seriously and truly listen to them; by attending to patient testimony, and to the broader context of that testimony, as well as to what is unspoken in that context, clinicians can avoid exacerbating structural violence and oppression.[7]

Patient testimony is taken up appropriately when the clinician listens actively for the sake of deeper understanding, pays attention to what is not said, holds a stance of being open to the truth of the patient's testimony, and attends to the testifier with empathetic understanding. Appropriate uptake involves listening for the sake of acquiring deeper understanding of the patient's perspective so the listener can respond appropriately to the patient, as opposed to trying to seek out defeaters that would test the truth or accuracy of testimony. Sometimes when we listen to others' testimony, we do so critically, wanting to test the truth of the testimony by seeing if there are any defeaters that would undermine it. When a clinician has a reason to suspect a patient's testimony is inaccurate, it may be appropriate for the clinician to seek out possible defeaters in this way; under normal circumstances, however, such a critical stance is not appropriate and can be harmful to the therapeutic relationship. Instead, clinicians should recognize that patient testimony usually reflects the truth as the patient sees it from their own perspective and acknowledge their primary responsibility as trying to understand it rather than as trying to engage with it critically by assessing its validity. The clinician should instead adopt a default attitude of trust toward the patient, particularly when there is little at stake in trusting. Through this, they hold an attitude of optimism that the testimony is true to the best of the patient's ability to recount it, and they want simply to understand it better so as to understand the patient's perspective more deeply.

Having one's testimony taken up appropriately is an important aspect of exercising agency. Uptake is a way of treating the person whose testimony one is taking up as an agent. When a person's testimony is taken up appropriately, this makes their action as a knower have an effect on the world, allowing them to exercise their agency more fully and completely. When a clinician takes up a patient's testimony appropriately, this allows the patient's action to have an effect on the world, demonstrating to the patient that their action makes a difference to what happens. This shows the patient that they have agency and helps the patient to see themselves better as agents. Uptake of a psychotic patient's testimony is especially beneficial as it strengthens the patient's sense of themselves as an agent, which is typically impaired in psychosis.

The therapist I initially saw when I was psychotic (discussed in chapter 5) did not take up my testimony appropriately, viewing me as an unreliable witness to my own experience, not accepting my interpretation of my experience as one of hearing voices. The therapist I saw later who became my regular therapist, on the other hand, took up my testimony appropriately by taking my interpretation of my experience seriously and helping me to identify my experience as psychotic so I could better understand it. By taking my account seriously, he helped me exercise my agency more fully, so I was an active participant in dialogue and not simply a passive receiver of ideas.

Power, Privilege, and Credibility

Giving testimony is one form of epistemic power or agency. Epistemic power is the capacity to participate in epistemic activities as a knower. Epistemic privilege is the liberty to be able to participate in such activities. Because of the power differential between them, there is a huge disparity in the epistemic privilege and power that clinicians have compared to patients as well as a striking imbalance in credibility and trustworthiness. As a result, patients have significantly less power and privilege compared to clinicians.

The epistemic power and privilege of mental health professionals, especially in the totalizing environment of a psychiatric hospital, is almost too obvious to state. Havi Carel and Ian James Kidd identify three related components of epistemic privilege.[8] One form of privilege is the authority to create and enforce the norms that govern epistemic practices, in other words having the power to determine the conditions for communication, inquiry, and other epistemic activities. A second form of privilege involves having an authoritative procedural role in epistemic practices, such as by acting as gatekeepers that determine who can participate in the practices and how and by enforcing norms and expectations about how participation should occur. A third form of privilege is decision-making power, which involves not simply giving approval for a course of action, but also such things as deciding what kind of evidence counts and how much evidence is sufficient, and how much attention and energy an issue deserves. Mental health professionals have all of these kinds of privileges, while patients have very little.

One place where patients do have epistemic privilege is in terms of their access to their firsthand experience.[9] Anastasia Scrutton argues that people with mental illness have epistemic power in two areas: they have firsthand knowledge into their own experience that is unattainable by others and thus can use that knowledge in informational exchanges, and they have knowledge of what is good for them; they know their own needs and what works for them best.[10] Şerife Tekin adds that patients also have distinctive knowledge about "orientational challenges" related to symptoms, what their responses are to different treatment methods, how mental illness affects various dimensions of their life such as interpersonal relationships, how the way their illness is framed affects what accommodations they can receive, and what psychological traits are needed to be able to deal with their illness.[11] The knowledge that people have of their own experience allows people to see certain aspects of their experience that others may not notice. In illuminating more angles of the experience, such firsthand knowledge allows people to see more that is salient and to see meaning where others may not. It allows for the possibility of expanding knowledge by creating new frameworks of meaning that better account for more of the experience.

While Scrutton and Tekin identify some important forms of epistemic power that people with mental illness have, this power is limited. As long as a person is positioned as a patient, as an object of treatment and as a recipient of care by mental health experts, a person's firsthand knowledge of their experience and what is good for them is only useful to the extent that mental health professionals care about these and decide to listen to a person's expression of their experience and needs. In settings where mental health professionals appreciate patient perspectives and incorporate this knowledge into their own understanding, first-person knowledge of experience and needs can play a valuable epistemic role in the construction of meaning and in decision making. In outpatient settings in particular, where patient input into their experience is seen as desirable for the goals of treatment, first-person knowledge of experience and needs is seen as valuable. In psychotherapy, for instance, patients and clinicians typically work together to develop frameworks of understanding in which a person can make sense of their experience; patient perspectives are crucial for creating such frameworks.

In more restrictive settings, such as hospitals, firsthand knowledge of experiences, needs, and interests is less valued and has less power. The power dynamics inherent to the structure of a hospital limit the ways such knowledge can be made available and used. Within the structure of a hospital, the epistemic privilege of people who have mental illness is often marginal because their contributions are not taken up appropriately. The reason for this disparity in how patient testimony is received is due to the different goals in inpatient and outpatient treatment. In outpatient treatment, patient testimony helps the patient develop agency and autonomy, allowing them to better manage their symptoms and to have greater control over their condition; in inpatient treatment, however, patient testimony is regarded as irrelevant, or even detrimental, to patient and staff safety and management.

While patients' special access to their firsthand experiences and needs and interests allows them the epistemic power to create and give testimony, therefore, such testimony is not always taken up appropriately and regarded as epistemically relevant and fruitful. Before I explain some ways that patient testimony is sometimes not taken up appropriately, let us consider the role that diminished credibility plays in uptake. A person's epistemic power and the ability for their testimony to be taken up well is greatly impacted by their credibility.

Credibility is a form of social power that allows a person to control their social world through epistemic practices such as information exchange, inquiry, and communication.[12] As Miranda Fricker observes, people are granted credibility when they seem like competent participants in epistemic practices and when they appear to be able to present reliable testimony.[13] Perception plays a role in how we grant credibility: we assign credibility to someone based on how they appear to us. When people appear untrustworthy or incompetent, we withhold credibility. Ideally, our perceptions of other people's credibility are based on evidence, including the person's past epistemic performance and the epistemic capacities they currently exhibit. In reality, however, our perceptions of credibility are influenced by a variety of factors, including social norms about complying with authority, emotional reactions, moral commitments, and other beliefs we hold.[14] Our unconscious beliefs, including any implicit biases we may hold, also play a role. Blatant and subtle stereotypes, including stereotypes about mental illness, affect how we perceive someone's credibility.

When we engage in epistemic practices, we have certain expectations of our fellow participants. These expectations govern the way we receive and give information.[15] One is that we assume our fellow participants have a capacity for salience, a sense of which ideas are worth taking seriously versus which are irrelevant or problematic. We also expect that our fellow participants have the ability to contribute meaningfully to the epistemic activity, such as by providing relevant information, corroborating or refuting an idea, or having sufficient background information to make sense of ideas. When people fail to meet these expectations, we are unable to see them as credible participants and unable to engage with them in epistemically meaningful ways. When we believe that people will not be able to meet these expectations, we attribute diminished credibility to them and view whatever epistemic contributions they do make as less legitimate, authoritative, true, or meaningful.

People who have mental illness, especially severe illness, and especially when they are known or presumed to be psychotic, are sometimes granted low credibility due to perceptions of their epistemic capacities.[16] This is based on awareness that people with mental illness may suffer an actual loss of epistemic competence due to their illness. Because of their potential to have diminished or distorted cognitive and rational processes, people with mental illness, especially psychosis, are sometimes regarded as unreliable testifiers and incompetent participants in epistemic practices. Whether due to delusions, poverty of thought, disorganized thinking, impulsivity, or manipulation, they are sometimes seen as incapable of providing reliable testimony and so their ideas are distrusted.[17]

When we know that someone is psychotic, we may assume that many of the person's statements must be, or at least may be, falsehoods. In such a case, our trust default position is the reverse of what it normally is. Normally our default position is to assume that someone's testimony is true unless we have evidence that suggests otherwise. In the context of severe mental illness, however, our default position is sometimes to assume that the testimony of the person with mental illness is false, unless we have evidence to suggest otherwise. Even if we do not adopt a default position of distrust, we typically maintain skepticism around the person's testimony. The person experiencing psychosis is positioned, by virtue of how people view their mental illness, as needing to prove the accuracy of their testimony in order to acquire credibility. This puts a major epistemic burden on people with severe mental illness whose illness makes epistemic participation more difficult to begin with.[18]

When people have actual mental impairments that interfere with their ability to participate meaningfully in certain epistemic practices, granting these people less credibility is justifiable. However, what we usually see and base our judgment upon is not people's actual impairments, but rather the potential impairments we expect them to have based on their mental illness. Our judgments of people are typically influenced by stigma that affects how we see people's epistemic participation. One of our common stereotypes about mental illness is that people with mental illness are globally incompetent, lacking an array of basic capacities that allow them to function in various areas of their life. Based on this stereotype, we sometimes assume that people who have mental illness, particularly severe mental illness, are incompetent in a range of ways that impact epistemic participation.[19] This assumption can lead us to grant people less credibility than their actual situation warrants, which results in them having an unjust credibility deficit based on their social identity, or what Fricker calls an identity-prejudicial credibility deficit.[20] This lack of credibility diminishes the social power of people with mental illness.

Mental patients are especially prone to experiencing an identity-prejudicial credibility deficit because of the way they are situated as sick people under the care of treatment providers. Being positioned as recipients of care, subject to the power of mental health professionals, disempowers mental patients, especially when patients are expected to comply with clinicians' recommendations and not given opportunities to participate actively in their treatment. Mental patients are assumed to have less credibility because of this lack of power. In hospital settings, where the totalizing nature of hospital management reduces a person's identity simply to being a patient (and roles the patient had outside the hospital, such as [in my case] mother, wife, and professor are treated as irrelevant), patients are seen as wholly lacking power, and this lack of power is seen to reduce credibility drastically. Clinicians see patients only in a series of disconnected fragments (pieces of behavior in a particular setting that itself affects behavior, as I explain below) and do not seek to understand their patients as individuals with particular backgrounds, interests, and needs, because this could detract from the goal of psychiatric hospitals to maximize patient and staff safety through careful management.

While clinicians have automatic credibility by virtue of their professional role and the expertise that accompanies the role, patients often have to establish and prove their credibility. Moreover, while clinicians are trustworthy to different degrees, they have an automatic *prima facie* trustworthiness based on their professional role; patients, on the other hand, are sometimes seen as untrustworthy, especially when they are judged to be incompetent. Credibility and power are co-constitutive, in that having more of one increases the other, and having less of one decreases the other. Having a lack of epistemic power, as mental patients do, diminishes a person's credibility; having diminished credibility, as mental patients do, reduces a person's power because it decreases opportunities to participate in epistemic activities meaningfully. Patients have diminished power and credibility due to their mental illness and to the way they are situated as sick people in need of treatment.

Uptake

When patients have diminished power and are seen to have reduced credibility, their testimony is often not taken up appropriately. Sometimes this results in testimonial injustice. There are several ways this can happen.

Epistemic Objectification

First, patient testimony can fail to be taken up appropriately when patients experience epistemic objectification, where they are valued as sources of information, yet, at the same time, they are excluded from participating in epistemic practices such as interpretation.[21] In this way, they are *objects* of epistemic processes, but not *participants* within them. Their testimony is accepted as credible, and it is taken up to be used for clinicians' purposes, but they are excluded from further epistemic participation. This exclusion disempowers patients, and the objectification of patients as mere sources of information results in what Gaile Pohlhaus Jr. describes as "truncated subjectivity," where their perspectives and experiences are valuable and meaningful only with respect to others' aims and not to their own.[22] In intake sessions, for example, patients' account of their own experience is regarded as credible and valued for providing the raw data that can be used to determine diagnosis and treatment plans but not necessarily valued for helping the patient determine or pursue their own needs and interests. Mental patients are vulnerable to having truncated subjectivity anyway, especially when they are in situations, such as hospitalization, that reduce their identity to the patient role. Their already truncated subjectivity can be exacerbated when they are seen as sources of information who are unable to participate meaningfully in epistemic practices.

People who have mental illness are sometimes seen as objects rather than participants in part because of the untrustworthiness accorded them based on their having a mental illness. In other words, because we believe that mental illness *necessarily* and *globally* impacts epistemic faculties, we believe that people cannot participate in meaningful ways and so can only be sources of data. Because they are not seen as participants in epistemic processes who can help create the frameworks by which experience should be understood, and therefore are not able to explain their experience to others in their own way, people who have mental illness tend to find their experience explained by others in terms of preexisting frameworks that may or may not be accurate or helpful.[23] The parts of their experience that fit the framework are accepted as salient while other parts of their experience that do not fit the experience may be regarded as irrelevant, or even untrue.

When we try to understand a person's experience solely within a preexisting framework, we reduce the person's experience, ignoring aspects that do not fit the framework and overemphasizing aspects that do. When the first therapist I saw after becoming psychotic refused to recognize my symptoms as psychotic because she believed I had too much insight, she tried to fit my experience within her preexisting framework of what constitutes severe illness instead of looking at my situation through my own perspective. She saw me as a source of information but regarded me as incapable of contributing my own interpretation of it. In addition, when mental health technicians in the hospital I stayed at refused to accept my understanding of my extreme agitation as going through withdrawal, they epistemically objectified me by fitting the information I gave them about being agitated into their preexisting framework of anxiety. Through this, they ignored what I saw as important aspects of my experience, thereby truncating my subjectivity even more than it already was.

People whose experience is superimposed on existing frameworks by others in this way often find that the meaning given to their experience is inaccurate or misguided. *They* want to determine which aspects of their experience are salient and to impose meaning on their experience in a way that accounts for all of the experience, not just preselected parts. This may involve creating new frameworks of meaning rather than relying on established ones.[24] But people need to have an epistemic voice in order to be able to do this. When people with mental illness are regarded only as objects of epistemic practices and sources of data, they are denied the epistemic voice that would allow them to make meaning of their own experience in a way that others would understand or pay attention to. This diminishes their agency in an important way and constitutes an epistemic injustice.

Participatory Prejudice

Second, and relatedly, patient testimony can fail to be taken up appropriately when patients experience participatory prejudice, in which they are seen as being incapable of providing relevant and meaningful epistemic contributions. Participatory prejudice occurs when people are excluded from epistemic practices because they are seen as lacking the capacities needed for having a sense of relevance due to prejudice.[25] In other words, they may make epistemic contributions, but, based on how they are socially located, those contributions are ignored, degraded, patronized, or otherwise not taken seriously because they are not seen as mattering. Participatory prejudice often accompanies epistemic objectification; when mental health technicians epistemically objectified me by interpreting my experience within their preexisting framework, for example, this was due at least in part to participatory prejudice. Excluding mental patients from contributing ideas about their treatment in treatment decision making, because they are seen as lacking the ability to make relevant contributions based on their status as mental patients, is an example of participatory prejudice. Exclusion from epistemic practices may be justifiable when there are good reasons to think that people do not have the relevant background and skills to contribute meaningfully, but it is unjust when people are prevented from participating based on inaccurate or unfair beliefs about their ability to participate, such as beliefs based on negative stereotypes. In such cases, exclusion is a result of identity-prejudicial credibility deficit.

In the informational perspective of epistemic justice, we evaluate whether someone is able to provide relevant information in a specific context, looking at the type of information or ideas that is offered and seeing if it is appropriate to the circumstances.[26] We can be prejudicial in our judgment of a person's ability to make relevant and useful epistemic contributions by refusing to acknowledge the significance of the information or perspective they offer or the inquiries they pose, or by refusing to consider alternative views about what counts as relevant information and how it is significant as credible. For example, clinicians might refuse to acknowledge the significance of the information that people who have mental illness can offer, believing that only those who have certain kinds of expertise have the authority to contribute relevant ideas. Patients' firsthand experience and perspective can offer a different but still salient dimension to whatever is being considered epistemically, however.[27] While clinician accounts of a patient's situation provide an important perspective, it is only one perspective;[28] patient accounts also in fact provide important perspectives that enhance knowledge of the patient's situation; for example, patients' interpretation of their own experience can be useful to determine accurate diagnosis and appropriate treatment.

Ignoring patient accounts can lead to many problems. Regarding only some types of epistemic contributions as relevant and useful and excluding others can lead to epistemic inefficiencies and ineffectiveness when such exclusion is not done carefully and justifiably. It may also be unfair and unjust toward those who are excluded when it results from the automatic downgrading of credibility that occurs with negative stereotyping. In addition, when patient accounts are regarded as irrelevant, patients are silenced in the testimonial exchange, which can lead patients to censor themselves, create a lack of confidence, and consequently impact treatment adherence.[29]

When patients are perceived as being able to offer relevant contributions, they are allowed to engage in epistemic practices like decision making; when they are not perceived in this way, they are not allowed to engage in such practices. In outpatient settings, patients are generally perceived as being able to offer relevant information, as their firsthand knowledge of their experience is regarded as a valuable perspective that must be engaged with in order to achieve treatment goals. This is because examining the patient perspective is seen as an important aspect of increasing the patient's agency in order to improve the patient's self-control, self-efficacy, and management of symptoms.

In a mental hospital, however, patients are typically excluded from decision making about almost all issues that directly concern them, including decisions about their personal course of treatment within the hospital and decisions about what daily activities are available to patients and how they will proceed. Patients are never invited into meetings with staff where decisions about the daily structure are made and often have very little voice in whatever meetings they are invited into about their course of treatment. Whatever opinion they have tends to be seen as simply a preference, something that they "like" or "do not like," not a vested view for which they can give meaningful reasons. Their opinion may be registered in that sense—the patient likes or does not like their medicine—but it often carries no weight in actual decision making. These decisions about the duration of

stay and date of discharge are made largely by psychiatrists and social workers. Psychiatrists determine what medication patients will take, and nurses
and mental health technicians make decisions about what structured activities patients are expected to engage in. Excluding patients from epistemic
practices when they are wrongly viewed as being unable to offer relevant
information is an epistemic injustice.

Lack of Reliability

Third, patient testimony can fail to be taken up appropriately when patients
are viewed as unreliable reporters due to assumptions that they are globally
incompetent and thus untrustworthy, based on negative stereotypes about
mental illness. In the informational perspective of epistemic justice, we
evaluate whether someone is able to provide reliable information. When
we assume that people are unable to provide reliable information based on
how they are socially situated, we downgrade their credibility and trustworthiness based on their identity. This results in them having an unjust
identity-prejudicial credibility deficit.

While patients are often seen as lacking relevant expertise to contribute
meaningfully in areas such as interpretation of experience, and so are rel-
egated to sharing only first-person knowledge about their experience, they
may be seen as having little to contribute with respect to this as well. They
may be regarded as unreliable witnesses to their own experience, unable to
contribute meaningfully even to a first-person perspective of their condition. For example, when staff in the hospital downplayed my roommate's
concerns about feeling disempowered in the hospital setting because they
saw her as delusional and uncooperative, they saw her as an unreliable witness to her own experience.

Because mental illness can affect people's cognitive processes, their view
of things may be seen as untrustworthy. People who have mental illness
can be seen, rightly or wrongly, as paranoid, overly anxious, high strung,
distraught, exaggerating, delusional, or complaining, all of which affects
how we perceive the trustworthiness of what they say. When we believe
that a person is cognitively impaired such as by being overly emotional or
delusional, or when we see them as simply difficult, we view their statements through that lens and interpret their meaning in light of this. When
this occurs, we treat the content of their statements as not entirely trustworthy. We may believe that a person's self-report of what they experience

is misguided or simply not true, that even if they believe their own account, they are misleading themselves, and that when they interpret their experience in a certain way they do so through a lens (such as of paranoia, anxiety, distress, etc.) that gives the experience meaning it does not really have.

Accepting the testimony of mental patients can be difficult even for people who are well aware of the dangers of assuming global incompetence. When I was hospitalized, despite knowing that I should not approach fellow patients with automatic skepticism, I had the same trepidation in accepting their testimony that others may have had in accepting mine, such as the nursing student who initially doubted whether I was a Regis professor. I never could tell immediately whether I could trust that what my fellow patients said was true. I had to look at the available evidence and the context in which they shared information and fit what they said with what else I believed to be true before I could determine whether what they said was true.

For instance, when my first roommate told me she was a librarian in a public library, I had to see if that fit with other information that she shared about herself and the way she talked about reading and knowledge. When her claim seemed to fit the available information, I believed her. One patient who was manic told me she was a peer support specialist who worked with mentally ill clients. This I believed immediately, because her statement followed a demonstration of remarkable skill at communicating with a patient who was otherwise in his own world, speaking of the "frequencies" of things in ways that made no sense to the rest of us. This woman communicated with him in his own language so effectively that I knew she had had to have special training and/or experience to develop such skill; she had adopted the young man's "language game," to use a Wittgensteinian expression, so she could dialogue with him on his own terms. One floridly psychotic patient who screamed frequently and was nearly incoherent when he spoke was reported to be a lawyer trained at Harvard who had become psychotic following a cancer treatment. I never knew whether to believe this. I never got enough evidence or had enough surrounding knowledge to be able to determine if this proposition seemed to be true.

Holding an attitude of automatic distrust toward any group of people seems *prima facie* unfair and usually unwarranted and can constitute testimonial injustice. Distrusting people with mental illness simply because they have mental illness or simply because they are patients receiving care from mental health professionals indeed seems unfair. Yet, skepticism may be appropriate in certain circumstances, especially when we have reason to believe that someone is delusional, and it matters whether their testimony is accurate or not. The nursing student who was skeptical when I told her I was a philosophy professor did not hold an inappropriate attitude toward me, since she had reason to believe—before even talking to me, based on where we were located—that I could be markedly delusional. Nonetheless, little was at stake with respect to how true my testimony was, so it would have been even better if she had held a position of default trust toward me. Holding an attitude of optimism that the patient's testimony is true, or at least seems true from the patient's own perspective, should be the default attitude to take. Clinicians should then see their role as trying to understand the patient's perspective as best as they can rather than trying to assess patient testimony critically for accuracy.

The fact that the nursing student was willing to give up her skepticism and replace it with trust when the evidence supported the truth of my testimony was helpful. Skepticism is most justifiable when we are easily willing to replace it with trust or distrust when there is evidence to suggest the truth or falsity of testimony. Maintaining skepticism even in the face of evidence of truth is unfair; maintaining skepticism in the face of evidence of falsity is naïve. In cases where a person's truthfulness and trustworthiness are uncertain, as when there is evidence that a person may be delusional, and when it matters whether their testimony is true or not, skepticism is the appropriate attitude to hold, as long as it is accompanied by a willingness to trust if evidence warrants it. However, clinicians have a special duty to hold a trusting attitude toward patients when there is little at stake.

Distrust of a person's interpretation and even self-report of their experience may be based on a couple of different factors. I discuss two here: strategies of expression and reducing behavior to symptoms.

Different Styles of Expression

Patient testimony can fail to be taken up appropriately when patients are regarded as having a style of expression that differs from the norm, or that is outside the boundaries of a range of suitable responses, so they are not accepted as credible participants in meaning making.[30] For example, people who are highly emotional—for example, distraught, angry, or anxious—may be regarded as irrational and not taken seriously in epistemic exchanges. Their style of expression may be so off putting with respect to the norms of the context that the content of their expression may be ignored.

The idea that style of expression impacts how seriously a patient is regarded shows up in how patients in a psychiatric hospital communicate with staff, especially staff whom they see infrequently such as psychiatrists. In my experience, except for the initial intake session, which might last ten to twenty minutes, doctors met with patients for only a couple of minutes each day. This gave precious little opportunity for patients to communicate their needs. A patient had to be careful and concise in what information they wanted to share in order to use those minutes effectively. Complaints were pointless; they were ignored, typically interpreted through symptoms (for example, not liking a medicine due to delusion, paranoia, or anxiety). In order to be taken seriously, a patient had to appear as rational and unaffected by their illness as possible. Thus, pleas to change treatment, such as to change medicines or doses, had to be presented as an argument supported by good reasons, without succumbing to emotion, without criticizing staff or treatment decisions, and without appearing paranoid, anxious, or distraught.

When I went through withdrawal after being taken off ziprasidone, I tried to appear as reasonable and credible as possible in order to make my case for going back on it. I documented my withdrawal symptoms on the day's check-in sheet and begged both the night staff and the morning staff to talk to the doctor about putting me back on ziprasidone. While the staff thought my extreme agitation was due to anxiety, not withdrawal, they told me I could talk to the doctor about it when he made his rounds on the unit. When I met with the psychiatrist, I explained how ziprasidone seemed to be effective and that the problem that landed me in the hospital was that I had not taken it at the prescribed dose, not that it did not work. I had the feeling that the doctor was skeptical of my account of the situation, but he did allow me to go off lurasidone and return to ziprasidone at the correct dose. My withdrawal symptoms subsided immediately after I started taking the ziprasidone again and I felt instantly better.

This exchange with the psychiatrist and the resulting decision occurred in less than five minutes. Conciseness and careful articulation were key. I tried to appear as rational and controlled as possible despite my agitation, as I knew that if I appeared too emotional the psychiatrist would chalk it up to symptoms and not take my request seriously. I spoke clearly and directly and made my request with as close to my professor voice (where I have authority and credibility) as I could muster. Not everyone who wanted a medicine change from what the doctor ordered got their request granted. I got my request granted because I appeared rational and controlled and spoke directly and concisely. I was able to self-regulate myself to come across with as much authority as possible given my situation.

Of course, few patients have the insight to be able to recognize how they come across to others and have the capability to control this. Most patients are overwhelmed by symptoms of their illness or simply lack insight. For these patients it may not be possible to control one's presentation to be concise, well articulated, well argued, and unemotional. When people cannot help their style of expression, it is unfair to expect them to self-regulate their expression in a narrow way. Discounting people's epistemic participation due to styles of expression they may have little or no control over is a clear epistemic harm that is unfair to people who lack the ability to self-regulate precisely and thus constitutes testimonial injustice.

Misinterpretation of Behavior as Symptoms

Patient testimony can also fail to be taken up appropriately when their behaviors and emotions are misinterpreted as symptoms. In some settings, especially in a hospital, where a patient's identity is reduced to being a patient and where all attention is focused on treatment (mainly for the purposes of crisis stabilization), all behavior and emotional expression may be seen through the lens of a patient's illness and interpreted as symptoms of their illness. Thus, when a patient reports a physical symptom, it may be viewed as symptomatic or psychosomatic of the illness, such as a physical manifestation of the mental disorder or a sensation that is "all in one's head" as a result of the disorder. Or when a patient voices a complaint, makes a request, or reacts emotionally, it may be discounted as the product of symptoms, or even a symptom itself, rather than viewed as a legitimate concern, desire, or reaction. When a patient is delusional, their concern may be ignored and discounted as "simply" (reductively) a delusion rather than a legitimate concern worth taking seriously. Yet patients can have legitimate concerns even if they are symptomatic or delusional. Delusions, moreover, should not simply be dismissed, as they sometimes reflect genuine concerns that the patients have about issues in their actual experience and so should be taken seriously.

When I made my request to go back on ziprasidone, I feared the psychiatrist would interpret me in one of these ways.[31] Such misinterpretation results from incorrect judgments about people's behavior and in some cases may simply constitute epistemic bad luck; more commonly, however, such misinterpretation is systemic and consequently unjust when people with mental illness are routinely reduced to their symptoms and not taken seriously due to their mental illness. Either way, misinterpretation is an epistemic harm to the people whose behavior is misinterpreted and sometimes an epistemic injustice.

Anyone with knowledge of a person's mental illness status can be prone to this kind of misinterpretation, not only medical and mental health professionals, but also family and friends. In fact, during or following an acute period of psychiatric illness, family and friends may be especially hypervigilant for symptoms and in this context prone to misinterpret behavior as symptoms. Mental health professionals who see mentally ill patients at their sickest and who do see patients behaving and reacting in particular ways due to their illness may be inclined to interpret much or all of their behavior as symptoms regardless of what specific behaviors a patient exhibits and the particular contexts in which it arises. Their experience working with patients at their sickest conditions them to view behavior through the lens of illness. As a result, patients sometimes find that their requests, complaints, emotional reactions, and so on are ignored, discounted, or patronized, chalked up to symptoms rather than worth paying attention to in their own right.

If psychiatric patients, especially when in an acute care setting such as a mental hospital, seem excessively emotional or anxious, there is good reason for this. Psychiatric patients may in fact be more emotional, anxious, and generally reactive than the average person, even compared to other people who have mental illness and to other people who are hospitalized for physical health reasons, because they are in particularly great distress.[32] This is in part because of the nature of what brought them to this level of care—symptoms of mental illness that warrant hospitalization, for example, are distressing indeed—and in part because the process of being hospitalized or otherwise treated is or can be itself distressing. Many people who are hospitalized for psychiatric reasons are hospitalized against their will, which can be traumatic. Whether someone has entered a hospital voluntarily or not, the process of being given a room with no frills, a roommate whom one does not know, a foreign schedule and structure, in a typically sterile white setting is disorienting, to say the least, and usually harrowing. When people in a hospital setting seem to be especially emotional, angry, distraught, anxious, delusional, or incoherent, these affective and cognitive effects must be understood at least in part as responses to their situation, not merely as symptoms of their illness.

People may react to their treatment, and especially to being hospitalized, with understandable emotions such as sadness, anger, and anxiety, yet have their emotions regarded as symptomatic, for example sadness as a sign of depression, anger as a signal of paranoid aggression, or anxiety as a disorder in its own right. In fact, people can be very sad being in a hospital and feeling isolated and alone, missing their family, being cut off from other aspects of their life. People can be angry that they were hospitalized against their will. Independent of any anxiety disorder, being hospitalized can make a person feel anxious because they do not have control over their experiences; they are out of their routine and home structure; they do not have control over things like when they can eat or get their medicine or what to do at various points of the day when the day is highly structured with activities in which they are expected to participate. Moreover, in the hospital a person has little to do besides think about one's current experience of being in the hospital; it is easy for the person to become fixated on whatever emotions they are feeling there. Any kind of treatment can cause these types of emotion, and acute treatment especially so.

Before I was hospitalized, I was not conscious of experiencing any anxiety, but I developed anxiety over the course of my hospitalization stay as I felt less and less like I had control over my surroundings and my ability to do what I wanted when I wanted. I was especially anxious about getting my medicine at the right time. Having little else to think about than my daily experience in the hospital, I focused intensely on my desire to get my medicine on time and got more anxious about it than I probably needed to be, all because I felt like I had little control over it. People develop many emotional reactions to being hospitalized that are completely reasonable responses to their situation, but which easily get misinterpreted as pathological symptoms stemming from illness.

In deciding how to respond to patient testimony, the difficulty for clinicians is in sorting out what testimony is the patient's own versus what testimony is unduly influenced by psychosis. Testimony that stems from psychosis may not be trustworthy, consisting of, for example, delusional beliefs or attempts of the psychosis to advance its own goals and perpetuate itself. While skepticism is appropriate when clinicians have reason to doubt a patient's testimony, and when it matters whether the testimony is true or not, clinicians should seek out further evidence that would support or undermine testimony by engaging in conversation with patients. Through dialogue, they can test potential defeaters. However, clinicians should generally adopt a default position of trust, where they understand their primary responsibility as trying to understand the patient's perspective from their own point of view rather than trying to evaluate it, especially when there is little at stake in trusting patient testimony. Clinicians should avoid automatically distrusting patients and be willing to shift whatever skepticism they hold to trust if evidence warrants it.

Sometimes patients do share testimony that is delusional or that advances the goals of psychosis rather than their own good. When this appears to be happening, clinicians should try to address this testimony through dialogue with patients, being open to patients' ideas about their own situations and helping patients to see when they are not thinking clearly or rationally within a framework that makes sense to the patient. Clinicians working with psychotic patients are in a difficult position of trying to discern the validity of testimony, but they treat patients best when they are open to the possibility that patients know, at least to some extent, what they are talking about.

Conclusion

The nurse who was skeptical when I claimed to be a professor was not sure whether I was credible and had good reasons for thinking I was not based on my status as a patient in a psychiatric hospital. As far as she knew, I could easily have had the type of delusions that would make me a discreditable participant in epistemic practices or an unreliable testifier. Being a patient in the intensive treatment unit of the mental hospital automatically called my credibility into question. For some people, it would have automatically downgraded my credibility so that I would not be believed. For the staff who attributed my severe agitation after going off ziprasidone to anxiety rather than withdrawal, my position as a mental patient automatically made me an unreliable reporter so that my ideas about my condition were not taken seriously. For most mental health professionals who work with patients when they are sickest, in hospitals or intensive outpatient settings, this automatic discrediting of patients is probably the norm. The fact that the nursing student who spoke with me was skeptical of my story but did not automatically discredit me speaks well of her ability to pay attention to the particular details of the actual situation rather than making global assumptions based on partial information. Hopefully, with time and experience, she will adopt a default position of trust, trying to understand how a patient's testimony seems true to them without needing to evaluate its validity.

In order to assuage her skepticism, the nursing student asked me questions about Regis to gain further knowledge that could help her in deciding whether I was telling the truth about my identity. She did not simply distrust me, as she could have, closing off conversation when it seemed to veer into the unbelievable. Rather, she continued to converse with me with the goal of trying to determine whether I was believable. She welcomed me into conversation. Possibly because she was new to the profession, she did not carry with her the typical script of how to interact with mental patients that clinicians tend to learn over time. Perhaps it would have been more noble if she did not have an ulterior motive in the conversation—to ascertain whether I was telling the truth about my identity—but the fact that she did have one did not detract from the value of the conversation to me. She thought I was worth talking to despite my epistemic position as someone who might not be believable. When she gained enough knowledge about my understanding of Regis that my identity as a professor made sense, she then believed me.

While many mental health professionals would have automatically ignored, discounted, or patronized me based on my mental health status and patient status (as the staff who worked with me did), she did not. She talked to me as if we were moral equals, with respect, courtesy, and interest. She wanted to go beyond a surface-level understanding of me as simply (reductively) a patient in order to understand me and my circumstances better. She treated me as an equal participant in testimonial exchange: we participated reciprocally, as in addition to her questioning of me, I asked her questions as well about being a nursing student. In this testimonial exchange, I was initially taken aback at no longer having automatic credibility and at the idea that a student whom I could have taught was the one with automatic epistemic power and privilege, while I had little of these.

But I was also impressed with the way she treated me given our respective roles as patient and nursing student.

Giving testimony is an important exercise of epistemic agency that helps patients own, understand, and exert control over their experience, all of which contribute to patients' general capacity for agency, autonomy, and recovery. Giving testimony is only effective when it is taken up appropriately: accepted with a stance of openness and responded to as fitting for the context. Clinicians can fail to take up patient testimony in many ways, causing epistemic harm, and in some cases creating epistemic injustices to patients. In order to avoid failed uptake, clinicians should take seriously patients' self-report and interpretation of their experience, respond to these as needed, and use these in decision making.

Clinicians should encourage patients to give testimony about their experience and show patients that they value the firsthand knowledge patients can share. They should invite patients to participate in epistemic practices related to diagnosis and treatment so patients have a say in how their experience is understood and have a say in what actions they should take in recovery. For example, clinicians should involve patients in recognizing symptoms, interpreting symptoms, naming experience through diagnosis, accepting diagnosis, situating experience within larger frameworks, seeking causes of symptoms, developing control over the causes or expression of symptoms, and integrating illness experience into the patient's identity. While including and valuing patient voice is easier in outpatient settings, where it is conducive to treatment goals involving increased agency, it is also important in inpatient settings. Psychiatric hospitals should augment their goal of patient and staff safety and management to include also the goal, so important in outpatient treatment, to increase patient agency and autonomy. In the restrictive setting of a hospital, patients' experiences should be ascertained on a daily basis through conversation or writing; staff should communicate and work with patients, so patients know that their testimony is heard and cared about. Patients and clinicians should work together to formulate treatment goals and determine together the means to achieve these.

Moreover, clinicians should always take patients seriously, even when they are excessively emotional, paranoid, or delusional. Patients' concerns should never be dismissed as mere symptoms and ignored. Realizing that the experience of various treatments, including hospitalization, can themselves be distressing and anxiety producing and conjure up different emotions for different people, clinicians should be accepting of the array of styles of expression that patients may have. Clinicians should adopt a position of default trust in patient testimony and put more effort into seeking out evidence to support or undermine testimony if there is reason to be skeptical. Trust is especially important in circumstances where there is little at stake if patient testimony is unreliable, for example by letting patients try out their own ideas about what treatment they should receive if the treatment is reasonable, such as entertaining my request to be put back on ziprasidone.

Clinicians have a responsibility to take up patient testimony appropriately by taking it seriously and attending to it sufficiently based on what the situation calls for. In this way, clinicians help foster patients' sense of agency, enabling their action to have an effect on the world. By being open to patient perspectives and by being willing to learn from patients, clinicians can use that knowledge to create better interactions with patients and help patients work on their recovery more effectively. In the next chapter, I explore how clinicians should encourage and guide patients in developing a specific kind of testimony, namely constructing a narrative that makes sense of their experience by putting it into a larger framework of meaning.

7 Meaning Making

Introduction

When I began having psychotic episodes without corresponding mood changes, I adopted a primarily biomedical explanation for my psychosis, believing that it was due to faulty neurotransmitter activity in my brain. While I could identify life stressors that precipitated or exacerbated symptoms, such as loneliness, none was significant enough to be a primary cause. Everyone experiences loneliness from time to time, and work and family pressures, but few people develop profound alienation as a response and retreat into the inner world of psychosis. Since I did not have particular life stressors that could satisfactorily explain the development of psychosis (no history of trauma, loss, difficult family dynamics, poverty, or significant social marginalization, for example), a biomedical explanation seemed obvious. The leading mental disorder diagnoses that account for episodes of psychosis without corresponding mood change that were psychologically unexplainable are schizophrenia-spectrum disorders. Thus, I assumed I had developed—that my bipolar disorder had turned into—schizoaffective disorder, which just means that, in addition to manic and depressive episodes, I can have episodes of psychosis without corresponding mood change due to biological changes in the brain.

I was not sure why my psychiatrist did not see my episodes of psychosis in the same way that I did, but he seemed to think there was something "underlying" (his word) my psychosis besides faulty brain chemistry; he just didn't know what it was yet. To me, this was mystifying, as no particular psychosocial explanation fit the facts of my experience as I perceived it. My psychosis did solve some problems for me, like loneliness, but there was no obvious explanation for why my reaction to loneliness resulted in psychosis, which seemed extreme, rather than simply depression or anxiety, for example. Since I had no strong psychosocial explanation that resonates, I felt that my primary explanation must be biomedical.

My psychiatrist was wary, however, of diagnosing me with a disorder that in his eyes reduced to a biological disorder because he thought that the implication of this was that only medication would be useful; individual therapy, group therapy, and other treatments would not be useful to an essentially biologically based illness. He wanted to hold out hope that various therapies can help me. Because of his caution around giving someone a diagnosis of schizophrenia, my symptoms had to meet a high standard of evidence in order for him to interpret them as schizophrenia.

I found it interesting that even though he was a psychiatrist he was reluctant to view mental illness symptoms as simply the product of faulty brain chemistry requiring medication. In other words, he rejected the common tendency within psychiatry to reduce mental illness experience to biological abnormalities. He thought the psychological dimension of experience played an important role in leading to mental illness symptoms and wanted to leave the door to that form of treatment open. Many patients would be grateful for this, but I found it frustrating as I simply did not see how my symptoms could *not* be a product of faulty brain chemistry.

Being a mental patient is a confusing experience. When a person has a mental illness, they experience a range of feelings, thoughts, and behaviors that do not seem to make sense and that may have no discernible cause. Like many mental patients, I wanted to understand what I had been experiencing and why. I wanted to be able to name my symptoms so that instead of feeling like I had a chaotic array of experiences, I could identify them as particular things, and so that instead of wondering if any of it was imaginary, I could recognize them as symptoms of a disorder. Since my diagnosis of bipolar I disorder did not account for my experiences of psychosis without corresponding mood change, I wanted to have a diagnosis that accurately reflected my experiences. In addition, I wanted to have a framework for making sense of my experiences and ideally for understanding what caused or contributed to my symptoms. I was desperate to engage in practices of meaning making so my confusing experiences could make some sort of sense. Consequently, I adopted a biomedical explanation of my illness as a way to make sense of my experience.

Patients are epistemic agents in various ways; one way is through the practices of meaning making in which they engage when trying to understand their mental illness experiences. Patients are often not *conscious* of being epistemic agents in this way, but they exercise epistemic agency nonetheless in their desire to gain greater understanding of their experience. Gaining a greater understanding of their experience allows a person to satisfy their curiosity about their experience and gives them a sense of control over their experience, providing a way to make sense of what would otherwise be experienced as random or chaotic events that happened to them irrespective of their will.

Patients are vulnerable to feeling like they are living a chaotic, meaningless life that is out of their control; to combat this vulnerability, they need to seek meaning in their experience and to try to understand it in a larger context. If a patient did not try to put their mental illness experience into greater context, it would feel detached from other aspects of their experience, and it would be harder to integrate it into their identity and their sense of agency, creating greater disunity of self. They would consequently feel passive to their mental illness experience, feeling as if they were victims of a force that they did not have control over and possibly did not understand. Putting personal experience in the context of a larger narrative, on the other hand, gives perspective for making meaning of the experience and often allows a person to feel like they have some control over their experience, in terms of both the course of illness and its meaning. Even in the context of a medical model of psychiatric disability, making meaning of one's experience is important, as what explanation(s) a patient adopts affects how they understand their identity and agency and how they participate in treatment.

The primary ways that patients try to gain greater understanding of their experience are by creating a personal narrative of their experience and by putting their personal experience in the context of a more global overarching narrative of mental illness experience. Developing a personal narrative of experience is a way of understanding and exerting control over one's experience by selecting what is salient and putting order on events. Putting one's experience in the context of a larger framework of meaning is a way of making sense of one's experience within an identifiable structure. Both are important aspects of meaning making. Developing a credible narrative of one's experience involves a negotiation of power between patient and clinician as the patient tries to understand their experiences in their own way and the clinician tries to guide the patient to think about their experiences in certain ways the clinician finds useful.

This chapter examines the epistemic agency that patients have when engaged in practices of meaning making, looking at some of the ways that patients negotiate power with their clinician to develop narratives that best explain and make sense of their experience. First, I start by exploring the ways in which patients have epistemic agency with respect to meaning making and consider how patients work with clinicians in therapy to develop plausible narratives that make sense of their experience. Then, I examine the creation of personal narratives and review how patients rely on larger narratives about mental illness as a way to situate their own experience. Next, I investigate the role that clinicians play in guiding patients on how to make meaning of their mental illness experience and look at the need to rely on epistemic trust. While in chapter 6 I argued that clinicians should trust patient testimony unless they have a good reason not to do so, here I examine what it takes for a patient to trust clinician testimony and different ways of understanding mental illness experience. Creating personal narratives and locating one's experience within a larger framework of meaning are important expressions of epistemic agency in which patients engage in the process of recovery.

The Mental Patient as an Epistemic Agent Engaged in Practices of Meaning Making

In their quest to understand their mental illness experience better, mental patients naturally engage in practices of meaning making, exercising their epistemic agency through an inherent desire for greater understanding. The desire to gain a greater understanding of one's personal experience is part of one's dedication to the epistemic virtue of conscientiousness, or the desire to attain truth.[1] Being conscientious is part of what it is to live a good life. The epistemically virtuous person, therefore, continuously seeks greater understanding—of the self, others, the world, and events—as a life goal.[2] They make seeking greater understanding a habit of mind.[3] This commitment to conscientiousness involves a continual pursuit of knowledge, which requires continuously assessing alternative views in order to determine what view is the best, meaning most fitting with the evidence or most likely to be true.

Many people with severe mental illness are not likely to view the continual quest for greater understanding as an overarching life goal, whether because their symptoms are too distracting, because they are preoccupied with practical matters and the daily tasks of day-to-day living, or because they lack the capacity for self-awareness. Even if they do not actively pursue knowledge with conscious awareness, however, they often still engage in activities that involve the pursuit of knowledge. Whether people are consciously aware of it or not, most people want to gain greater understanding—of themselves, others, the world, and events. Most people with mental illness care about being engaged in epistemic activities, whether or not they have insight about this.

Making meaning of one's experience is a form of pursuing knowledge; the creation of personal narratives and the attempt to fit our personal experiences within a larger narrative framework are processes of seeking truth and understanding of our experience. Engaging in these activities involves entering a deliberative frame of mind of determining what we ought to believe.[4] It is easier to enter a deliberative frame of mind when a person has some self-awareness of their epistemic states, but self-awareness is not necessary for evaluating different views and for determining what one ought to believe.

Determining what one ought to believe does require testimonial sensibility, however, or sensitivity to reasons for and against a view.[5] Such sensibility includes sensitivity to information that could either support or cast doubt on the credibility of information or testimony.[6] Because testimonial sensibility is shaped through our participation in epistemic practices with others, people who are largely isolated, as many people with severe mental illness are, may have difficulty developing robust testimonial sensibility. People with severe mental illness may also have cognitive problems that make examining and evaluating reasons for and against a view difficult. Nevertheless, even if people have some difficulty with examining and evaluating a view, they will do the best they can when they are invested in trying to gain understanding. As most people with severe mental illness want to understand their situation and themselves better, they do the best they can to engage adequately in epistemic practices involved with gaining greater understanding, despite whatever impairments they may have.

The pursuit of knowledge can take different forms. For instance, the pursuit of knowledge may involve defeating alternative narratives until a person is left with just one undefeated framework that seems like the best or only way to understand their experiences.[7] When there is conflicting evidence, very little evidence, or a wide range of disparate evidence, however, defeating all alternative frameworks may be difficult or impossible to achieve. The pursuit of knowledge may instead involve a probabilistic process of considering the likelihood of alternative views and settling on the view that is most likely or least unlikely. This process may lead to a plausible result more easily than trying to defeat all alternatives. Often, finding a narrative that best explains one's personal experiences involves considering the relationships that different narratives have with each other, seeing where they are compatible and where they are contradictory. The meaning framework that best accounts for one's experience may in fact be multiple compatible frameworks that provide different kinds of insight that are complementary to each other.

However, the pursuit of knowledge here is understood; it requires many abilities and skills and is enabled by having certain epistemic virtues which are truth conducive. For example, Christopher Hookway points out that defeating alternative views requires certain abilities, including the ability to identify whether something is an alternative, whether it is relevant and whether it is "live," the ability to determine what evidence is required to defeat alternative views, and whether that information is available, and the ability to determine that no relevant alternatives, upon being defeated, are "live."[8] Other abilities that can be important for the pursuit of knowledge include the ability to weigh and compare alternative accounts, the ability to distinguish different kinds of evidence and to discern what constitutes good evidence, the ability to consider alternative interpretations of evidence and to weigh and compare evidence, the ability to distinguish and examine different reasons for an argument and to weigh and compare them, and the ability to recognize where accounts are compatible with each other and where they are contradictory. Seeing where narratives are compatible or contradictory requires the ability to think through what different views entail and how they may or may not fit with each other.

Mental patients may have difficulty exercising these abilities. In chapters 1 and 2, I explained that mental patients often have various reduced epistemic and moral capacities due to their psychosis. This can make the pursuit of knowledge difficult for mental patients and is a primary reason why mental patients are more likely to have problems acquiring knowledge. Nevertheless, even though patients may struggle with acquiring knowledge well, they still actively engage in epistemic activities as they try to do so because they have a natural inclination to want to understand themselves and their situation better. With guidance, patients can develop their epistemic and moral capacities by engaging in epistemic activities in deliberate and intentional ways.

The pursuit of knowledge and the construction of meaning found in the quest to gain greater understanding of one's mental illness experience also involves exercising various epistemic virtues. These include curiosity, or the desire to learn more, conscientiousness, or the desire to attain truth,[9] diligence, or putting in effort to understand alternative views, and attentiveness, recognizing what is salient in considering a view and paying due attention to it. Other epistemic virtues that are important include open-mindedness, which is the willingness to take distinct novel standpoints seriously,[10] impartiality, or the willingness to consider and weigh evidence without bias and to adopt views as evidence warrants and not based on personal interests,[11] intellectual sobriety, which is the dedication to consider evidence carefully and evaluate and weigh it before developing or changing a belief,[12] intellectual courage, the willingness to change one's beliefs if evidence warrants it,[13] and perseverance, the willingness to see the epistemic project of trying to gain greater understanding of one's personal experience through to a tentative conclusion.[14] The quest to gain greater understanding also requires epistemic humility, or the recognition that one is fallible and that one's ideas may be wrong, so being always open to considering new evidence and ideas and revising one's ideas when evidence warrants it. These epistemic traits are virtues because they are truth conducive;[15] having these virtues helps a person develop knowledge and create meaning. On a reliabilist account, these virtues are virtues because possessing them aids a person's epistemic projects more reliably than not possessing them.[16]

Patients have these virtues to different degrees, but they can develop them more when they are guided in their epistemic quests by people who can help them participate in epistemic activities well. Clinicians, especially therapists, play an important role here. When therapists help patients try to articulate what happened to them and what causal factors seem relevant, patients can investigate evidence and reasons to see what holds up under scrutiny and what accounts of mental illness experience that evidence and reasons support. When therapists help patients reason about what is in their interests and how their illness experience supports and challenges what is in their interests, patients can pursue different paths of reasoning, compare different reasons, and develop their own conclusions based on well-thought-out reasoning. Through these kinds of activities, patients can practice the epistemic virtues identified above. Guiding patients through the practice of these virtues helps patients indeed to develop these virtues.

In looking at different narratives that might explain their mental illness experience, a patient must adopt various epistemic skills and virtues that will help them. They must try to understand a given narrative deeply and on its own terms and try to see the reasons and evidence that would suggest that narrative to be truthful. They must consider how well the narrative fits the facts of their experience as they understand them and how deep the explanation can go. They should think through the practical consequences of accepting that narrative and consider the effect the narrative would have on how they see the future, how they see themselves in relation to their illness, and how they can exert some control over their illness in order to affect its future course.

Conditions for Meaning Making in Therapy

Patients typically engage in these epistemic practices of meaning making in the context of therapy, where a common goal often involves the patient attaining greater understanding of their experience, which will help them in gaining insight and exploring issues of identity and agency. Developing an understanding of the patient's experience through therapy requires that a patient and therapist work together to construct a personal narrative of what happened and why and to consider alternative meaning frameworks that could explain and make sense of the experience, ultimately settling on the narrative or narratives that account for the person's experiences best. Settling on a narrative(s) requires negotiating power through engaging in epistemic activities together. Patients must develop the tools to consider different narratives on their own terms; clinicians must guide patients in these queries to help them develop these tools.

Many epistemic practices go into the process of developing such a framework. Both patient and therapist should do a lot of questioning and not let assumptions go unchallenged. They should examine together a range of accounts and ideas that could explain the illness experience and think about the practical consequences of one account versus another, as well as consider what other ideas or beliefs a given account entails. They need to consider together whether an account fits the facts of experience as they are understood, but also examine whether the facts can be interpreted differently.

Carrying out these epistemic practices requires a range of epistemic skills and virtues. Both patients and clinicians need to engage in deep listening in order to truly hear the ideas of the other. They must approach this endeavor with due diligence, willing to do what it takes, epistemically speaking, to be successful in trying to come to develop the best account they can. Listening can be challenging for therapists if they think their professional expertise usurps any position the patient may have regarding their illness. Therapists sometimes hold beliefs that thwart open-minded and charitable listening, such as beliefs that expertise always trumps first-person experience, that it is the role of therapists to answer rather than to ask questions, and that a sane person, especially a clinician, should never collude with the delusion of a mentally ill person by taking their delusion seriously.[17] These beliefs can be obstacles to good listening because they reinforce a one-sided power dynamic where the therapist has considerable epistemic power and the patient has very little. At the same time, patients sometimes hold beliefs that first-person experience always trumps professional expertise, making it difficult for patients to take seriously the professional perspectives of clinicians.[18] Good listening requires humility, accepting that one does not have all the answers and realizing that one has a lot to learn from others.

Listening can also be challenging for patients who have mental illness symptoms that make concentration, reasoning, and interacting meaningfully with others difficult. Therapists who work with patients who lack some of the cognitive capacities required for good listening can feel frustrated that patients do not seem to understand or accept their views. Considerable practice, patience, and negotiation may be necessary as the patient and therapist each try to help each other to improve their listening skills.

Both parties must listen with open-mindedness, willing to change their own ideas if the evidence presented warrants it. In order to be able to do this, they must adhere to evidential norms about revising ideas based on evidence. This can be a challenge for patients, especially psychotic patients who do not necessarily reason correctly. After all, patients with psychosis in particular often have reasoning deficiencies and cognitive biases that impact the conclusions they draw. Cognitive biases include the bias against disconfirmatory evidence, a bias of discounting evidence that does not support one's views;[19] jumping-to-conclusions bias, a bias of accepting preliminary explanations of events without paying attention to doubt;[20] and jumping-to-perceptions bias, a bias of accepting a perceived experience as it initially seems without entertaining doubt.[21] Psychotic patients also commonly experience cognitive deficits such as the inability to suspend the impulse to prioritize first-person experience in order to evaluate beliefs about that experience based on other sources of information;[22] the inability to experience one's thoughts as one's own;[23] and the decreased ability to filter out unrealistic explanations (lowered decision threshold), making it easier to take seriously outlandish ideas.[24] Psychotic patients also have affective biases that influence their beliefs, including greater confidence in false beliefs (and a lack of belief flexibility)[25] and decreased confidence in true beliefs.[26] When patients seem incapable of revising their ideas appropriately based on evidence, therapists may need to try to be more persuasive, or they may need to recognize that coming to a shared understanding of the patient's experience may be impossible.

Developing a shared understanding may require some persuasion, particularly when the best account is not obvious to both parties. Each party will need to be able to give reasons for their view so that the other person can try to understand why they adhere to their view. Each should also try to empathize with the other so they can see the situation from the other's perspective. In chapter 5, I emphasized the importance of therapists developing empathetic understanding of their patients; the reverse is also true, however: patients should try to see the situation from their therapist's perspective as well. This would help them get outside of the possibly solipsistic mindset in their own head, where they may be able only to see things from their own narrow point of view.

We might wonder why patient and therapist should come to a shared understanding of illness experience; in other words, why would it matter if each explained the illness experience differently? Developing a shared account confers legitimacy on whatever account is ultimately chosen. The account is granted authority from two different but equally important sources, as the therapist lends professional authority to the account, while the patient offers first-person authority to the account. When the patient verifies that the professional's meaning framework fits the facts of their experience, they provide first-person confirmation of the account. When the therapist affirms the patient's account of their experience as plausible, they grant the account professional legitimacy. Each supports the truthfulness of the other. Neither *proves* the truthfulness of the account, as there is no single account that can be objectively verified. But in supporting its truthfulness from their respective points of view, the patient and therapist together determine what account is more likely and better fits the facts as they are understood. Together, the patient and therapist determine the best account given the epistemic resources they have, knowing that their account is always open to revision based on further evidence and reasoning.

Being in agreement on how to understand a patient's experience can be crucial for a positive therapeutic relationship, leading to shared goals for treatment and a shared idea of what means are appropriate for reaching these goals, thus contributing to therapeutic alliance. Being in agreement on how to understand a patient's experience can also contribute to more productive therapy sessions. Not seeing eye to eye can lead a patient to feel misunderstood and hinder whatever work a therapist and patient can do together. This difference in understanding can occur in any place where therapist and patient do epistemic work together, including recognizing relevant symptoms, deciding how symptoms ought to be interpreted, determining likely causes of symptoms or reasons for symptoms, and assessing how symptoms can be managed. Through this work, patients demonstrate conscientiousness and pursue knowledge of their condition in relation to a professional expert and not simply in their own head. This work can thus be very valuable in patient's epistemic pursuits in attempting to gain greater understanding of themselves. Feeling misunderstood at any place in the process of meaning making can undermine the whole experience of receiving care from a mental health clinician.

I have worked with therapists who were able to be on the same page as me, and I have quickly ended relationships with therapists with whom I could not negotiate a shared understanding. For example, I have had clinicians who seemed to think that all my problems revolved around anxiety and framed all my experiences in those terms; this felt very reductive and invalidating, as I did not see my own experiences in this way, and it truncated my subjectivity, as I described in chapter 6. The therapist I saw briefly when I was psychotic who thought I had too much insight to have psychosis was another example of a therapist with whom I could not negotiate a shared understanding. These clinicians' dismissal of my experiences and of my interpretation of my experiences exacerbated my symptoms, as they made me feel profoundly misunderstood.

The therapist I later saw who became my regular therapist validated my perspective on my experience. As I described in chapter 5, he was the first clinician I have ever had who recognized my symptoms as psychosis, and by labeling it and talking about it as psychosis in therapy, I was able to work through a lot of issues related to my experience. We did not see eye to eye on everything. As I tried to fit my experience into a broader narrative framework, I found that understanding my symptoms as chiefly biological in nature made the most sense; he at times seemed to have adopted my psychiatrist's view that my symptoms have some unknown psychological cause. We sometimes argued over how to understand my condition. But at least we had enough of a shared understanding of *what* I was experiencing and enough respect for each other to be able to entertain these arguments and take each other seriously. Some basic shared understanding and mutual respect is absolutely required for the clinician-patient relationship to be positive and productive.

Constructing a narrative is a means of giving testimony, and it is best done through dialogue between patient and clinician. Both clinicians and patients must be willing to engage in appropriate uptake of the narrative that they create together. They must attend to the working narrative with care in order to comprehend its greater context, grasp its meaning (especially to the patient), be open to learning more that might support or undermine it, and be willing to work with each other to revise the narrative as appropriate given the evidence. Appropriate uptake requires that each party adopts empathetic understanding toward the other in order to understand their point of view as deeply as possible. In order to work together fruitfully, both the clinician and the patient must trust that the other is a generally reliable testifier who can participate meaningfully in epistemic activity.

In constructing a narrative, the clinician helps the patient to make choices about how to understand events, which events have salience, which events to include in the story, and how to order events. Part of the role of the clinician is to help give present events context through the narrative by connecting present events to both past and future. The clinician also helps the patient recognize what aspects of interpretation are their own and what aspects arise from their psychosis, as well as recognize when psychosis is taking over the story so they can reassert their control in reframing the story more appropriately. Enabling the patient to identify what goals and actions are their own and what goals and actions belong to psychosis helps patients exert this control. The narrative should explain what events have already happened, and how these came to be, and point to goals of recovery and the steps needed to achieve these. Helping the patient articulate their conception of a meaningful life and identify the steps needed to achieve this flourishing are key to being intentional in what meaning a narrative has.

Let us now look more closely at some of the epistemic work that patients engage in, sometimes in therapy and sometimes on their own. This involves developing personal narratives and locating their experience within larger frameworks of meaning.

Personal Narratives

Patients frequently construct personal narratives of their experience as a way of trying to understand what happened to them, what causal factors were relevant, and how they ended up where they are. Psychotic patients often experience narrative impoverishment because they tend to lack coherence, language fluidity, temporal structure, self-reference, and a sense of agency. Constructing a personal narrative in therapy can help a person externalize their problem, seeing it as separate from themselves, by naming it and mapping its effects. Therapists can help patients deconstruct problem stories, where they explore totalizing descriptions of themselves, such as seeing themselves as a failure, and look at causes of their feelings. When developing a narrative of their experience, patients can reauthor alternative and preferred accounts, where they reject totalizing descriptions of themselves and instead look at outcomes that occur when the patient resists their identified problem.[27] In developing a personal narrative in a therapeutic setting, a patient can explore their intentions, motivations, values, and general reasons for action, as well as examine their own desires for the future. In the process, they can develop future goals for themselves, including treatment goals. By helping a patient examine and set ends for themselves, the process of constructing a personal narrative in therapy can help a patient increase their autonomy.

Patients may construct multiple narratives with different themes and genres to try to make sense of their experience. David Lumsden notes that we all have different narrative threads within us that do not have to be combined into an overarching narrative in order to make sense of our lives; rather, each thread can make sense of a certain subset of our experiences that can be ordered and integrated into a coherent whole.[28] We adjudicate between different narrative threads through conversation with others who help us create, shape, and evaluate the various narrative threads we construct.[29] The role of a therapist is to guide the patient in creating and assessing various narratives that help the patient see their experience in different ways so they can examine their values and develop future goals.

In constructing personal narratives, patients typically draw on certain narrative genres, describing their experience in terms of escape (from illness or from the mental health system), enlightenment (framing their personal stories as quests, conversion, or growth), or endurance.[30] Narratives about mental illness sometimes fit typical genres of illness narratives, including restitution narratives, which tell a story that a person was well, became sick, and then became well again; chaos narratives, which tell a story that lacks coherence, causality, and/or a neat ending; and quest narratives, which tell a story that there is something gained from having illness.[31] Narrative arcs for these personal narratives vary, as some patients' narratives focus on being unwell, some on "getting by," and some on getting well.[32] Some people attribute causes of their mental illness to psychological or social factors, and some people situate themselves and their recovery within a community, but narratives generally depict the experience of the individual undergoing the prototypical process of recovery.

As studies of narratives of psychosis show, people with psychotic disorders tend to understand their experience in terms of personal recovery narratives that emphasize particular themes of illness experience. One study describes a typical narrative arc of a person with schizophrenia with several parts or "chapters," beginning with the memory that one was "normal," competent and healthy, with goals and a sense of being in control of one's life.[33] When psychosis hits, it seems as if the brain "shuts down" and replaces what once made sense with clutter that one cannot see through. The psychotic break that occurs here as the initial break from reality, and the resulting paranoia and loss of self, are predominant themes in a person's illness narrative.[34] As psychosis takes over, a person disengages with the activities they were once involved with, such as school, work, or family life. As apathy, disinterest, fatigue, and passivity settle in, the person finds themselves doing "nothing"; even simple tasks of daily living seem too hard. At some point this "coasting" becomes unsatisfying, and a person works on trying to regain their life by setting new goals that reflect the reality of their situation, by regaining abilities, and by finding activities or hobbies of interest. Ideally the person is able to move beyond the uncertainty and unpredictability of psychosis, able to look forward and envision a future for themselves that they can work toward.[35]

Other themes that commonly show up in personal narratives about psychotic experience include social isolation, difficulties with social interaction, and an unmet need for connecting with others.[36] People also focus on the therapeutic relationships they have with their clinicians, on stigma that they experience or expect to experience, and on methods of coping and engagement in the process of recovery. In narratives that focus on the process of recovery, patients talk about falling into crisis, getting diagnosis, getting treatment, coming to terms with their illness, learning and practicing coping strategies, making meaning of their experience, and trying to avoid future crises.[37] Personal narratives can either internalize or externalize (or both) root problems involved with psychosis depending on how the individual understands their experience.

Besides exploring what happened to them and what lessons they learned from their experience, patients often explore in their personal narratives what comes after being sick, examining what life after psychosis consists of and what recovery looks like. In addition to whatever concrete losses they may endure, a person has to deal with what can be a profound loss of hope and possibility. When their illness makes it impossible for them to live the life they did before getting sick, they have to reevaluate the goals and dreams they once had and accept that their life may not be the same as what they once thought it would be, or even as what it was before they got sick. This requires having some degree of autonomy, for it involves reflection on values and goals. In place of their previous aims, patients have to identify realistic goals that reflect their lived reality. They have to accept the indeterminism and uncertainty that now constitutes their life and find a way to move on despite it. In other words, they have to find a way to give their lives the structure that psychosis broke asunder, and they have to address the existential questions about how to live a good life despite enduring illness. Constructing a personal narrative requires some degree of autonomous reflection about values and gives patients a way to explore what life after illness can be like. Therapists play an important role in helping patients to do the necessary reflection to be able to construct such a narrative.

Larger Narratives of Mental Illness

In addition to constructing personal narratives that try to make sense of what happened and that explore future goals and steps, patients commonly try to situate their experience within larger narrative structures that give a greater meaning context for understanding that experience. Here patients generally have to work within available narrative structures, choosing from various narratives that are presented to them from different sources, evaluating the narratives to see which best fit the available evidence and which best explain their experience. This process of situating one's story within a larger narrative structure is a process of pursuing knowledge for the sake of gaining greater understanding. When patients participate in this epistemic work, they are acting conscientiously as epistemic agents desiring to attain truth and knowledge. They act with diligence, trying to understand the different available frameworks, and attentiveness, paying attention to what is salient. They seek greater understanding of their experience as part of their life goals.

Patients are usually presented with certain frameworks for understanding their experience. The two leading narrative frameworks used to explain a patient's experience are biomedical narratives and psychosocial narratives. They are often presented as dichotomous narratives that are exclusive of each other, even though in actuality they often complement each other. These narratives are frequently espoused by therapists and psychiatrists treating the patient, but they are also dominant narratives within American culture and so are easily adopted simply through acceptance of cultural norms about how to understand mental illness. Alternative narratives are also available, but they are much less common and not usually put forth by or endorsed by mental health professionals. Patients sometimes encounter these alternative narratives through social media, the internet, or social support groups, or in certain cases their cultural or religious group. Let us look at these narratives more closely, starting with the two dominant narratives.

Biomedical narratives. Biomedical narratives treat mental illness as a brain disease, explaining mental illness symptoms as the product of faulty brain processes or abnormal brain structures. The idea that mental illness stems from malfunctions in neurotransmitter activity is a very common example of a biomedical narrative. In schizophrenia, excessive dopamine and glutamate transmission[38] and deficient GABA activity[39] are thought to play roles. Other biomedical narratives may attribute mental illness to structural problems in the brain, such as decreased gray matter[40] or disorganized glial cells[41] in the case of schizophrenia.

According to biomedical narratives, the causes of brain malfunction or abnormality are varied; brain malfunction or abnormality may arise from genetic abnormalities, from exogenous agents such as psychotropic drugs (whether recreational drugs or prescribed drugs), from viruses, from developmental abnormalities that occurred when the brain was forming in the womb, or from various psychosocial stressors that "rewire the brain," so to speak, changing its structure and operation in response to stressors. Biomedical narratives thus explain what occurs in the brain when a person experiences mental illness symptoms, but they do not assume any particular causal factor as being more relevant than another; in other words, any causal factor that has a biological component (such as changes the brain in some way) may be relevant. It is important to emphasize that biomedical narratives are compatible with psychosocial explanations that seek to identify psychological and social factors that underlie mental illness symptoms, only they explain them in terms of their effect on the brain rather than in terms of behavioral response.

Psychosocial narratives. Psychosocial narratives treat mental illness as a maladaptive response to psychological and social problems. For example, mental illness symptoms may arise as a way to deal with stress, as either a coping mechanism or avoidance mechanism, as a way to process or avoid stimuli, or as a way to meet one's needs. In this view, mental illness serves various functions in a person's psychological development and response. The idea of mental illness as a response to psychological and social problems goes back to Adolf Meyer, who in the 1930s described mental illnesses as reactive types, or sets of maladaptive reactions developed in response to environmental stress.[42] Examples of psychosocial narratives include the idea that psychotic symptoms such as hearing voices develop as a way to not be present during difficult situations (enabling avoidance), as a way to distract a person from their environment (allowing one to avoid stimuli in particular), as a way to feel close to a loved one who died (enabling a person to meet their needs), as a way to process trauma (acting as a coping mechanism), or as a way to deal with a person's fears about themselves (allowing a person to process emotions). Some of the difficult situations that people may be responding to in developing symptoms like psychosis may be trauma,[43] loss,[44] difficult family dynamics,[45] social marginalization,[46] or poverty.[47] Narratives focusing on social marginalization and poverty can sometimes constitute social justice narratives, which empower individuals and situate them within a larger community from which they can draw political power.[48]

Psychosocial narratives explain why a person experiences particular mental illness symptoms in terms of psychological and social factors. They are compatible with biomedical explanations of what occurs in the brain when a person is dealing with these stressors, but they treat the psychological/sociological explanation as more meaningful or fundamental than the biological/medical explanation.

Although psychosocial and biomedical explanations are compatible with each other, they have very different foci and lead to different emphases in treatment. Psychosocial narratives are typically examined in therapy, where some of the therapeutic goals include developing insight and developing some control over mental illness symptoms. Understanding the psychological explanation can help a person address existential questions about identity, agency, and their future and help a person to gain insight into their behavior so they can make changes and exert control over their illness. Biomedical narratives are typically put forth by psychiatrists, who frame illness in terms of symptoms arising from faulty brain processes that can be treated by medications. Accepting a biomedical narrative enables a person to accept drug treatment as a feasible treatment option, increasing their willingness to take medications and put up with potentially undesirable side effects for the sake of overall health improvement. Psychiatrists and therapists typically work in tandem, each respecting the professional expertise and perspective of the other, recognizing that psychosocial and biomedical explanations both shed light on different aspects of illness and can be complementary to each other.

Critics of biomedical narratives sometimes argue that biomedical narratives reinforce stereotypes about people with illness as being defective or as having an internal weakness that they have no control over, making their illness seem inevitable, and leaving people vulnerable to stigmatization.[49] Even if this defect or weakness is understood as not being the person's fault, making the person not blameworthy for it, it still invites feelings of (or expectations that one should feel) shame. These critics find psychosocial narratives more empowering because they locate the cause of illness in events external to the person. While this is true, however, psychosocial narratives can also suggest personal weakness if they are read in a certain way, not in terms of a defect in the brain, but in terms of an inability to cope with life circumstances or to get one's needs met appropriately; this may be understood as victim blaming. When the patient is a female, this narrative reinforces feminine stereotypes of women being weak and unable to cope with stress.[50] I worry that psychosocial narratives may be used to stereotype women and blame them for being weak and unable to cope. We must be careful not to use narratives to support stereotypes, stigmatization, or unfair blame. Whatever narratives are adopted must be based on the best fit of evidence and not on our preconceived ideas about what people with mental illness, women, or other groups of people are like.

Both biomedical narratives and psychosocial narratives are compatible with a "DSM culture" in which individuals learn to identify their experiences as symptoms of their disorder as delineated by the *Diagnostic and Statistical Manual* (DSM) that is used in diagnosis. Şerife Tekin worries that understanding one's experiences mainly in terms of symptoms is reductive, ignoring interpersonal factors and leading to hyponarrativity, a very thin narrative reflecting impoverished self-insight.[51] Ginger Hoffman and Jennifer Hansen believe that women are especially prone to understanding their experiences in this reductive way.[52] Tekin associates primarily biomedical narratives with this hyponarrativity, but the DSM is neutral on causes of mental disorders and thus is compatible with psychosocial narratives as well. The real problem is not in how we understand the causes of disorder but rather in how reductive a symptom-based narrative can be.[53] Biomedical narratives can be as resourceful for patients as psychosocial narratives can be, when they give patients tools to deal with their illness;[54] either type of memoir can be either reductive or resourceful, depending on the richness of insight that underlies it.

The way to avoid creating a reductive narrative is to increase epistemic resources so the patient can develop greater insight into their condition and not rely solely on DSM criteria to understand their experiences. Having patients read other patients' memoirs and talking through different narrative frameworks in therapy can help provide these epistemic resources.

(Gaining greater cognitive function can also help, as hyponarrativity can also result from cognitive difficulties caused by mental illness.[55]) The goal is to gain greater insight so one can develop a thicker narrative that is rich and resourceful, giving the patient tools to work through their problems so they can grow as a person.[56] Investigating various dimensions of the self is one way to do this. Tekin identifies five dimensions of a multitudinous self: the ecological self (the physical body), the intersubjective or relational self, the temporally extended self that has past memories and future goals, the private self that is the subject of first-person experience, and the conceptual self, where a person has self-concepts about who they see themselves as that are action guiding.[57] Developing alternative narratives that go beyond the two dominant narratives can be one way to explore how these various aspects of self are affected by illness.

Mohammed Abouelleil Rashed identifies three alternative accounts that he calls "Mad narratives," created not by scientists or therapists but by people with mental illness themselves as ways to explain their experience outside of the dominant paradigms. These narratives include the following:

Spiritual transformation. Some people with mental illness regard their mental illness experience as one of spiritual transformation.[58] These people regard the experiences and behaviors they have that others identify as mental illness experience instead as part of the process of spiritual transformation. While less common in a globalized society, this framework is more acceptable in indigenous cultures throughout the world where experiences like hearing voices are viewed as evidence of spirit possession, whether they be good spirits or bad spirits.[59] In globalized society, people might see their experience as a process of being broken down through suffering and then reborn into a new life, all cast in a spiritual context. They might see their travails as the result of God or gods who are testing them, seeing how much fortitude, patience, or obedience they have or testing their faith. They might see themselves as personally chosen by God or gods to have a unique and special experience. In globalized society, spiritual transformation narratives are difficult to take on their own and tend to be accepted in conjunction with other narratives that are made compatible with it.

Dangerous gifts. Some people with mental illness regard their mental illness experience as a dangerous gift, dangerous in the sense that it creates impairments and causes much suffering, but also a gift in the sense that it is the basis for creativity and vision.[60] Such a narrative sees value in mental illness experience rather than seeing it as purely needless suffering. For example, the vision statement of the Icarus Project, an online support network aligned with the antipsychiatry movement, which is critical of dominant understandings of mental illness and dominant treatment methods (particularly medication), states: "We are members of a group that has been misunderstood and persecuted throughout history, but has also been responsible for some of the world's most extraordinary creations. Sensitivities, visions, and inspirations are not necessarily symptoms of illness, they are gifts needing cultivation and care. When honored and nurtured, these gifts can lay the foundation for a wiser and more compassionate society."[61] In the dangerous gifts narrative, people discern value in their mental illness experience and find such experience as worthwhile even though it may also involve much distress and difficulty. This narrative does not identify any particular source for a person's mental illness experience. Such a narrative is compatible with biomedical and psychosocial narratives that regard mental illness as stemming from abnormal biological processes or psychosocial problems. Dangerous gifts narratives are able to explain the appeal of mental illness symptoms such as mania, but they do not describe mental illness conditions that do not involve discernible value, such as dementia-like states brought on by psychosis.

Healing voices. The healing voices narrative applies specifically to people who hear voices. According to this narrative, voices are not the random expression of abnormal biological processes but rather serve important functions for a person, functions that must be recognized in order to gain some control over the experience.[62] While voices can be berating and belittling, accepting one's voices and talking back to them can lead one to exert some control over them. Voices can then be healing, allowing for personal growth as their meaning and function are discerned. This narrative is compatible with psychosocial narratives that attribute symptoms like hearing voices to psychosocial triggers; it is not as easily compatible with biomedical narratives that locate their source in abnormal biological processes. This is because biomedical narratives do not see symptoms like hearing voices as serving any particular function, whereas psychosocial narratives can easily accept that symptoms serve functions.

Alternative narratives can be helpful ways for people to process their experience when their experiences do not easily fit one of the dominant paradigms. Like biomedical and psychosocial narratives, when they are seen as the exclusive explanation of a person's experience, they can be too reductive. As studies of personal narratives of patients with psychosis show, patients typically understand their experiences within the context of one or both of the dominant narratives, framing their personal recovery story in terms of a biomedical and/or psychosocial narrative.[63] Nevertheless, alternative narratives can be useful frameworks for understanding other facets of experience besides biomedical and psychosocial factors. Feeling like their experience is too complicated to reduce to a single explanation, many people, I believe, find their experience more satisfactorily explained in terms of multiple narratives that are compatible with each other rather than simply a solo narrative.

Settling on Larger Narrative Frameworks

Patients need to navigate these different larger narratives to find what larger narratives seem the most plausible and best explain their experience. We might wonder why patients have to choose among different narratives to try to explain their experience. Does it really matter if the patient believes their mental illness results from brain abnormalities, psychosocial stressors, spirit possession, or other sources? There is a place, after all, for epistemic restraint, when seeking out more knowledge is not appropriate or necessary.[64] But we need to be able to discern when restraint is appropriate and when it is important to develop knowledge so we can construct beliefs and make judgments. In this case, it is important that a person gain greater understanding of their mental illness experience, and it does matter which narrative(s) they adopt in forming that understanding. This is because the narratives we use to understand our personal experience are action guiding.

What account a patient believes about the development and nature of their mental illness affects how they think about their future in relation to the illness, what kind of control they have over what happens to them, what kinds of treatment options are acceptable, and how they think about taking medicine and participating in various therapies. When I adopt a biomedical narrative of my illness, for example, I accept that medication is a necessary treatment and I commit myself to the idea that medication will play a significant role in my life. To the extent that I understand my illness in psychosocial terms, I need to examine the psychosocial stressors that seemed to play a role in my symptoms and become committed to managing them as best as I can. The different narratives imply different forms of agency in relation to the illness and indicate different treatment options that would help manage the illness. Whatever narrative(s) a person adopts affects how they feel and think about their illness and what they do in relation to their illness, thereby affecting its course and treatment. It really is important for a person to evaluate different narratives and adopt the one(s) that best fit their experience as they understand it.

Developing a personal narrative and developing greater understanding of one's experience by situating it within a larger meaning framework fit many of the goals that patients have in therapy. Patients see counseling therapists for a variety of reasons, including both practical and existential reasons. In therapy, patients might learn coping and mindfulness skills (such as through acceptance and commitment therapy or dialectical behavioral therapy), how to recognize and deal with their thoughts and emotions (such as through cognitive behavioral therapy and dialectical behavioral therapy), how to identify and avoid or address triggers that cause or exacerbate symptoms, and how to deal with stress constructively. Patients also see therapists for more existential reasons, such as to help them better understand themselves so they can choose to act differently in the future (gaining insight), to make sense of their experience (developing a meaning framework), to figure out who they are in relation to their illness (exploring questions about identity), and to help them identify where they have agency to change things (exploring questions about agency). Making sense of one's experience underlies many existential goals: whatever account a person gives of their experience also affects how they understand themselves in relation to their illness, what kind of future they see for themselves, and where they see themselves able to make changes that affect the course of their illness. By making sense of their experience, patients are also able to implement the practical skills learned in therapy more effectively. Working with a therapist to develop a greater understanding of their experience can thus help a person address many of the other goals they may have in therapy as well as satisfy an innate curiosity and desire for understanding.

A good therapist does not tell the patient how they should understand their experience but rather acts as a guide helping the patient to determine their own understanding. A good therapist helps the patient see the various frameworks that are available for understanding experience and helps the patient think through both the evidence that the frameworks explain and the ways that the frameworks do and do not fit their experience. Ultimately, the patient has to determine for themselves what the best way to understand their experience is. But their explorations with their therapist can be very helpful in guiding and expanding their understanding. Clinicians—not only therapists, but also psychiatrists and other mental health professionals—play an important role in helping patients to frame and understand their experience.

Navigating different frameworks of meaning requires in part deciding where to place one's epistemic trust. Patients have to decide whose epistemic authority they trust in determining what narratives seem the most plausible. This involves both assessing the credibility of the authors of various narratives—for example, the scientists who espouse biomedical narratives and the psychologists who recommend psychosocial narratives—and assessing the guidance they receive from clinicians who help them navigate these meaning frameworks. In navigating the different narratives by which patients might understand their experience, patients must have epistemic trust in the clinicians who help them. They must trust clinicians to have relevant information and knowledge and trust that they will engage with patients properly, taking patient ideas seriously and maintaining reciprocity in dialogic engagement. Patients must trust that clinicians will both use their expertise to help guide the patient and respect them as epistemic partners at the same time.

Epistemic Trust

Trust is essential to knowledge. We need to rely on others' knowledge because we cannot do all the epistemic work of developing knowledge on our own.[65] We are unable to gather, interpret, and assess evidence for every view that we might consider adopting, nor can we evaluate all reasons for and against every potential view ourselves, nor can we adopt all available perspectives to see all sides of an issue. Instead, we must rely on experts who have specialized knowledge that we are unable to acquire ourselves,[66] as well as other trustworthy people who can provide information and testimony that we can trust, including individuals who have unique perspectives to bear on an issue. As explained in chapter 6, this means that medical professionals should seek out patient testimony to understand perspectives based on firsthand experience that can aid in diagnosis and treatment. This also means that lay people should seek out expert testimony and trust it when there are no defeaters present that would undermine it.

Trusting someone to give accurate knowledge and reliable testimony involves several components. It requires that the person whose knowledge or testimony is trusted, the testifier, communicates what they know; that the person who is trusting that the knowledge is accurate or the testimony is reliable believes that information based on what they know about the person; and that the person trusting the accuracy of knowledge has confidence in the person being trusted.[67] Trusting one's clinician requires that the clinician communicates what they know, that the clinician is trustworthy, and that one has confidence in the clinician.

When we trust the knowledge of another, we are epistemically dependent on the other and thus vulnerable to the other.[68] Despite this vulnerability, we all have to trust others for much of our knowledge. Even experts have to trust other experts in their own field, as no one has the ability or means to gather all of the evidence that can be gathered.[69] When trust is developed appropriately, it is truth conducive, meaning that it leads a person to develop knowledge and create meaning in a reliable way. On a reliabilist epistemology account, the epistemic goodness of a belief is based on the reliability of the process by which the belief is formed;[70] when other people demonstrate to us repeatedly over time that they can provide accurate and reliable testimony and information to us, we are able to trust them to continue to do so and, in so doing, to aid us in our own epistemic projects. As a patient works with their clinician over time, and the clinician demonstrates that they have the knowledge that they are expected to have, the clinician exhibits trustworthiness, and the patient develops greater trust of their clinician.

What is it that we trust when we trust the knowledge of others? We trust that those who have knowledge to share have gathered evidence and acquired their knowledge with the same epistemic virtues that we find valuable. We assume they have curiosity, conscientiousness, and attentiveness; we trust that they are open minded, impartial, intellectually sober, intellectually courageous, persevering, and epistemically humble. If they attained their knowledge in the same general ways that we would have, then we believe we can trust the outcome of their process. Just as these virtues help us in gaining knowledge and making meaning more reliably, we trust that they will help others do the same. When a patient trusts their clinician, they assume the clinician has the epistemic virtues that allow them to have the same approach to knowledge seeking and meaning making that they do.

How do we know whom we can trust? Depending on the context, we may adopt default trust, trusting the information or testimony of others to be accurate or reliable unless presented with some reason why we should not.[71] For default trust to be reliable, we need to have a sensitivity to defeaters, able to discern what counts as a reason against accepting information or testimony or a reason against the trustworthiness of the person presenting these, and able to weigh such reasons against one's default trust position to determine an epistemic judgment of trustworthiness. If we do not have this defeater sensitivity, we will not know when to let go of our default trust and will be prone to gullibility, believing information or testimony when it is unwarranted.

In other contexts, we may adopt default distrust and remain ever vigilant, not ready to trust information or testimony until it has been vetted. Our default here would be to withhold trust until we find positive reasons to believe a view is correct or to believe the person espousing it is trustworthy. For vigilant trust to be reliable, we need to be sensitive to reasons that count for and against a view, and we need to have the capacity to judge the trustworthiness of testimony or information based on how the person presenting these is epistemically situated, what competence and authority they have, and what cues they give. If we do not have these capacities, we will not know when it is appropriate to relax our vigilance and will be prone to suspiciousness and paranoia, distrusting others and disbelieving information and testimony even when there is reason to trust and evidence for belief.

When making a credibility judgment about the veracity of a view, we typically draw on several sources of information, including information about the person espousing the view (helping us to form judgments of their trustworthiness), the ways that a view is put forth (for example as an assertion or a question, or with confidence or tentativeness), background knowledge about the content of the view (what else we know to be true, and how the view under examination fits within that), and structural features of the way the view is put forth (its format—for example a scientific study versus an opinion piece).[72] Ideally, determining the trustworthiness of a person presenting information or testimony involves monitoring testifiers to determine their credibility, judging their reliability by looking at their past experience with gathering and relaying information. This requires cognitive processes and skills of epistemic competence, which we develop through epistemic practice in community with others.[73]

In reality, however, most people do not interact with others in a way that allows them to monitor testifiers;[74] frequently we trust or distrust people's testimony based on factors that have nothing to do with past experience. Factors such as the epistemic position and expertise (if any) of the person offering testimony or information and our ability to discern good reasoning and sound arguments are relevant and tend to be helpful in epistemic assessment; other factors also play a role but may be idiosyncratic or prejudicial and can produce less reliable results. These include our own previous beliefs and prejudices, our own past history of trusting others epistemically, our internalization (or not) of norms of compliance and conformism, social norms, social reputational cues, our emotional reactions, and our moral commitments.[75] To the extent that we are able to develop epistemic competence through epistemic practices in community with others, we are often able to rely on common sense in assessing whether someone's testimony or information is accurate or reliable.[76]

People with severe mental illness may have difficulty making credibility judgments that are accurate and reliable, whether these lead to trusting or distrusting others, as they may have reasoning and cognitive deficits that interfere with their ability to assess information about interlocutors, discern how views are espoused, fit a given view within a context of other knowledge, or assess the nature of the view based on its format. Especially if they are socially isolated or have little advanced education, they may lack relevant background knowledge, never having had the opportunity to acquire it; if they are socially isolated, they may not be able to develop sufficient epistemic competence to make common sense judgments reliably. They may fail to understand social norms or read social reputational cues that would indicate someone's trustworthiness (such as professional expertise), or they may fail to recognize defeaters that call into question trustworthiness (such as claims based on shoddy evidence). They may be motivated more by prejudicial beliefs (such as prejudices against the medical system) than by reasoning about the actual case at hand. Their beliefs, emotional reactions, and moral commitments may be formed through bad or questionable processes, such as generalizing from one bad experience with a clinician to develop distrust toward clinicians in general or generalizing from their own privileged position in which they have always had positive experiences with clinicians to believe that clinicians can do no wrong. Such biases can lead people to make inaccurate credibility judgments, so that they are either overly distrustful or overly trusting of clinicians and the narratives that can help them understand their experience, without considering other relevant factors.

While all people are prone to biases in making credibility judgments, people with cognitive difficulties stemming from mental illness may be more likely to rely on such biases for their epistemic judgments because they have less capability for making cognitive judgments about the worthiness of evidence or the reliability of the process through which evidence is gathered. Relying on biases to make epistemic judgments rather than examining and making judgments about the specific features of a given situation leads to judgments that may be inaccurate or unreliable. As a result of lacking the epistemic competence to judge credibility accurately or reliably, people with mental illness may lack the ability to be critical and discerning and thus be too trusting of others, or they may fail to develop the capacity to trust at all and be overly suspicious of others. In the former case, their default trust becomes a permanent stance that cannot be outweighed by potential defeaters; in the latter case, they adopt such a high level of vigilance that no considerations in favor of trust can relax it. Consequently, they may be gullible to information that is not accurate or reliable or may be unable to acquire knowledge that would be gained through trust.

People with severe mental illness who are evaluating narratives that help explain their mental illness experience can be vulnerable to both of these problems. Excessive suspicion aimed at one source—for example, scientists and psychiatrists who put forth biomedical narratives—may result in gullible acceptance of accounts from another source—for example, various alternative narratives. Scientists, psychiatrists, and therapists may be judged suspiciously for a variety of reasons, including the fact that, as professionals and experts, they have expertise over knowledge that seems far removed from everyday experience. Narratives that are alternatives to the dominant frameworks for understanding mental illness experience may seem more interesting simply because they are unusual, arise directly from patient experience rather than from professional expertise, and avoid whatever qualms one may have over the dominant frameworks. The opposite can also happen: a person may distrust fellow patients whose experience seems very different from their own, or who seem like they have an axe to grind, and thereby reject patient-generated alternative narratives and instead trust scientific narratives that seem safer and more comfortable because of their familiarity and expertise. Clinicians can help patients recognize these biases where they occur and work with patients to correct their biases so they can develop the tools needed for accurate credibility judgments and appropriate trust.

At the same time that people with severe mental illness may be prone to distrust or overly trust clinicians and particular narratives due to epistemic impairments, they also often have a wealth of experience and first-person knowledge upon which they can draw to develop their credibility judgments. Having experience with different treatment modalities can provide insight into which treatments work for them, which can shed light on which larger narrative frameworks seem to make the most sense for understanding their experience. First-person knowledge about their needs and interests and the effects of their illness can also inform what frameworks make the most sense. Even as they recognize the possible epistemic impairments people with severe mental illness may have, clinicians should also recognize and value the knowledge they have and encourage patients to use that knowledge to develop greater understanding of their condition. With this encouragement, clinicians can help empower patients to use their own hermeneutical resources to increase their epistemic agency.

In order to help patients most fruitfully, it is crucial that clinicians be as trustworthy as possible. This involves not only sharing all their relevant knowledge to help the patient make the best treatment decisions, but also having the epistemic humility to acknowledge what they do not know or can only surmise, as it is easier to trust a clinician who is open to learning more and revising their ideas than it is to trust a clinician who claims to have the final and conclusive word on a patient's situation. The clinician's perspective is powerful, as it helps shape the patient's understanding of their situation; it is important for clinicians to recognize their power and to be careful not to abuse it by approaching interactions with patients with honesty, humility, open-mindedness, and conscientiousness.

In addition, acquiring trustworthiness also involves treating the patient with respect as a fellow interlocutor. This requires taking seriously all of the patient's ideas, including whatever biases they have for or against authority, seeing these as worth addressing rather than simply dismissing. Whatever meaning a patient gives of their illness experience must be taken seriously and assessed carefully through dialogue with the patient. If the clinician throws around their expertise as if it trumps all the patient's ideas and fails to listen to the patient's concerns, the clinician will lose the patient's trust of them. If they treat the patient as a fellow interlocutor whom they respect and take seriously, on the other hand, they will gain the patient's trust.

Moreover, it is important that the clinician work with the patient to develop a shared understanding of the patient's experience to which both can agree. Adopting the other-oriented perspective of empathetic understanding helps with this. In order for the patient to find the clinician's perspective to be trustworthy, the clinician must base their perspective of the patient's situation on an understanding of the patient's experience—gained through empathy and dialogue—that coheres with the patient's self-understanding.

Epistemic trust helps us deal with the uncertainty inherent to trying to make sense of mental illness experience. There is no single correct way of understanding why events happened to a person and how the person became the way they are; different accounts can be given that make more or less sense of the facts of the situation and that account for reasons and evidence in better and worse ways. Finding the narrative(s) that best explain a person's experience is a matter of finding the right fit between the facts as they are perceived and the explanations that can be given. Patients often need help in determining this fit and figuring out how best to understand their experience; clinicians play an important role in guiding them. In order for the patient to be guided effectively in participating in epistemic practices, it is important that they are able to trust their clinician.

Epistemic trust does not always lead to positive results, but when we have the epistemic competence to evaluate the trustworthiness and credibility of testifiers, it can often guide us well. While various factors can affect our ability to trust when and only when it is warranted, epistemic trust is necessary to some extent simply because we cannot acquire and assess all the information and evidence necessary to make all epistemic judgments oneself. Developing the competence to judge credibility accurately and reliably is key to being able to gain knowledge through epistemic trust.

Conclusion

In the beginning of this chapter, I discussed how I have adopted a primarily biomedical narrative with a secondary psychosocial narrative to explain my mental illness experience because it seems like the best explanation of my experiences. Since my psychosis does not have significant psychosocial causes that I can identify, a narrative that explains my psychosis primarily in terms of faulty brain chemistry and secondarily in terms of solving certain psychological problems seems most fitting. Adopting these narratives leads me to conclude that antipsychotic medication is essential to treating my psychosis, and it provides motivation for me to take medication as prescribed. Indeed, some of the evidence I have for believing that the biomedical narrative is true is my response to medication: when I take antipsychotic medication, I feel so much better that it is like being a different person. Moreover, I know from reducing my prescribed medication so many times that even a small decrease in antipsychotic medication creates noticeable effects in functioning, leading to significant impairment. The dramatic role that medication plays in treating my symptoms is proof to me that my psychosis has a fundamentally biological component. My psychiatrist's inability to see this stymies me.

My psychiatrist's belief that if I have a biologically based schizophrenia-spectrum illness, then I will not benefit from therapy, is false. Even in a biomedical narrative of mental illness, there is room to address psychosocial issues that contribute to or result from faulty brain chemistry. Therapy still plays an important role in my treatment even if my illness is at root biomedical. I need therapy in order to address the practical questions that arise with chronic illness, such as how to cope with my symptoms, how to avoid triggering symptoms, and what kind of control I have over my illness, as well as existential questions about who I am, who I can be, who I want to be, and how I see my future. To address these questions, I need to try to understand the nature of my illness and put it into larger frameworks of meaning. I also need therapy to address the psychosocial issues that do seem like relevant triggers or complicating factors, such as to explore my sometimes deep sense of loneliness.

In constructing a narrative of my experience, I need to see how what has happened in the past has led to my current situation and examine what ends I ought to pursue and the means to achieve these ends. This requires me to distinguish what my psychosis values from what I value, and what goals the psychosis has—namely to be self-perpetuating—from what goals I have, and to recognize the role that health and well-being play in achieving my goals. With the guidance of my therapist, I explore these practical and existential questions as I try to make meaning of my experience.

The fact that therapy plays an important role even within a primarily biomedical narrative does not detract from the fact that medication is critical for treating psychosis; therapy and medication are both essential. Addressing psychological issues will help me manage my psychosis and possibly avoid worsening symptoms, but by itself it cannot eradicate psychosis. Only when the psychosis is under control with medication can I even look at these issues in a meaningful way. Without medication, all of my experience, including my experience in therapy, is filtered through psychosis; this changes the meaning of these practical and existential issues so that they are moot, or mean something entirely different that is accessible only to myself, making it so I cannot genuinely address them at all.

While I perceive my psychosis to be chiefly biomedical, the issue of the nature of my psychosis is not settled, especially for my psychiatrist. He is open to the possibility that I have schizoaffective disorder but needs more evidence to warrant the diagnosis. (What kind of evidence he needs, I am not sure. The decisive evidence would be progressive deterioration of functioning in areas such as work and family life, a fate I am terrified of and hope never happens. If this is the only evidence that is sufficient to prove I have schizoaffective disorder, I guess I have to hope that he never has reason to diagnose me with this disorder.) I am open to the possibility that I do not have schizoaffective disorder, but I still want to have *some* account of my psychotic episodes that seems to explain what they are and why they arise. If I had an alternative explanation that seemed to fit the facts of my experience as well as or better than schizoaffective disorder, I would be satisfied. My psychiatrist needs to wait for time to pass to see if I continue to struggle with psychosis and, if so, what course it takes; I need either to remain open to other possible explanations or learn to live with the fact that I may never have a satisfactory explanation.

My primarily biomedical understanding of my experiences is no more than a tentative conclusion, a belief that I can hold for now as long as the evidence available to me warrants it, but one that is revisable if I learn of new evidence that justifies revision. I must remain open minded and diligent, working to seek the truth continuously even if it threatens my self-understanding. My belief that I have schizoaffective disorder—or that my bipolar disorder has somehow shifted to schizophrenia, that what used to be chiefly a mood disorder is now predominantly a psychotic disorder—is provisional, as I cannot have certainty that this is the right way to understand my experience, at least not with the evidence I have right now. In this narrative, antipsychotic medication is essential for treating my condition, but so is therapy. If my condition does worsen to the point that my psychiatrist is comfortable diagnosing me with schizoaffective disorder or schizophrenia, I will consider that to be evidence in favor of that I do indeed have a schizophrenia-spectrum disorder: if he, with his high standard of evidence, believes I have this disorder, then that will seem to confirm my belief.

Psychiatric patients engage in many epistemic practices as part of their outpatient treatment, including meaning making. Patients want to understand their experiences to make sense of them. Some of the ways that they do this is to by constructing personal narratives that explain what happened to them and by putting their experiences in the context of a larger framework of meaning. Biomedical and psychosocial narratives are the leading narratives of mental illness in our contemporary culture, but alternative narratives also exist. It matters what narratives patients adopt in making sense of their experience, as this affects how they deal with issues of identity and agency, which are typically addressed in therapy, as well as their attitude toward treatment. Patients need to assess the evidence for the narratives they are presented with and choose the narrative(s) that are supported by the best available evidence and that fit the experience of the patient.

In this chapter and chapter 6, I examined two ways that patients must exercise their agency in order to develop their agency and autonomy more fully: giving testimony and making meaning of their experience. In the next chapter, I explore an additional way that patients exercise their agency and participate actively in their recovery: by making choices, both choices to engage in treatment and choices to show up and participate in life.

8 Choices

Introduction

In July 2019, I found myself attending a philosophy conference in San Francisco. While traveling always gives me anxiety, conferences had become much more difficult since my psychotic break two years earlier. It was hard to stay present, concentrate on what I was hearing, and follow people's trains of thought. Worse than following talks I heard in the conference was dealing with everything related to traveling. I always worried that I would forget how to do the things one needs to do while traveling—flying on an airplane, getting a taxi, checking myself into the hotel. With my stress level increased due to being out of my daily routine, I found it challenging to figure out how to do each step. It was always a relief to be alone in my room at night and in between sessions where I didn't have to worry about interacting with others and didn't have to stress out figuring out what to do.

It was the third day of the conference, and I was not feeling okay. Paranoid, I found it painful to be around other people. The noise in my head grew loud and confusing. Everything had become creepy again, and I felt isolated and alone in a world I didn't fully understand. Every time there was a break in the conference schedule, I walked across the campus back to my room where I could pace by myself for a few minutes before having to head back for another session.

Although I was feeling psychotic again, I was also a little proud of myself. I had made it to the third day before I began feeling so awful. The first two days I had felt relatively "normal" and had enjoyed myself at the conference, even going out of my way to talk with colleagues. That was amazing. I had only started taking risperidone a week or so earlier, so its relief from psychosis was new to me. A month earlier, in June, I had been so psychotic that I did not think I could return to work come fall. Immersed in a fog of confusion, I couldn't understand anything that was going on around me; the noise in my head was too loud to perceive the world outside my head, and a voice was telling me to kill myself. At the time, I felt utterly hopeless. I figured that once the semester rolled around, I would have to go on disability because there was no way I could teach like that. But then I tried risperidone, and suddenly my head quieted down, and I stopped hearing the voice telling me to kill myself. It was easier to understand what people said and to pay attention to what was happening outside my head. In this better state of mind, I went to San Francisco, hoping I could maintain this equilibrium. Having two good days before I started feeling sick again felt miraculous. Even though I had run up against my limits, I had done better than I had done at a conference in over two years. I couldn't believe it.

The following months were challenging, as I was at a crossroads. My head remained quieter, so it was easier to stay connected to the world and easier to interact with people, but psychosis seemed only an arm's length away. I remained simultaneously tempted by psychosis and terrified of it. Trying to pay attention to the world outside my head and trying to interact with others appropriately took so much work that I longed to escape into psychosis, where I didn't have to care about anything outside of my head. At the same time, I remembered all too vividly what it was like not to be able to function at all and to feel like I was going to lose my job and my family, and the possibility of returning to that state of mind scared me.

While the idea of going down on my antipsychotic medication was tempting, therefore, I knew where it would lead me, and I knew that the consequences would only be bad. Every time I took my medication during this period, I had to deliberate about whether I should take the prescribed amount or whether to take less. Each time, ever since I was so sick that I thought I would not be able to return to work, I ended up choosing to take the prescribed amount. But it always involved a debate about whether it was worth it.

There were so many things I didn't want to do. I was too tired from struggling so hard to stay sane and connected to teach, to make dinner, to socialize. Often all I wanted to do was to sleep, to escape. But I made myself show up and participate. While I didn't go out of my way to socialize, I made myself have normal conversations with colleagues at work. Every night, I made dinner, even if I ended up taking many shortcuts. Sometimes my husband helped me. Once a week, I drove my daughter to violin lessons. Every week, I made it to the grocery store. Each afternoon, I picked up my daughters from school. When they got home, I tended to their needs. Instead of shutting down, I talked with my husband regularly about how things were going. Day after day, I chose to show up and did the things expected of me. When I was in need, I asked for help. Even though everything felt very hard, I chose to keep trying.

Still distrusting myself, I always felt like I was on the verge of becoming psychotic again. Worried that I would forget what to say or not be able to understand and respond appropriately to my students, I maintained high anxiety about going into the classroom. Everything I did, I had to do slowly, to stay on track. It was hard to stay sufficiently mentally organized in order to be able to function as I ought. My mind always threatened to disintegrate. Sometimes the noise in my head grew louder, and psychosis tried to pull me back in. Knowing that I would be too tempted to go down on my medication, I had to increase the risperidone a few times to lessen the pull of psychosis. It was a real struggle to not become psychotic again, and a real struggle to keep myself from making choices that would pull me back into it.

Yet, somehow, I did it. Week after week passed, and I kept making choices to take my medication and to show up and participate in life activities. In October, I went to another conference and had a much harder time there, spending most of my time alone in my room or walking. But in January, I attended another conference and had a much easier time, not only attending sessions all day but even intentionally socializing with colleagues. As time passed, everything became easier and more manageable. The things that had seemed like so much work months earlier now were doable. I still had to slow down and take it easy to keep my mind organized, but I could do it. Eventually six months passed since I started taking the risperidone, and through that time I managed to remain free of psychosis. No longer distracted by my inner world, I was able to connect with others and with the world outside my head to a much greater degree. I continued to see my therapist and psychiatrist regularly, but I did not need intensive treatment during this time. No longer was my life dominated by illness or treatment; I was finally able to just live my life.

Making continuous choices to engage in treatment by taking my medication as prescribed and attending therapy and to show up and participate in life activities were central to my recovery. Had I continued to make poor choices, I would have fallen back into psychosis and threatened my ability to function again. By making positive choices, I changed the trajectory of my illness. What I chose to do mattered to what happened to me. I was able to make good choices when I could recognize and be motivated by what was truly of value: my ability to function, my health and well-being, my ability to feel good subjectively. Only since I started taking risperidone was I able to perceive what I valued, because only at a sufficiently high dose of antipsychotic medication did the clutter of my mind clear up enough for me to be able to think for myself without letting the psychosis rule me. When I made these choices, I countered the influence the psychosis had over me. By making positive choices, I was able to have some control over my condition and able to make change possible, so I could live a different life than the life I lived while I was sick.

Making choices about treatment is one of the important expressions of agency in which a patient can participate in the process of recovery, countering the passivity of illness. Due to their psychosis and treatment, a patient is generally positioned to be passive: passive to the force of their illness and passive to the dictates of treatment. Psychosis imposes its own choices on the patient, taking over the choice process (such as by making some options for action appear better than others) in order to advance its own goals (such as staying sick). Treatment can impose choices on a patient, too, when clinicians determine what options are available to a patient, and especially when clinicians decide for a patient what they need without seeking out their perspective.

A patient who participates actively in their treatment, however, makes deliberate, intentional choices about which advice to follow, and how, countering both the force of psychosis and the imposition of clinician determinations. They learn to see their clinicians as providing guidance for their recovery that they can use in their growth and development, but which is ultimately up to them to accept. Through this active participation, they can come to see that their actions have some effect on their condition, that what happens to them is at least partly in their control. When a patient makes decisions about what kind of life to live and what steps they need to take in order to live that life, instead of simply obeying the dictates of psychosis or the determinations of their clinicians, they overcome the passivity of their situation, asserting their voice and participating actively in their recovery.

Making decisions about treatment can be a one-time event when a person deliberates about whether to follow advice and how and then follows through with their choice. Or it can be a reoccurring event when a person makes choices continuously about whether to follow recommendations and how to take action, for example each time they are supposed to take their medication. Whether active participation in treatment involves a one-time choice or reoccurring choices depends on the meaning the choice holds for the person engaging in it. In my case, I had to deliberate almost every time I made a choice about taking my medication or doing what was expected of me.

Making choices about treatment or recovery in general always occurs in a context of great uncertainty. Patients never know for sure what the consequences of treatment or any particular action in their recovery will be, or what the consequences of refraining from treatment or a particular action will be, and so they can never make fully accurate judgments about whether engaging in treatment or performing a particular action is on the whole better than not engaging or performing. Patients can only make educated guesses about the consequences of participating versus not participating in treatment based on research, clinician expertise, other patients' experiences, and their own past experience. Decisions based on consequences are thus always tentative conclusions based on the best available evidence but open to revision should new evidence become apparent. A person can change their mind when they learn new information. Since they can never have conclusive information about consequences, their choice is never absolute. And this is where trust comes in: patients have to trust that treatment or a particular action will "work," that it will have the desired effect on them and not cause worse problems.

There are several kinds of treatment that mental patients can make decisions about, but the primary treatments are medication and therapy (counseling). In this chapter, I focus on the decision to take medication as prescribed. This is because the standard treatment for psychosis is antipsychotic medication, yet adherence to medication treatment is a problem for many psychotic patients, as it was for me. In this chapter, I explain both rational and irrational factors that play a role in a person's decision making about whether to take medication as prescribed, arguing that both rational and irrational factors must be taken seriously and addressed by clinicians. Then I situate making choices about treatment within a larger context of making choices about participating in life in general and show that, by making choices continuously to engage in treatment and to show up in life, a person exercises their agency and autonomy, and, through this, they gradually learn to take responsibility for themselves.

The Choice to Take Medication as Prescribed

A common recommendation is for patients to take antipsychotic medication for one to two years following the remission of a psychotic episode in order to restore brain functioning fully. Studies examining relapse rates of patients support this proposal, as relapse rates after achieving remission from psychotic symptoms are very high when patients stop taking their antipsychotic medication.[1] At the same time, however, this common recommendation is not universally endorsed,[2] as not all patients benefit from taking, or seem to need to take, antipsychotic medication after their psychotic episode ends. Given that antipsychotic medication has strong effects and causes changes in brain structure, some researchers caution clinicians about having patients take antipsychotic medication in high doses or for a long period of time.

Adherence to treatment involves following prescribed treatment; medication adherence consists of taking medication as prescribed by one's psychiatrist. Medication nonadherence, therefore, consists of not taking medication as prescribed,[3] whether willfully (on purpose) or unintentionally (such as through forgetting), and may involve a complete discontinuation of medication or a partial continuation of taking less than the prescribed amount, or taking the prescribed amount less frequently than is prescribed. Nonadherence rates are estimated to be at least 50 percent[4] in people who have psychotic disorders, possibly as high as 70 to 80 percent.[5] Nonadherence can lead to many problems, including relapse of psychotic symptoms, (re)admission to hospital, greater use of psychiatric emergency services, poorer life satisfaction, increase in substance use problems (often in an effort at self-medication), and suicide attempts.[6]

For some people, taking their medication as prescribed or not is not something they think about; they just do it, or they don't. When they don't take it, this is either because they forget to take their medication (sometimes aided by the psychosis that encourages forgetting), or because they make a choice not to take it because they don't think it is worth it. For other people, however, taking their medication as prescribed or not is a choice they make after some deliberation. They actually think about the pros and cons and make a choice based on their weighing of relevant factors.

Some people who contemplate their choice deliberate for a while and then make a choice to which they are committed; after their initial cogitation, they might not put further thought into it. Other people who deliberate about their choice, however, do so on a more regular basis, perhaps even every single time they ought to be taking the medication. For these people, whether to take their medication as prescribed is always a live choice during which they could choose a different option than the one they have previously chosen. In these circumstances, taking medication can be agonizing because they have to put themselves through this deliberation every time they are supposed to take their medication. This agony of perpetual decision making can itself be enough of a problem to cause a person to give up and make a regular habit of not taking their medication. Sometimes it is just too hard to have to decide to take it.

People make choices based on what options they believe they have. Making a choice typically involves considering the pros and cons of an option and weighing them against each other. As Jon Elster explains, a rational choice is one that is in the right kinds of relationships between our desires, beliefs, and information.[7] Minimally rational choices are sensitive to rewards; a person is minimally rational when they are willing to change their action based on the likely outcomes of that action (pursuing positive outcomes and avoiding negative outcomes). Most action is at least minimally rational. Choices are more rational when they stand in the right relationship to desires, belief, and information. There are three levels of optimality here. Rational choices satisfy a person's desires, given their beliefs. When their beliefs are grounded in the information available, the choices that a person makes are more robustly rational. When beliefs are grounded in an *optimal* level of information, choices are maximally rational.[8]

Sometimes people with severe mental illness are able to make choices about whether to take their medication based on rational factors, grounding their desires in beliefs that are based on a reasonable amount of information. Usually this involves a calculation of benefits and losses.[9] Many factors may be relevant. Whether a medication is perceived as effective or not matters,[10] as does the severity of side effects from medication.[11] Increased functioning and generally feeling "better" without significant side effects count in favor of taking medication, while negative effects without corresponding benefit understandably count against it.

For some patients who are able to think about the long-term future, long-term effects of medication can be a relevant factor. The cortical thinning caused by antipsychotics,[12] for example, is concerning, leading some scientists to conclude that antipsychotics should not be used for long periods of time;[13] occasionally, antipsychotics can also cause rebound psychosis through dopamine supersensitivity,[14] which is also concerning. Having family support makes taking medication easier,[15] while practical obstacles like lack of sufficient access to healthcare and pharmacy make it harder.[16] The psychological meanings that taking medication has is also significant;[17] fears of dependence on medication or feeling like taking medication is a sign of weakness can affect a person's choice to take medication. When patients experience losses such as a perceived loss of control, a loss of their identity, changes in personal meaning, or decreased functioning such as that due to sedation or grogginess, these losses count in favor of discontinuing medication.[18]

On the other hand, people with severe mental illness may have rational impairments and deficits in epistemic capacities that prevent them from reaching higher levels of rationality when making a choice, whether that choice involves taking or not taking medication. They may not have the patience, diligence, or self-awareness to acquire basic information, never mind optimal levels of information. They may have false beliefs based on misinformation, for example ideas that medication should only be taken when one is symptomatic, or ignorance, for example not understanding the consequences of not taking medication. When patients seek out information on their own, such as on the internet, they may find false information and may have misplaced epistemic trust in sources that do not warrant such trust. Psychosis can interfere with the ability to recognize and assess evidence that would support or undermine claims, leading to gullible acceptance of false claims or vigilant distrust of true claims.

Patients may make choices based on delusional beliefs, such as the belief that medication is poison or the belief that clinicians are always right. They may have biases that prevent them from calculating losses and benefits accurately. Inaccurate beliefs about health,[19] distrust or misplaced trust in clinicians, and negative (or positive) experiences of and attitudes toward the medical system[20] all affect choices about adhering to medication, as do the amount of knowledge a person has about their condition[21] and the amount of knowledge they have about how to take their medication.[22] Symptoms like disorganization, hostility, and paranoia can impede a person's ability to make a rational choice about whether the benefits outweigh the costs in taking their medication,[23] as can negative symptoms that lead to decreased motivation.[24] When patients make choices that are only minimally rational or not rational at all, their decision is based more on poor judgment or bias than on rational considerations.

Patients vary in their ability to recognize, reason about, and calculate losses and benefits of taking medication appropriately. For some patients, the meaning of medication changes at various times, and so the same patient may make disparate choices about how they take their medication. The more psychotic I am, for instance, the less I can reason rationally about relevant factors and the more I base my choice on poor judgment, mainly the dictates of my psychosis. In this situation, psychosis supplants the normal decision-making process with a process of choice making of its own through which it advances its own ends. In this condition, I value the wrong things and cannot form appropriate desires as the basis for my choice and action. When I am less psychotic, on the other hand, I am better able to reason about relevant factors and to value my health and well-being, my ability to function, and my ability to feel good, enabling me to make rationally informed choices. Ironically, the more that a person needs antipsychotic medication, the less able they tend to be to make a decision about taking it based on rational factors; when their psychosis is under control, and they are in less need, they have an easier time thinking through the relevant considerations rationally.

Factors in Choosing to Take Medication

Many factors go into my decision making about medication. My belief that the medication I am prescribed is effective is a significant factor, as I see little reason to take medication that will not help me. As everyone who has tried taking psychiatric medication knows, however, believing in a medication's effectiveness requires a leap of faith and trust in one's psychiatrist and in the medical system that supports medication taking. Desired effects of medication often do not manifest until weeks after a person begins taking a medication, while side effects—which tend to be most pronounced when a person starts a medication, before their body and brain get used to it—tend to emerge immediately. Thus, a person has to endure undesirable side effects for a length of time before they can even tell if the medication is "working" to produce the desired effects. And, of course, the desired effects are rarely perfect: rarely does a medication eliminate all of a person's symptoms as if they are cured; usually it dampens some of the symptoms, so the symptoms are more tolerable. Once in a while, a medication will work exactly as desired; when its effectiveness is clear, this makes the decision to take it easier. When a medication does not work exactly as desired, and/or its effects are not immediately apparent, however, deciding to stay on the medication requires a great deal of trust that it will eventually work as desired.

The trust involved with believing and hoping that a medication will work as desired is a trust of one's clinicians and their professional expertise, of the medical system in which they operate, of the science that supports medication taking, and even of oneself. When a person decides to take medication they are prescribed, they are trusting that their psychiatrist has the clinical expertise required to make a judgment about which medication might work to address the patient's symptoms and that their clinicians can provide accurate testimony about the effects of medication. They are trusting that the mental healthcare system that supports medication taking is set up in such a way as to produce positive outcomes for patients—that is, to help patients get better. They are trusting that the scientific studies that support medication taking are accurate and reliable. In addition, they exhibit self-trust, trusting themselves to be able to provide accurate testimony about the effects of medication and to ascertain their needs and interests appropriately. Trust in all of these areas is necessary for a person to believe and hope that a prescribed medication might work for them.

A more existential type of trust is necessary, too. A person has to believe that something good will come of their actions even if they are not currently in a position to be able to see what that good is. Jonathan Lear calls this conviction "radical hope."[25] In addition, a person has to believe that it is possible for them to get better, and they have to have reason to think that choosing to take medication will help them achieve this goal of getting better. In other words, as discussed in chapter 2, they have to be able to see themselves in the future and to be able to see that their action has an effect on the world, that through their action they are able to change their situation so that it can be different in the future. Moreover, they have to want to get better: they must believe that they are deserving of a better life in order to have the motivation to work on getting better. Only in possessing these aspects of agency can they make an autonomous choice about whether it is worth it to take medication.

When a person distrusts clinicians or the medical system in general because they have been subject to abuse, trauma, or coerced treatment, or because they are likely to be subjected to systemic oppression such as racism, they might not be able to summon enough trust to try a medication or to stay on a medication. If they have been victims of violence, trauma, or oppression, they may not believe their choice will be respected by others. This can lead them to feel like they have no agency around treatment decisions, and they may silence themselves as a consequence rather than actively participating in treatment decisions. When a patient distrusts clinicians or the medical system in general, clinicians need to work extra hard to regain the patient's trust in order to give the patient greater opportunities to make autonomous decisions about taking medication.

In addition to effectiveness and trust, side effects play a big role in most people's calculations. For most people, the decision to take medication is based on weighing the effectiveness of the medication against its undesirable side effects. When side effects are too difficult to bear, the effectiveness of a medication may become irrelevant as the negative side effects heavily outweigh any positive benefit. In the past, I have tried some medications that made me too lethargic and apathetic to function, or that gave me undesirable neurological effects, and I was unable to stay on those long enough to see if they even "worked."

A cost-benefit analysis of effectiveness versus side effects of my current antipsychotic medications, however, leads me to conclude overwhelmingly that these medications are worth taking: they are effective at keeping my psychosis under control, and I can deal with their side effects (tremor, tics, sleeping nine to ten hours a night, etc.). I can think much more clearly on these medications, and I can make connections, recall details, and analyze ideas, which I cannot do when I am not on these medications. When taking a sufficiently high dose of my antipsychotic medications, I do not see things in the world as "special," and I am not distracted by hallucinations or strange ideas. These medications allow me to function in all areas of my life in a way that I am simply unable to do when I am not on them. Taking antipsychotic medications should be, for me at least, a no-brainer. When I weigh the benefits of taking antipsychotics medications against their side effects, it is clear to me that I ought to take them as prescribed.

I do experience some losses as a result of taking antipsychotic medication. Before taking this medication, I used to be especially attuned to the weather, the quality of daylight, and the appearance of the sky (which in Colorado is always breathtaking). These colored my mood and determined if I felt "normal," creepy, closed in, exhilarated, and so on. Since taking the medication, however, I feel more detached from the weather, daylight, and sky, and these no longer affect my mood. Sometimes I miss the attunement I used to feel. Sometimes I also miss the way certain experiences felt like they held special significance and the way I used to be able to hear secret messages in music. Now music is bland, and experience is ordinary. Being able to function in various areas of my life is more important than these things, and taking medication is worth these relatively minor losses I experience. But I have to acknowledge that the losses exist.

When the benefits of taking a medication do not outweigh the costs, as when side effects are too difficult to bear relative to whatever positive effects might exist, it is important that clinicians look at other treatment options and other ways to address psychosis with a patient. When rational considerations count against taking a medication as prescribed, patients need to know that other options exist and can be utilized; otherwise, they may feel despair. Other treatment options can include different medications and different ways of taking a medication (for example, different dosages at different times of the day), as well as other treatment modalities such as therapies like cognitive behavioral therapy, dialectical behavioral therapy, and acceptance and commitment therapy. Lifestyle changes such as eating, sleeping, and exercising differently can help, as can changes in how a person interacts with others. It is important to explore a full range of options so patients do not feel stuck with only bad options.

Long-term effects can also factor into a person's cost-benefit analysis, which can complicate matters. In order for these to be relevant, a person must be able to see themselves in the long-term future and to care what happens to them. A person stuck in a constant present, as commonly occurs when one is stuck in the throes of psychosis, is unable to care about long-term effects, but a person who is rational, coherent, and able to think about their future is. When I have been more rational, I have worried that taking antipsychotic medication would worsen my symptoms over the long term by causing a rebound effect, which would cause me to need to take greater amounts of medication to be able to function. When I talked with my psychiatrist and therapist about potential long-term effects, my psychiatrist tried to reassure me that the majority of studies show that antipsychotic medication reduces symptoms and improves functioning, even in the long term; he was not concerned about the possibility of cortical thinning. His response did not console me; while I wanted him to be right, I did not have enough evidence to know whether I could believe him or not.

My therapist's approach was different; he argued that the long-term effects are irrelevant. He pointed out that we do not make decisions about taking medication based on what they will do in the far future; we base our decisions on our immediate needs. If I cannot teach or take care of my children when I am off of my antipsychotic medication, it doesn't matter what the long-term effects are that I am avoiding by not taking the medication; what matters is my need to function, now. If the side effects of the medication were to cause me to not function in some important ways, however—for example, if I were too sedated or muddy headed to think clearly enough to teach or to care for my children adequately—I may decide it is better for me not to take medication. But in such a case, my decision not to take medication will still be based on a consideration of my immediate needs, namely my immediate need to function in various areas of my life.

My therapist was correct. The potential long-term consequences of taking antipsychotic medication are ultimately irrelevant in my decision whether to take this medication. I cannot afford to consider long-term effects because my immediate needs are so pressing. Thus, I worry in an abstract way about cortical thinning and the possibility of antipsychotic medication actually worsening my symptoms in the long term, but there is nothing I can do about these possibilities. I need to be able to function, now, or I will lose my job, my family, my home, and all other facets of my life. If these medications somehow shorten my life, or the parts of my life where I can function adequately, they at least allow me to function for some duration of time. The alternative would be *not* to take the medication and to have no life to speak of, to be unable to carry out my work duties, take care of my family members, and take care of my home, thus potentially losing all of these. That is not a live option; that is an option that no one who is rational could choose. When I am rational, the fact that antipsychotic medication enables me to function is the only thing that matters in determining whether to take the medication.

For many patients, decisions about taking or not taking medication are acts of control that help them feel like they are directing their lives instead of feeling like they are passive recipients of the dictates of their illness and treatment.[26] When patients feel like they are subject to the demands of their clinicians, not taking medication as prescribed can be experienced as an act of agency and an expression of autonomy. Since psychosis can sometimes persuade a patient not to take medication in order to advance its own ends, however, this control may be largely illusory; the person may in fact be in the control of their psychosis and not realize it or not care about it. Nonetheless, for patients who feel like their illness and treatment are largely out of their control, the control they believe they have in not taking medication can be significant.

In order for patients to value appropriately the choice to adhere to medication, when the benefits of medication outweigh the costs, they may need to feel like taking their medication as prescribed is also an expression of self-determination. One important way that this can happen is for patients to see that their health and well-being is in their control. Clinicians can play an important role in addressing this need by showing patients that patients have control over what decision they make, and what will happen as a result of that decision, so they can see that they have some control over their condition. Examining past choices and the consequences that resulted from them can help patients see this. Identifying future goals and the steps needed to achieve those goals can also help patients see what control they have. Constructing a narrative that highlights the relationship between past actions and consequences, and the relationship between future goals and steps needed to achieve these goals, can help illuminate the control that patients have over their condition.

Another important way that patients can experience taking medication as an act of self-determination is when patients are presented with a range of treatment options from which they can choose. Having a choice of different medications to try, or a choice of different ways they can take their medication (different doses, at different times of day, etc.), can feel empowering. In a variety of ways, the patient needs to feel like what happens in their treatment—and whether they get better, worse, or stay the same—is at least partly up to them, especially when their illness so often feels like it is out of their control.

For a long time, I struggled with feeling like my ziprasidone was ruling my life, and it made me feel like I had no control over the situation. In order to get its full effect, I must take the ziprasidone with a meal, but, because it makes me very tired two hours after taking it, I have to time my dinner exactly, so I get sleepy for bedtime at the right time. This need to time my dinner correctly has caused me a lot of problems, and many times this has made me take less of my medication so it wouldn't make me so tired so early at night. This rationale for taking less medication fed the desire of my psychosis that I take less medication so it would remain present, and I used this as a justification for allowing my psychosis to fester.

My psychiatrist was very unhappy that I did this, and we finally struck a compromise: when I needed to stay awake later at night, I would take only some of my medication with food and the rest of it later, without food. Negotiating this was a huge deal, as it satisfied both my psychiatrist's desire for me to take all my medication regularly, and it satisfied my need to live my life without being ruled by my medication. This helped me to feel like I had more control over my medication taking and over my illness in general. It is important that clinicians work with patients to find ways of taking medication that work for the patient so the patient can experience medication taking as an expression of self-determination. Then, the choice to engage in treatment feels like an act of agency and the patient doesn't feel like a victim of forces outside of their control.

Difficulties with Choosing to Take Medication as Prescribed

While in my case rational considerations weigh heavily in favor of taking my antipsychotic medication, I have sometimes struggled to do so. When I was less rational and my illness was more in charge of me, I felt doubt about the value of taking medication in general, but especially my antipsychotic medication. For reasons I do not fully understand, taking this medication sometimes involved intense deliberation as what ought to be a no-brainer became a very difficult decision to make. I found myself experiencing a combination of temptation, compulsion, and punishment that led me to decide against taking it. When I was feeling less rational, I believed that

I did not deserve to feel well or to function adequately, and I sometimes punished myself by not taking my medication (usually my antipsychotic medication but sometimes my antidepressant and/or antianxiety medication as well).

Moreover, when I was feeling less rational, I missed the way I used to see the world as "special" and I missed the extraordinary experiences and ideas I had when I was psychotic. Functioning well became irrelevant compared to the way I saw and interacted with the world. The voice emerged and told me that the world outside my head did not matter, and I found myself unable to be motivated by the rational considerations that ought to move me. Instead, I was both simultaneously tempted and compelled by my psychosis to free the psychosis from the medication straitjacket so I could see and interact with the world in all its extraordinariness. When I was less rational, I heard commands from a voice telling me to go down on my medication so that the voice could remain ever present and take control of me entirely. I did not know what the consequence of defiance was, but when I perceived such commands, I did not dare to disobey.

At one point, knowing that I could not rely on myself to take my medication regularly as prescribed, I tried to implement strategies that would help me. Figuring it would be hard to say no to a friend, I asked a couple of close friends to email me once a day and remind me to take my medication. But the grip of the psychosis was stronger than my self-consciousness about what my friends might think of me, and I found myself going down on my medication despite their reminders. Soon I stopped asking my friends to do this, because I realized it put them in an uncomfortable position. It was not their responsibility to make me choose to take my medication as prescribed; it was my responsibility. My inability to take responsibility for myself ought not to be their problem, so I quickly stopped putting them in this position.

The temptation to go down on my medication was something I had to address in therapy. Although my choice to go down on my medication was in my case always based on poor judgment, based on irrational factors, my clinicians took my reasons for decreasing my medication seriously. They treated these as reasons worth addressing no matter how irrational they were. In other words, they took up my reasoning appropriately; appropriate uptake occurs not only in relation to testimony, but also in relation to reasons.

By talking through my concerns, my clinicians tried to show me places where I was irrational and helped me to reason more clearly. They did not ignore or discount my reasoning; instead, they treated it as important because it was important to me. They helped me to respond to the voice that compelled me not to take my medication. And they helped me to see more clearly the harms and losses that accrued if I did not take my medication as prescribed and to weigh these more appropriately against whatever benefits I perceived come from psychosis. When I raised rational concerns about long-term effects, they addressed these directly. If I had not found the benefits of taking medication to outweigh the costs—if the side effects had been too difficult to bear relative to the positive effects—I am sure that they would have helped me look at other options—other medications or even other therapies—as they had in the past when I had tried other medications that didn't "work."

In addition, my clinicians helped me to see more clearly what my needs and interests were and the value of health and well-being in my ability to live the kind of life I wanted to live, and they helped me set goals in relation to this value. By helping me to reason more clearly, they helped me to make better decisions based on rational considerations. Although when I failed to take my medication as prescribed, I was irrational, my clinicians treated me as if I were an agent capable of reasoning and worked with me to improve this capacity. In doing this, I was able to make better choices.

Furthermore, in helping me to make better choices about taking medication, they gave me the tools to make better choices in all areas of my life. As I became better at making choices in my best interests related to medication, I also became better at making positive choices in general. As my decision-making capacity improved, it became easier to make the everyday choices to show up and participate in life and thus participate more actively in my recovery.

Choices

Participating actively in recovery is more than just deciding whether to take medication or attend therapy, in other words whether to consent to treatment. Consent to treatment is relevant when treatment is seen as necessary to fix a person's problem by alleviating their symptoms. But recovery from psychosis is not just about eradicating hallucinations and delusions. Rather, it is about changing a person's meaning structure, so the world makes sense to them again. This involves many aspects, including restoring thought organization and addressing the various related cognitive difficulties, relearning how to connect appropriately to the world and to others, and understanding one's experiences within a greater context (as explained in chapter 7). Changing meaning structure does require consent to treatment: a person has to be willing to engage in relevant treatments in order for this restoration of meaning and coherence to occur. But this also requires more than just consent to treatment: it additionally requires a person to make many kinds of choices in directing their life in an ongoing manner. In addition to engaging in recommended treatments, participating actively in recovery means making choice after choice about how to live one's life and choosing over and over, at least most of the time, to pursue goods that are connected to health and well-being.

Sometimes recovery is about the big decisions: the choice to call the crisis hotline, the choice to see a psychiatrist or therapist for the first time, the choice to walk into a crisis center and ask to be hospitalized. And it is definitely concerned with the decisions related to treatment: in my case, the choice to see a therapist regularly and a psychiatrist as needed, the choice to make myself vulnerable to mental health professionals and to lay bare my soul, the choice to answer the suicidal screening worksheet truthfully, the choice to be honest to my clinicians about the over-the-counter medication I had hidden in my car "just in case" I decided I needed to overdose, the choice to take medication as prescribed despite hearing a voice telling myself not to do so. These choices require significant courage, trust, self-empathy, and humility.

But recovery is also about the small choices a person makes on a daily, even hourly, basis: in my case, the choice to go into work and face the difficult moments when I was in charge of the classroom, the choice to ask for help making dinner when my thoughts were too disordered to conceptualize each step, the choice to talk to my husband instead of shutting down, the choice to help my daughters get ready for bed even though all I wanted to do was to go to bed myself, the choice to hug my daughters and tell them I love them. When a person is sick with psychosis, all of these little actions become very difficult if not impossible. Choosing to do them anyway, despite their difficulty, involves making courageous choices that are necessary to recovery. Making choices like these seems so small and insignificant, but it changes the course of one's trajectory. Choosing to show up to life and to participate in the activities that are expected of a person makes it so that the person *can* do these things. It changes what had seemed like an impossibility into something that is now possible, and, as one continues to do show up and participate, and gets better at it, it becomes manageable.

Participating actively in recovery involves being willing to put in the work involved with making continuous choices no matter how much struggle it involves. Often it requires that a person have radical hope, trusting that show-ing up in life and participating in the activities in which they are expected to participate will lead to some good, even if they are not in a position to be able to see what that good might be. A person has to trust that no matter how hard it is to show up and participate in life, it is worth doing.

When a person is in the throes of recovery, they usually do not feel like they have much hope. Nor do they usually have the strength and resilience required for recovery. But they build that strength, resilience, and hope one step at a time, through each individual small choice they make about whether to show up and participate. A patient does not start off strong, or resilient—they would not be so sick if they did start off that way—but they develop strength and resilience until eventually, at some point, they become capable of looking back and seeing how strong and resilient they have become. In the early days of recovery, they often feel hopeless, as if nothing can ever change, yet each time they make the choice to show up and participate in life, they are making change happen. After a while, they are able to see the change, and they develop more hope and confidence in themselves as well.

When I was in recovery, two huge roadblocks stood in my way: the feel-ing of desert and the feeling of impossibility. Feeling like I deserved to be sick, I often tried to punish myself for my illness by making myself more ill: by engaging in self-harming behavior, by pursuing the psychosis, by not taking my medication as prescribed. Since I did not feel like I deserved to be well, this made it hard to work on getting well. The feeling that I deserved to be sick removed what motivation I might have to recover. It piggybacked on the self-perpetuating nature of psychosis and overdetermined my actions so that they were aimed at staying sick rather than working on getting better.

Another huge roadblock was the feeling of impossibility I had regarding recovery. At some point, I had been sick for so long that it felt like I would always be sick. At that point, I could only see myself as a sick person; I could not remember what it felt like to be well. A feeling of impotence engulfed me: I felt as if there were nothing I could do to change my situation. After being in treatment for a long time, it felt like nothing was working, and no matter what I did, I managed to stay sick. And so, I believed that I would always be sick, that I had no power to change my circumstances. Here I lost hope, I lost faith in myself, and I even lost trust in the mental health system that didn't seem to be working.

Two things countered these roadblocks. First, I started taking risperidone, which immediately made me feel better: less psychotic, more connected to reality. After I began to feel better, I could develop some hope that recovery was possible. When my outlook changed as a result of being less psychotic, I no longer saw myself as deserving to be sick. With an improved mindset, and with the help of my therapist, I saw that health and well-being were goods for which I ought to strive, that they were possibilities I could achieve, and that they were goods that I deserved.

Second, I kept making the small choices to show up and participate in life. Each choice I made added to the other choices, and eventually I was able to see that, slowly but surely, I had changed my circumstances. After enough time had passed, I saw that I was not as sick as I used to be. I was able to do more things in life. Because I had made the effort of showing up even when it was very, very hard, I had, over time, made it easier to show up, enabling me to do more things. No longer stuck in the mental world my mind had constructed, I was able to connect with the world and with other people in a way that had once seemed impossible. The world outside my head made more sense and held more meaning and value that I could draw upon and connect with. By making continuous choices to participate in life, I was able to change the meaning structure that conditioned my experience and to restore meaning, coherence, and organization in my mind.

Making choices to show up and participate in life consistently was only possible for me once I was taking risperidone and feeling better and less psychotic. When I was more psychotic, I could only make these kinds of choices intermittently, without conviction, commitment, or consistency. When I became less psychotic, I was able to value these choices more and it became easier to make these choices. Once I was on adequate medication, I was able to comprehend my situation better and both to see more clearly what was worthwhile and meaningful and to reason about it in an appropriate way, thus enabling me to exercise both autonomy and agency. This helped me to see why showing up was important and helped me to figure out how to show up and participate in the right way. Since medication was necessary for me to make these choices consistently, it was important that I regularly chose to take my medication as prescribed. I was able to do this because risperidone was immediately effective at helping me to feel better, providing motivation to continue taking it, and I trusted that continuing to take the medication would continue to make me feel better. Trust in my clinicians, the mental health system, the future, and myself enabled me to make choices that helped me regain control over my life.

Taking Responsibility

When a person learns to make choices that are in their best interests, including choices to engage in treatment and take medication as prescribed (when the benefits outweigh the costs) and choices to show up and participate in life activities, they practice taking responsibility for themselves. Taking responsibility means taking ownership of one's actions. John Martin Fischer and Mark Ravizza argue that taking responsibility is a process of recognizing one's agency and seeing that one is a fitting subject of reactive attitudes of praise and blame based on one's actions.[27] To take responsibility for oneself, therefore, a person has to see themselves in a certain way. They have to see that their choices and actions make a difference in the world, that certain things in the world happen as a direct result of their choices and intentional action. This comes in part from recognizing themselves as capable of giving intelligible reasons for their actions, in other words as being motivated by reasons that are intelligible to others. A person has to see that, in guiding their action, their reasons for action cause certain events to happen in the world.

Seeing that their choices and actions have an effect on the world requires that a person is connected to the world in the right sort of way. As Fischer and Ravizza note, their recognition of themselves as agents must be based on evidence. To take responsibility for oneself, a person has to recognize the source of action correctly. Seeing that their ideas and actions come from themselves, they don't believe themselves to be acted upon by an external force such as the FBI or their psychosis itself. They also don't take responsibility for events that they did not cause; they recognize correctly which events they do have a causal influence on and which events they do not and attribute causes accurately.

The second part of taking responsibility involves seeing oneself as a fit candidate for reactive attitudes. To take responsibility for themselves, a person has to accept that they are appropriate subjects of praise or blame, that their actions can be evaluated by others and that their character—as the source of actions—can be assessed. They have to see that they are situated with respect to others in a certain way: as members of a shared moral community in which they are moral equals. In other words, a person has to recognize that other people see them as agents and assess their action and character accordingly.

One way that patients learn to do this is through therapy. Michelle Ciurria regards therapeutic engagement as a distinctive type of reactive attitude involving evaluating a patient in terms of their participation in therapy, for example praising them for trying out techniques recommended by the therapist or blaming them for not making the effort.[28] Reactive attitudes are therapeutic when they increase agency and thus justified in a therapeutic setting where they can be efficacious in motivating a person to act. Holding reactive attitudes toward a patient in a therapeutic context helps the patient see themselves as a fit candidate for reactive attitudes in general and thus helps them to see themselves as agents capable of taking responsibility and being held responsible.

Critics argue that seeing oneself in a certain way, and believing oneself to be an agent, is not necessary for actually having moral responsibility.[29] Fischer and Ravizza dispute this, arguing that responsibility is a subjectivist notion and that one's self-reflexive belief is relevant for responsibility.[30] Regardless of whether believing oneself to be an agent is necessary for having moral responsibility, it does seem necessary for *taking* responsibility. Taking responsibility involves accepting that responsibility applies to one's actions, that others may evaluate one's action and judge its moral character. In order to take responsibility for one's actions and oneself, a person has to regard themselves as capable of agency and as appropriately being regarded by others as an agent.

Since psychosis can erode a person's sense of themselves as a subject and agent, psychotic individuals sometimes have particular difficulty taking responsibility for themselves. When this happens, recovery must involve restoring this sense of subjectivity and agency so a person can take ownership of their actions. This can require both taking medication that restores brain functioning so a person can sense that their actions come from themselves rather than from an external agency and participating in therapy so a person can gain insight and self-understanding that they can then use in perceiving their action properly.

Taking responsibility for oneself can also be understood in terms of having care and concern toward one's different selves, including the self that acted badly while psychotic, and responding appropriately.[31] Jennifer Radden agrees with Fischer and Ravizza that this involves developing ownership of one's actions by learning to identify one's action with oneself. In addition, not only does a person have to see themselves as a fit candidate for reactive attitudes by others, but they also need to develop appropriate reactive attitudes toward themselves, in particular adopting agent regret toward actions that they have done that cause unintended harm.[32] Developing agent regret is a way of accepting responsibility for an action with bad consequences that one can identify as one's own without wallowing in shame or guilt, which would not be productive. Agent regret is a feeling of disappointment in what has happened as a result of what one has done, which can create motivation to change one's behavior in the future so as to avoid causing the same problems later. In accepting responsibility in this way, a person responds to the part of themselves that acted badly while psychotic with care and concern.

Adopting ends is also an important part of taking responsibility. As Gary Watson says, "To adopt an end, to commit oneself to a conception of value in this way, is a way of taking responsibility."[33] Taking responsibility for oneself and one's actions involves accepting certain values as governing one's choices and action and setting goals for oneself in accordance with these values. It is a way of setting commitments for oneself and, by doing so, making oneself answerable to others for those commitments. Setting ends for oneself is a way of taking ownership for one's choices and actions because of the way they are expressive of one's values. When a person's choices and actions are truly their own, they are attributable to the person and the person is answerable to others for them. In taking responsibility, a person invites others to assess their action and, insofar as the action expresses their values, their character. The process of adopting ends, including values and goals, thus involves being answerable to others for those ends.

Determining what a worthwhile life consists of even when one is ill, and setting goals for different sorts of wellness, are ways that a person adopts ends in the process of recovery. In recovery, a person learns to recognize that health and well-being are in their best interests and that they ought to care about these interests. They develop that concern and formulate desires and goals based on these interests. They must be capable of envisioning a life for themselves that is different than the life they are currently living, and they must be capable of recognizing that their action can influence what happens. In recognizing their agency, they must be able to see that they have some control over what they do, what outcomes they bring about, and more globally, what kind of life they live. When a person is capable of determining what a good life for them can be and figuring out how to achieve that kind of life, they are capable of taking responsibility for themselves. They can set ends and make choices that are attributable to them and for which they are answerable to others. They can give reasons that are intelligible to others of why they do what they do. When they develop this capacity, which is a moral capacity, they develop their autonomy.

Determining what is of value and creating goals for oneself are not actions that a sick person can simply, suddenly, do. When a person is sick from psychosis, they might have to learn (as I did) to distinguish their own aims from the aims of psychosis and learn how to set ends for themselves that are truly their own. It takes practice to determine what is of value, to create goals for themselves, and to act on these choices and pursue these goals before they can do these things well. The main way that they do this is by making all the everyday choices they have to make about how to act, including the choices about whether to show up and participate in life activities, as well as making regular choices to engage in treatment. Each time a person makes such a choice, they both express and develop their idea of what they value. Each time they make a choice, they have the opportunity to work toward a goal. Thus, when a person makes choices about whether to engage in treatment, and whether to show up and participate in life, they practice setting ends for themselves, thereby exercising their autonomy.

Through the practice of making a choice, a person exercises their agency. This makes them vulnerable to assessment by others. A person makes themselves a fit candidate of praise or blame when they make choices about how to act. Moreover, when they are capable of giving reasons for their choice that are intelligible to others, they become answerable to others. As a person makes deliberate choices over and over again, making these choices to show up and participate becomes easier over time, and they become good at setting ends for themselves. Through making choices about how to act in each moment of their life, a person develops the capacity to take responsibility for themselves.

Taking responsibility for oneself requires that a person is able to recognize when their action is their own, at the same time accepting that others will hold them responsible for actions that are perceived to be their own whether or not they are so. Thus, it is important to the person recovering from psychosis to be able to distinguish the goals and actions their psychosis created (such as not taking medication in order to remain sick) from the goals and actions they have independently of the psychosis (such as being present to the world outside their head so they are able to take care of their children or work at their job). This way they can perceive more clearly what they ought to do and not fall victim to their psychosis again. Constructing a narrative of their experience that enables them to see these distinctions helps with this. Answerable only for their own actions, they do not necessarily need to, and they probably cannot, justify the actions caused by psychosis except to say that these actions were out of their willful control.

Acknowledging that other people may not be able to distinguish their own goals and actions from that of psychosis, however, they may need to make amends for actions they committed under psychosis. As members of a moral community, they must see themselves as fit candidates for reactive attitudes. They may be partially responsible for actions that were not truly their own if others perceive those actions to have come from them and if psychosis is not regarded as sufficiently excusing. Despite this possible need for atonement, the person recovering from psychosis is not blameworthy for actions that were not meaningfully their own and ought not engage in self-blame for what they did while psychotic. Accepting responsibility for actions that were not wholly in one's control can be a sign of moral maturity, but this acceptance does not make one morally blameworthy for such actions.

When I was recovering from psychosis, I tried to make amends for bad choices I made while I was psychotic, mostly by being committed to making better choices in the present and future. Although I may have been a poor mother and teacher while psychotic, I could be a good mother and teacher from this moment forward. This commitment would not erase all the bad actions I had performed, but it would help make amends. Knowing

I was not fully responsible for actions I performed due to psychosis, I did not waste time in self-blame. Wallowing in self-blame would not be effective for making amends. Instead, I was committed to making up for the bad choices I made while I was psychotic by making better choices in the present and future.

Conclusion

In a way, recovery is all about making choices. Since the options available to a person are at least partly framed by the person's setting, recovery has to involve countering the forces that influence choices. When a person is sick from psychosis and subject to mental health treatment, their choices are framed for them by their illness, which attempts to advance its own goals by circumscribing what options are available to a person, and by their clinicians, who determine what treatment is in the patient's best interests. Psychosis and clinicians each have their own goals for the patient and each, in their own way, try to persuade the patient regarding what to value and how to act.

Recovery involves trying to assert one's voice in the midst of this to determine for oneself what one ought to care about and do in relation to what one has decided are good influences. A patient in recovery may need to learn to distrust their psychosis, which does not care about the patient's well-being, only its own, and to trust, at least to some degree, their mental health professionals, whose role is to foster the patient's health. A patient may need to learn to discern when external influences have too much power in shaping their values, beliefs, and actions, as in the case of psychosis, and when external influences, such as clinicians, can be helpful in guiding the patient to take care of themselves. In recovery, a patient develops these skills as they make choices about how to act, learning how to exert their agency and power in response to forces that try to shape the patient's choices for them.

Every action involved in treatment and recovery involves making a choice. Treatment choices include seeking out help, accepting the medicalization of one's experiences when it seems appropriate, selecting one or more treatment modalities, assessing how much to trust one's clinician and recommended treatments, considering whether a clinician is effective and whether to continue seeing the clinician, deciding whether it is worth trying to engage in dialogue with a clinician who may or may not believe the patient, and determining how to value a clinician's perspective and how to incorporate that into a narrative of one's illness. All actions involved with carrying out the activities of daily living involve choices about whether and how to perform the action. Since psychosis may try to frame choices by omitting certain options for action and by persuading the patient to find other options for action appealing, patients in recovery must learn to recognize how this framing occurs and to assert their own voice in response to it.

Clinicians make choices throughout the treatment process as well, choosing how to interact with patients, how much effort to make in trying to understand a patient, whether to trust patients, how much choice and responsibility they can give patients in their treatment, whether and when to believe patient testimony, and how to guide patients to have deeper understanding of their condition and their values and choices. Clinicians play important roles in guiding patients regarding how to think about their experiences and their recovery, and they make choices about how to guide patients well. Although coercive treatment is sometimes justified, this has great costs to the patient that must be weighed carefully. The choices that clinicians make set what options are available to patients and thus influence patient choice; patients then must make choices about how to respond to all of these choices of clinicians. Recovery is a complicated dance of continuous choices.

The choice to engage in treatment is one kind of choice that a person in recovery must make over and over again. Each time they have the opportunity to take medication, attend therapy, or do homework, they have to make a choice about whether to participate or not. Sometimes they may not be able to make the choice to engage in treatment, as when I chose to reduce my medication all those times. When this results from the undue influence of an external force like psychosis, the person is not in that moment acting autonomously and not in that moment capable of acting as a moral agent. But sometimes they can make the choice to engage in treatment. Sometimes they can do this because they know it is good for them and can help them to live a better life: they see its positive effects, or at least they can perceive its potential to benefit them. Capable of imagining themselves having a future that is different than their present state (or a past state in which they were sick), they feel deserving of having a better life. At such times, a person is capable of setting ends for themselves and pursuing those ends through their choices; they are capable of autonomy and agency.

Other times, a person might make the choice to engage in treatment only because of radical hope: believing that something good may come of it even though they are not in a position to understand yet what that good is. Trust in the potential effects of medication, in one's clinicians, in the mental health system that sets the parameters for treatment, in the future, and in oneself all enable this hope. The capacity for imagining future goals and feeling deserving of achieving goods also enables this hope. The key to recovery is being able to make these choices consistently: to be able to choose to engage in treatment and to participate in life activities over and over. Eventually a person learns that these are in their best interests and will improve their life, and they can then use this to motivate their action.

After a while, these choices add up, and the person is no longer sick (or at least *as* sick) but instead is working toward their wellness. At this point, they may no longer need to be a mental patient under the watchful eye of mental health professionals. They may graduate to being a client of mental healthcare services, someone who consults professionals for help with a problem rather than having their life dominated by their illness and its treatment.

In the past couple of years, I have graduated to being a client, at least for some amount of time while my psychosis is in remission. Because my illness seems to be cyclical and episodic, I expect I will become very sick again someday and will once again become a mental patient dominated by my illness and its treatment. But for now, I am not really sick; I just consult with professionals to help me stay on track.

Being a mental patient does not need to be a career. It is an important place for a person to be in when they are sick enough to be able to benefit from intense mental healthcare treatment. But it is a transitory state, one that makes the journey from illness to health possible. Only because I spent a lot of time as a mental patient was I able to overcome my illness, at least for a while, and develop health and wellness. And for that, I am grateful.

Conclusion

Those of us with chronic and severe mental illness will be psychiatric patients or at least clients for long periods of time, possibly our whole adult lives. Many of us will be in recovery for all of that time, never "cured" of our symptoms but always trying to live the best life we can given our situation. We will often struggle with our symptoms, with our ability to function in various areas of our lives, and with getting better. We will have reprieves where our symptoms are decreased and our functioning is better, interspersed between periods when we are highly symptomatic and barely functioning. For many of us, it may not be possible to defeat psychosis entirely, but with medication and therapy we can try to contain and control it. If we work actively on our recovery, we may be able to make the periods of being well last much longer than the periods of being sick.

Recovery is best understood as a process, not a goal, and it requires engaging in many different kinds of activities over time. It involves developing agency, autonomy, trust, empathy, choice-making ability, voice, testimony, and narrative. Patients develop these skills and virtues by engaging with the practices involved with these processes, in whatever way they can, until they become better at doing these practices and eventually the practices become habit. For patients recovering from psychosis, developing these skills and virtues requires engaging in meaningful dialogue with clinicians who can help them discern what they value and help them determine what actions they need to take in order to live out those values, leading them to care about their own health and well-being and to act in ways that foster these goods. Patients develop the agency and autonomy required for managing their symptoms and taking control of their life when they learn to recognize the guidance that clinicians can provide while making the ultimate decisions for themselves about where to place their trust.

In my own recovery, I am very fortunate that I have many resources and much support upon which I can draw. Married for over twenty years to a wonderful man who is as supportive as any spouse can be, I also have a teenage daughter and a preteenage daughter who both give me great joy and meaning. My stable professional job as a philosophy professor affords me joy, meaning, respect, flexibility, and enough money to be able to pay my bills. My colleagues are generous, kind, caring, and understanding, and I think of many of them as friends. My supervisors try to support me in any way they can. I have good-quality, relatively affordable health insurance, and the clinicians I have through my health insurance are excellent, helping me with their professional expertise while being empathetic and trustworthy, making it easier for me to work with them. I have more resources and support than most people who have my mental illnesses (bipolar I disorder and psychotic disorder) do, and this puts me in a better position to be able to be successful in my recovery.

I also have more insight and education than most people who have my illnesses do. I understand my condition quite well and can tell when I am experiencing various states. This helps me identify when I am in need, which makes it easier for me to ask for help. Privileged by my educational background, I am able to understand (to some degree) the scientific articles I read and the scientific theories underlying certain aspects of psychosis. My unique social position—as someone who has severe mental illness but is also a professional philosopher—has allowed me to reflect on being mentally ill in a way that relatively few with severe mental illness can do. This gives me a particular perspective on recovery and the benefits of medicalizing psychotic experience, which may not be shared by all mental patients, especially those with different backgrounds than I have. Nonetheless, I do believe that my analysis is relatable to at least some other people who have experienced psychosis.

Narratives about psychosis written from a first-person perspective have different kinds of credibility depending on how the author is situated in relation to their psychosis. Narratives about psychosis that are constructed while one is psychotic can *illustrate* psychotic thinking, when they show the delusory worldview of the author,[1] but they cannot shed light on the nature of psychosis; only a narrative constructed by someone who has sufficient distance from their psychotic experience to be able to recognize it for what it is and to be able to reflect on it can provide insight into the nature of psychosis. People who are in the midst of psychosis are often not able to think clearly enough about their psychosis—to be able to take a step back from their psychotic experiences and evaluate them, to be able to have the distance to be self-reflective—to have something accurate and insightful to say about it. Those who are presently psychotic possess first-person credibility about the phenomenological experience of what it is like to be psychotic, but they frequently lack insight into their condition and thus lack credibility to interpret and make meaning of their condition due to their partial or global incompetence.

In contrast, those who have participated in the journey of recovery have the requisite first-person experience to speak with authority on such issues and are distanced enough from it to not be hindered by incompetence.[2] Early drafts of this book, which were written when my psychosis had just begun to recede, illustrate the way a person can describe their first-person experience and chronicle their symptoms, if they have enough insight to recognize their symptoms as symptoms, without having the deeper insight to make meaning of them. This book took its present shape only after enough distance passed between my present state and my psychotic experience, and after I received various forms of feedback, to be able to engage with my experience critically.

This is not to say that a person should not write or talk about their psychotic experience while psychotic. Constructing a narrative while psychotic is essential for helping a person to gain understanding and insight into the nature of their condition and to give them tools to deal with their condition and perhaps overcome it. Engaging in the process of narrative construction is a way of engaging in meaning making, which I argued in chapter 7 is not only important for healing, but also natural to people wanting to better understand their condition. But the more that a person is in the grip of their psychosis, the more that such a narrative will be colored by the psychosis. A narrative develops deeper meaning that is intelligible to others as the author gains insight and the ability to be adequately self-reflective. A narrative constructed while psychotic can be resourceful to the person who can use their narrative to better understand themselves and to grow from their experience, but it will not have significant credibility *to other people* until the person is capable of being sufficiently self-reflective about their experience to be able to engage with it critically. The value of this book as philosophical literature lies in its ability to contribute something meaningful to philosophical discourse, not simply as an illustration of a certain type of experience, but also as an interpretation of that experience that can be critically engaged with both by myself and by others.[3]

Writing this book has enabled me to construct a narrative about my own psychosis and to offer my own interpretation of it, which I hope has philosophical value, but which also has been therapeutically beneficial, as I have used this opportunity to make sense of my own mental illness experience. In the process of writing, I have had to make many choices about what aspects of psychosis and recovery to focus on and what stories to include to move along the narrative. Many stories about my experiences did not make it into the final draft of the manuscript because they did not make the points that I wanted to make about psychosis and recovery. I wrote earlier chapters of the manuscript that were deleted from the final draft of the manuscript because, while they included interesting commentary about various academic approaches to psychosis, they did not advance a philosophical argument. Making continuous choices along the way about what to include and how to structure and order my stories and philosophical points, I exercised my agency and autonomy as I constructed this narrative about my experiences. In doing this, I was able to come to terms with the power my psychosis used to have over me.

Writing this book also served many pragmatic purposes. During the writing of this book, I learned a tremendous amount about psychotic disorders that I did not know before, which has given me an even deeper understanding of what I have experienced with my illness. I thought more deeply about what a good therapeutic relationship looks like and what the process of recovery involves. This helped me to understand my relationships with my clinicians better and helped me to comprehend what I am doing in recovery, giving me fresh insight to what my own recovery process looks like.

For those of us with chronic, severe mental illness, having positive therapeutic relationships with our clinicians is essential. Having clinicians whom we can trust, and be trusted by, helps us to be more invested in our recovery. Working with clinicians who find ways for us to have epistemic and moral agency is crucial for us to develop our voice, our ability to make good choices that are truly our own, and our sense of self. Having clinicians who empathize with us, knowing that they cannot fully understand us but being committed to trying to understand us as best as they can, helps us feel less alone and more like we have partners in our recovery. When our clinicians help us understand our illness more deeply, and ourselves in relation to our illness, we have better insight and can be more effective in working on our recovery. When our clinicians take us seriously and address what concerns us no matter how irrational it may be, we have an easier time coming to agreement about what we need to do in our treatment. Having clinicians who work with us in productive, compassionate ways helps us to stay motivated and to continue working hard in our recovery.

For some psychotic patients (like myself), psychosis has agency and power of its own, dictating to the patient what to care about and what to do, overpowering the aims, interests, and desires of the patient themselves. Recovery from this type of psychosis requires countering that power by distinguishing carefully what the aims of psychosis are compared to the aims of the individual and by increasing agency and autonomy so the patient can determine for themselves what they ought to value and how they ought to act. Good clinicians guide patients to develop their agency and autonomy, influencing patients in a positive way to care about and act on their health and well-being in opposition to the sickness the psychosis perpetuates. In recovery, patients work on making consistent choices to engage in prescribed treatment as well as to show up and participate in life activities. They exercise their voice and agency by giving testimony of their experience and making meaning of their illness. When patients work actively on their recovery, they take the necessary steps to manage their illness and take control of their lives.

I am currently in the middle of the longest reprieve from my illness that I have experienced in a long time. For over two years now, from the time I started taking risperidone along with my ziprasidone, I have been mentally stable. Since then, I have not heard messages to reduce my medication or to kill myself. I do not currently even think of myself as a "sick person." For over two years before this period of wellness, I had thought of myself as *primarily* a sick person and only secondarily a wife, mother, and professor; my illness and its treatment had completely dominated my life. To be able to focus in recent months on other aspects of my life besides being sick has been amazing. While I know that this reprieve may not last indefinitely and that I will probably get sick again, I treasure the time I have had being well enough truly to have a life outside of illness.

Notes

1 Psychosis

1. For the sake of gender neutrality, I use the pronouns "they, their, theirs" in referring to singular persons. These pronouns are becoming more acceptable to use as singular pronouns, particularly since the *New York Times* now uses these pronouns in the context of transgender individuals. My reason for using gender-neutral pronouns is to avoid invoking gendered stereotypes, including stereotypes of women having mental illness because they are weak and of men with mental illness as being violent. I find the traditionally plural, third-person "they, their, theirs" to be less troublesome to use than other ways of attempting gender neutrality such as "he/she" (or "she/he") "s/he," and "he or she" (or "she or he") or alternating male and female pronouns (all of which reinforce gender binaries). Third-person, traditionally plural pronouns that are used to reference singular hypothetical persons may strike some readers as "wrong," but they are smoother to read and avoid raising gendered issues that arise through language.

2. Longden, Corsten, and Dillon, "Recovery, Discovery and Revolution"; McCarthy-Jones, *Hearing Voices*, 315–331; Romme et al., *Living with Voices*; Romme and Morris, "The Recovery Process with Hearing Voices."

3. Brosnan, "Power and Participation"; Cox and Simpson, "Cultural Safety, Diversity and the Service User and Carer Movement in Mental Health Research"; Minett, "User Participation in Mental Health Care"; Rush, "Mental Health Service User Involvement in England"; Sayce, *From Psychiatric Patient to Citizen*, 14.

Roe and Davidson point out difficulties for both user and clinician that arise from the user movement, including problems with generating, assessing, and respecting different forms of knowledge, and difficulties with trust and respect between users and clinicians. Roe and Davidson, "Destinations and Detours of the Users' Movement."

4. Longden, Corsten, and Dillon, "Recovery, Discovery and Revolution"; McCarthy-Jones, *Hearing Voices*; Romme et al., *Living with Voices*; Romme and Morris, "The Recovery Process with Hearing Voices."

5. Beaulaurier and Taylor define "consumers" as "persons with basic rights and the capacity to understand and even control the course of their treatment." Gill, Kewman, and Brannon describe "consumers" as participants "in decision making and policy setting affecting their lives." Beaulaurier and Taylor, "Social Work Practice With Disabilities in the Era of Disability Rights," 59; Gill, Kewman, and Brannon, "Transforming Psychological Practice and Society," 40–41.

6. Speed, "Patients, Consumers and Survivors."

More confusingly, Judi Chamberlin describes "consumers" as individuals "who accept the medical model of mental illness" in contrast to "survivors" who are critical of the medical model. The term "survivor" is used more commonly, however, to mean individuals who have been scarred by their experience in the mental health system and feel that they are "survivors" of the ordeal. Chamberlin, "User-Run Services," 283.

7. According to Liz Sayce, "consumer" is an unpopular term in the United Kingdom because of its connotation to purchasing power, which seems misapplied in the context of receiving mental health services. Sayce, *From Psychiatric Patient to Citizen*, 14.

8. For example, patients who have been given intravenous shots of antipsychotics involuntarily during acute psychosis retrospectively feel mixed about having been coerced to take medication; some feel powerless, affecting treatment outcomes, but many are appreciative. Patients who have been given long-acting injectable antipsychotics to address medication nonadherence feel mixed about these too, with many patients grateful to not have to decide on a daily basis whether to take their medication. Coercive measures are not always viewed negatively; very often patients are grateful for receiving care even when they thought at the time (in the throes of psychosis) that they did not want it. See, for example, Das, Malik, and Haddad, "A Qualitative Study of the Attitudes of Patients in an Early Intervention Service Towards Antipsychotic Long-Acting Injections"; Iyer et al., "A Qualitative Study of Experiences With and Perceptions Regarding Long-Acting Injectable Antipsychotics"; Patel et al., "Are Depot Antipsychotics More Coercive than Tablets?"

9. Liz Sayce claims that "in the U.S., people who are, or have been, diagnosed with a mental illness tend to define themselves as consumers, survivors or ex-patients" and she abbreviates these as "c/s/x." Sayce, *From Psychiatric Patient to Citizen*, 14.

Contra Sayce, no mental patient whom I have encountered sees themselves as anything other than a patient or client. To whatever extent these terms are popular, they are so only within a minority community of academics and members of user-run organizations like Hearing Voices Network (HVN), which are not terribly popular in North America (but which may be more popular in Great Britain, where HVN was founded). In North America, people are more likely to connect with peer support groups through mainstream mental health organizations such as National Alliance on Mental Illness or the Depression and Bipolar Support Alliance. Academics are enamored by these terms because they like to focus on the arguments of more extreme critics of the medical models of mental illness and disability, as I discuss later in chapter 3. I think it is more useful, however, to focus on the ordinary experiences had by the vast majority of patients.

Mike Slade identifies even more terms that could be used, including "mental health consumer," "psychiatric survivor," "person labelled with a psychiatry disability," "person diagnosed with a psychiatric disorder," "person with a mental health history," "person with mental health issues," "consumer/survivor/eX-inmate (CSX)," "person who has experienced the mental health system," "person experiencing severe and overwhelming mental and emotional problems, such as 'despair,'" and "person our society considers to have very different and unusual behavior, such as 'not sleeping.'" Many of these terms complicate rather than clarify the issue of how to identify patients who have mental illness. Slade, *Personal Recovery and Mental Illness*, 5.

10. Another approach to delineating these terms is to focus on where treatment is provided, where a "client" is treated in the community while a "patient" is treated on an inpatient unit in a hospital. Heard and Swales, *Changing Behavior in DBT*, 6.

In contrast, I construe "patient" more broadly to include all who are treated for mental illness, regardless of *where* they are treated or whether the treatment is voluntary or not, in contrast to a "client" who consults professionals of their own volition to treat a mental disorder that may or may not be disabling or making one "sick."

11. American Psychiatric Association, *Diagnostic and Statistical Manual of Mental Disorders*, 20.

12. For comparison of mental disorder versus mental illness, see Bolton, *What is Mental Disorder?*, 165, 277.

My analysis of mental illness is inspired by Lennart Nordenfelt's distinction between *disease* and *illness*. Disease and illness describe different aspects of a problematic condition in which a person's ability to meet their vital goals is impaired. While disease involves the biological aspect that underpins that condition, illness is the subjective part of that condition, involving how the condition is experienced by a person; disorder describes the cluster of symptoms that arises from the biological problem. In other words, disease is the biological problem that gives rise to symptoms and that underlies the experience of illness. Nordenfelt, *On the Nature of Health*, 109–111; Nordenfelt, *Rationality and Compulsion*, 54–59.

13. This is not to say that psychosis and other impairing conditions are *wholly* negative; some aspects of the experience can be positive, as I explain below. What matters for my claim that impairments reduce a person's quality of life is that they are negative *overall*, reducing a person's quality of life in general or on the whole, even if in some specific respects they improve it or change it in a neutral way.

14. In discussions of psychosis both in the academic literature and in the media, psychosis is often equated with schizophrenia, and the two terms are sometimes used interchangeably even though they have different meanings. ("Psychosis" refers

to a set of symptoms, while "schizophrenia" refers to a diagnostic category, the disorder most paradigmatically associated with psychotic symptoms.) In this book, I am mostly focusing on psychosis, the set of symptoms described here, rather than a specific diagnostic category. When discussing the scientific literature, however, I follow the literature and refer to schizophrenia where it does.

15. In the salience model of psychosis, the excessive dopamine transmission that seems to occur with psychosis creates extra, irregular feelings of salience that draw a person's attention to stimuli to which they would not otherwise pay attention. As a result, they assign meaning to those stimuli and develop beliefs and goal-directed behavior around their experience of the stimuli. This assignation and construction of meaning results in the "positive" symptoms that are hallmarks of psychosis: delusions, hallucinations, and paranoia. Hallucinations reflect the abnormal perception of salience, while delusions and paranoia are a person's way of explaining or describing their abnormal experience using culturally available frameworks (hence stereotypic stories about law enforcement going after a person, being mind read by a radio or television broadcast, or having one's body moved by alien forces). Kapur, Mizrahi, and Li, "From Dopamine to Salience to Psychosis"; Kapur, "Psychosis as a State of Aberrant Salience"; Moritz et al., "A Two-Stage Cognitive Theory of the Positive Symptoms of Psychosis."

16. Martin, "Hearing Voices and Listening to Those That Hear Them"; Moritz et al., "The Other Side of 'Madness'"; Nixon, Hagen, and Peters, "Recovery From Psychosis," 630–631.

17. Mauritz and van Meijel, "Loss and Grief in Patients with Schizophrenia," 254.

18. One of the losses that people experience is the loss of contact with shared reality; for example, Simon McCarthy-Jones notes that when people begin to hear voices, they lose "the sense of living in the same world as everyone else." McCarthy-Jones, *Hearing Voices*, 136.

19. Mauritz and van Meijel, "Loss and Grief in Patients with Schizophrenia," 258.

20. McCarthy-Jones, *Hearing Voices*, 136–140.

21. Saks, *The Center Cannot Hold*, 12–13.

22. I acknowledge that I am assuming a logocentric view of epistemic agency in relation to knowledge that is propositional. Other types of knowledge can also be the object of epistemic agency, including practical, tacit, embodied, and affective knowledge. Catala, "Metaepistemic Injustice and Intellectual Disability." I am focusing on propositional knowledge because it is the knowledge we have that is guided by reason that most impacts our moral agency and autonomy, which are my concern in this book.

23. I use the term "moral agency" broadly, as some might use the term "agency," to refer to the general capacity to make choices and to act based on reasons, for all choices to act in certain ways and all actions that consist of behaviors have a

normative context in the sense that choices and actions can be good or bad choices or actions, depending on what a situation calls for. I refer to choices and action in a behavioral sense as "moral" partly in order to distinguish these from epistemic action, which is undertaken in the context of being a knower. In contrast, I use the term "agency" to refer to action in general, including both epistemic action, in which one acts as a knower, and moral action, in which one makes choices about how to act.

24. Hamm, Buck, and Lysaker, "Reconciling the Ipseity-Disturbance Model with the Presence of Painful Affect in Schizophrenia"; Nelson, Parnas, and Sass, "Disturbance of Minimal Self (Ipseity) in Schizophrenia"; Sass, "Self-Disturbance and Schizophrenia"; Tekin, "Looking for the Self in Psychiatry," 249–266.

25. Stephens and Graham describe this distinction in terms of ownership versus agency. I find their language confusing, however, for in the ethics literature "ownership" usually refers to a conscious acceptance of one's actions as one's own, not an acknowledgment of experience as happening to a person. In this manuscript, I use the term "ownership" in relation to this conscious acceptance of one's actions as one's own, especially in chapters 7 and 8. Stephens and Graham, *When Self-Consciousness Breaks*.

2 Autonomy

1. Hoffman and Hansen observe that dependency is one of the two dominant themes in women's memoirs of depression, the other being a lack of creativity. Hoffman and Hansen, "Prozac or Prosaic Diaries?"

2. For example, see Kozuch and McKenna, "Free Will, Moral Responsibility, and Mental Illness," 92–93.

3. Szmukler, "Coercion in Psychiatric Treatment and Its Justifications," 132.

4. Egonsson, "Hypothetical Approval in Prudence and Medicine," 251.

5. See discussion in Gaylin and Jennings, *The Perversion of Autonomy*, 203–216; and Earley, *Crazy*, 147–159.

6. Halpern, *From Detached Concern to Empathy*, 101.

7. Halpern is explicit that she draws on Immanuel Kant's understanding of autonomy in developing her own conception. My own view is heavily influenced by both Kant, in the sense that autonomy involves choosing ends for oneself in a way that is guided by reason, and Aristotle, in the sense that autonomy involves formulating a conception of a meaningful life that is objectively good.

8. Oshana, "How Much Should We Value Autonomy?," 100.

9. In this paragraph, I am thinking specifically of *moral* agency, which is the power to choose and to act in a behavioral context as a response to given situations.

However, epistemic agency—the power to act as a knower—also involves practical reason. As I suggested in chapter 1, some people would call the power to choose and to act simply "agency," reserving "moral agency" to refer to choice and action in a specifically moral context. I call the power to choose and to act "moral agency" in part in order to distinguish it from epistemic agency, which is the power to act as a knower, and in part because all choices and actions occur in a normative context in the sense that choices and actions can be good or bad depending on what a situation calls for.

10. Halpern, *From Detached Concern to Empathy*, 107–110.

11. My understanding of what consists of a "conception of the good" draws from Aristotle's conception of *eudaimonia*, which can be understood as flourishing or well-being, or an objective sense of happiness. Aristotle, *Nicomachean Ethics*.

12. Dworkin, *The Theory and Practice of Autonomy*, 20.

13. Holyrod, "Relational Autonomy and Paternalistic Interventions," 325.

14. Edwards, "Beyond Mental Competence," 275.

15. Incompetence can be understood here as lacking practical wisdom or being unable to carry out actions requiring practical wisdom. Pepper-Smith, Harvey, and Silberfield, "Competency and Practical Judgment"; Widdershoven et al., "Competence in Chronic Mental Illness."

16. Halpern, *From Detached Concern to Empathy*, 103.

17. Kim, "The Place of Ability to Value in the Evaluation of Decision-Making Capacity," 190–193.

18. Feinberg, *Harm to Self*, 104.

19. Feinberg, "Legal Paternalism," 7.

20. Dworkin, *The Theory and Practice of Autonomy*, 20.

21. Frankfurt, "Freedom of the Will and the Concept of a Person."

22. Watson, "Free Agency."

23. Scoccia, "Paternalism and Respect for Autonomy," 320.

24. Dworkin, *The Theory and Practice of Autonomy*, 21.

25. Westlund, "Rethinking Relational Autonomy."

26. Oshana, "The Misguided Marriage of Responsibility and Autonomy."

27. Owen Flanagan notes that memoirs about alcoholism indicate that alcoholics often identify deeply with a lifestyle centered around drinking, so their desire to drink, rather than being contrary to their second-order volitions, are actually

consistent with their second-order volitions: having a desire to desire to drink. This complicates recovery, as recovery must then involve changing the deep self that has these second-order volitions and not simply changing the person's first-order desires. Flanagan, "Identity and Addiction."

Psychotic experience can appear to mimic this when a person seems to identify deeply with their psychosis and wants to hold onto it. However, in my case at least, I would argue that this is an appearance only, the product of false consciousness: in reality, it is the psychosis that wants the person to identify with it and hold onto it, not the person's own will. When psychosis is in remission, and not clouding their judgment, a person is able to think clearly and see that being psychotic is not what they truly want at all. Recovery then is not a matter of changing the deep self that identifies with psychosis but rather revealing the deep self underneath the psychosis.

28. Ted Zenzinger helped me clarify this point.

29. Brock, "Paternalism and Promoting the Good," 238–239.

30. Gary Watson discusses the way we make choices from options for action that appear on our deliberative screen, which can be shaped by coercive influences that circumscribe what options for action appear to be available to a person. Watson, "Volitional Necessities."

31. Joseph Demarco interprets Joel Feinberg as supporting a sliding scale of competence based on the difficulty of determining competence. Since competence is difficult to determine, incorrectly allowing an incompetent person to accept great risk can be disastrous; thus, we should raise the bar to be on the safe side and compensate with a high standard of competence in order to avoid mistakes. I support this view. Demarco, "Competence and Paternalism."

32. Scoccia, "In Defense of Hard Paternalism," 362–363.

33. Dworkin, *The Theory and Practice of Autonomy*, 32.

34. Darwall, "The Value of Autonomy and Autonomy of the Will," 268.

35. Darwall, "The Value of Autonomy and Autonomy of the Will," 268.

36. Regan, "Paternalism, Freedom, Identity, and Commitment."

37. Scoccia, "Paternalism and Respect for Autonomy," 333.

38. While hard paternalism uses coercion to interfere with fully voluntary choices, soft paternalism uses coercion to interfere with nonvoluntary choices. Dworkin, "Paternalism: Some Second Thoughts," 107; Scoccia, "In Defense of Hard Paternalism," 355.

39. Wikler, "Persuasion and Coercion for Health."

40. Aristotle, *Nicomachean Ethics*, 26–27 (1103a27–1103b25).

41. Frank, *The Wounded Storyteller*, 156.

3   Patient

1. Conrad, "Medicalization and Social Control," 216.

2. Gosselin, "Global Gender Injustice and Mental Disorders," 105–109; Pilgrim and Bentall, "The Medicalisation of Misery"; Ussher, "Are We Medicalizing Women's Misery?"

3. Reiheld, "Patient Complains of . . . ," 89–91.

4. Knaapen and Weisz, "The Biomedical Standardization of Premenstrual Syndrome."

5. Reiheld, "Patient Complains of . . . ," 79–83.

6. Gosselin, "Global Gender Injustice and Mental Disorders," 109–115.

7. Diller, "The Run on Ritalin"; Harre, "The Logical Basis of Psychiatric Meta-Narratives," 300–301; Schermer, "The Dynamics of the Treatment-Enhancement Distinction."

8. Boyle, "The Persistence of Medicalisation"; Moncrieff, "Neoliberalism and Bio-psychiatry"; Timimi, "Children's Mental Health and the Global Market."

9. Gosselin, "Global Gender Injustice and Mental Disorders," 105–109; Pilgrim and Bentall, "The Medicalisation of Misery"; Ussher, "Are We Medicalizing Women's Misery?"

10. Timimi, "Children's Mental Health and the Global Market."

11. Wardrope, "Medicalization and Epistemic Injustice," 345.

12. Reiheld, "Patient Complains of . . . ," 82–83.

13. Jutel, *Putting a Name to It*, 63–65.

14. I owe this point, and the point that diagnosis enables hermeneutical justice, to an anonymous reviewer.

15. Pitt et al., "Impact of a Diagnosis of Psychosis," 421.

16. Pitt et al., "Impact of a Diagnosis of Psychosis."
Diagnostic labels can also be problematic as they are expected to do too much normative work when they are used to identify a person's status rather than describe how well they are functioning. Szmukler, "When Psychiatric Diagnosis Becomes an Overworked Tool."

17. See discussions of the difference between the "bad difference" and "mere dif-ference" views of disability in Barnes, "Disability, Minority, and Difference"; and Barnes, "Valuing Disability, Causing Disability."

18. Chapman, "Neurodiversity Theory and Its Discontents"; McWade, Milton, and Beresford, "Mad Studies and Neurodiversity"; Perry, "Neuropluralism."

19. Longden, Corsten, and Dillon, "Recovery, Discovery and Revolution"; McCarthy-Jones, *Hearing Voices*, 315–331; Romme et al., *Living with Voices*; Romme and Morris, "The Recovery Process with Hearing Voices."

20. Cole, "The Body Politic"; Morris, "Impairment and Disability"; Pfeiffer, "The Categorization and Control of People with Disabilities"; Sayce, *From Psychiatric Patient to Citizen*, 129–130; Tremain, "On the Government of Disability."

21. Sayce, *From Psychiatric Patient to Citizen*, 129–130.

22. Amundson and Tresky, "Bioethics and Disability Rights"; Tremain, "On the Government of Disability."

23. Modern rehabilitative approaches take into account the concerns about autonomy and empowerment that social model of disability activists have raised. See Beaulaurier and Taylor, "Social Work Practice With Disabilities in the Era of Disability Rights"; Lutz and Bowers, "Understanding How Disability is Defined and Conceptualized in the Literature"; Nemec and Gagne, "Recovery From Psychiatric Disabilities"; Smart and Smart, "Models of Disability."

24. One model of psychiatric disability distinguishes between three different kinds of impairment, all of which are relevant when considering the ways that people can be disabled by their illness. These include functional impairment as deviation from statistical norms, impairment as deviating from personal ideals, and impairment as disrupted self-creation. Rudnick, "What is a Psychiatric Disability?"

25. One way to understand the objective harm involved in a medical model of disability is in counterfactual terms: a person would have been better off had they not been impaired. Brown, "Is Disability a Neutral Condition?"

It is not clear whether such a judgment ought to be subjective, up to the individual concerned, or objective, a judgment that can be made by others. On either type of judgment, severe mental illness, such as psychosis that produces dementia-like effects, causes impairment that one would be better off without.

26. Some theorists object to the social model of disability on the grounds that some health problems truly are impairments caused not by society but by one's illness; nonetheless, they recognize the important contributions that the social model of disability has made with respect to empowering individuals and seeing the ways in which impairments have social dimensions that can be addressed through structural change. They argue, however, that the social model of disability does not adequately take into account the ways that we are embodied and relational, and the ways that we are both limited and enabled by our (dis)abilities independently of social structures. DeVidi and Klausen, "No Mere Difference"; Shaw, "Towards Disability Ethics"; Terzi, "The Social Model of Disability."

27. Coles, "Meaning, Madness and Marginalisation"; Midlands Psychology Group, "Manifesto for a Social Materialist Psychology of Distress."

28. Gosselin, *Humanizing Mental Illness*.

29. Potter, *The Virtue of Defiance and Psychiatric Engagement*, 37.

30. Parsons, *The Social System*, 436–437.

31. For example, see discussions in Hannan, "Depression, Responsibility, and Criminal Defenses"; Hauptman, "Justice without Moral Responsibility?"

32. King and May, "Moral Responsibility and Mental Illness."

33. De Mamani et al., "Free Will Perceptions and Psychiatric Symptoms in Patients Diagnosed with Schizophrenia."

34. There are four predominant stereotypes we hold about people with mental illness: that they are incompetent and in need of treatment; that they have a character flaw like weakness of will; that they are dangerous and potentially violent; and that they are permanently defective and can never get better. The first three stereotypes are identified in Corrigan and Kleinlein, "The Impact of Mental Illness Stigma," 16; and Rusch, Angermeyer, and Corrigan, "Mental Illness Stigma," 530. The stereotype of people with mental illness as permanently defective, with a condition that is chronic or lifelong, potentially degenerative, and ultimately incurable, is described by Eminson, "Personal Responses to a Lack of Shared Perception," 123. See also discussion in Gosselin, "Mental Illness Stigma and Epistemic Credibility," 78–80.

35. This is one reason why early intervention services for first-episode psychosis can be so valuable: they strive to address the psychosis therapeutically while helping the person to transcend the sick role so they may not experience later bouts of psychosis.

36. Radden, *Divided Minds and Successive Selves*, 13–35.

37. The idea of narratives as "resourceful" comes from Tekin, "Self-Concept through the Diagnostic Looking Glass."

38. Radden, *Divided Minds and Successive Selves*, 195–211.

39. Radden, *Divided Minds and Successive Selves*, 110–113.

4 Trust

1. Collins and Kuehn, "The Construct of Hope in the Rehabilitation Process," 430.

2. Annette Baier understands trust as a relationship with three parts: A trusts B with thing C, where B has discretionary powers over C and A is vulnerable to B. Baier, "Trust and Antitrust."

3. Reyre et al. also connect trust to promises. Reyre et al., "Care and Prejudice," 186–187.

4. Hawley, "Trust, Distrust and Commitment," 10.

5. Trust and distrust can be regarded as participant reactive attitudes, attitudes that we hold in response to other people's actions based on our assumption that they are agents like us. Wendy Rogers regards trust as a reactive attitude, on par with love, gratitude, and praise, while distrust is a negative reactive attitude like anger, blame, and resentment. Rogers, "Is There a Moral Duty for Doctors to Trust Patients?," 77–78.

6. Jones, "Trust as an Affective Attitude." See also Rogers, "Is There a Moral Duty for Doctors to Trust Patients?," 77–80; Rogers and Ballantyne, "Gender and Trust in Medicine."

7. Miller, "The Other Side of Trust in Health Care," 59.

8. Reyre et al., "Care and Prejudice," 187.

9. Reyre et al., "Care and Prejudice," 185.

10. Reyre et al., "Care and Prejudice," 187.

11. While we can trust someone without believing that our trusting them will result in the person carrying out what is expected of them, we do need to believe our reliance on someone will result in a positive outcome in order to rely. This is because reliance is predicated on belief, while trust is primarily affective, though connected to belief. Jones, "Trust as an Affective Attitude," 15–16.

12. Miller, "The Other Side of Trust in Health Care," 52–53; Buchman, Ho, and Goldberg, "Investigating Trust, Expertise, and Epistemic Injustice in Chronic Pain," 32.

13. Reyre et al., "Care and Prejudice," 185.

14. Miller, "The Other Side of Trust in Health Care," 52–53.

15. Reyre et al., "Care and Prejudice," 187.

16. Miller, "The Other Side of Trust in Health Care," 52.

17. Rogers and Ballantyne, "Gender and Trust in Medicine," 49.

18. Eriksen et al., "Challenges in Relating to Mental Health Professionals."

19. Browne et al., "The Relationship between the Therapeutic Alliance and Client Variables in Individual Treatment for Schizophrenia Spectrum Disorders and Early Psychosis," 52.

20. Browne et al., "The Relationship between the Therapeutic Alliance and Client Variables in Individual Treatment for Schizophrenia Spectrum Disorders and Early Psychosis"; Shattock et al., "Therapeutic Alliance in Psychological Therapy for People with Schizophrenia and Related Psychoses."

21. Despite changes in the practice of medicine and access to healthcare treatment over the past few decades, patients' trust in doctors has remained steady. Ninety

percent of patients possess some level of trust for their doctors, and fully two-thirds have strong trust for their doctors. Moreover, there is a good deal of resiliency in the relationship of trust between patient and doctor; patients show a strong willingness to forgive mistakes or accept negative outcomes; only when doctors are seriously negligent or abusive do patients feel a betrayal of trust. Hall suggests that this resiliency in the relationship of trust between patient and doctor occurs for two reasons. First, a patient is in a condition of vulnerability in virtue of being a patient; being vulnerable makes a person more inclined to trust those who are helpful to them in their vulnerability. Second, even if a particular doctor does not live up to expectations, or actually violates trust, the practice of doctoring is itself seen as trustworthy, and this make patients inclined to trust most doctors despite the untrustworthiness of a few. Hall, "The Importance of Trust for Ethics, Law, and Public Policy," 159–162.

22. Buchman, Ho, and Goldberg, "Investigating Trust, Expertise, and Epistemic Injustice in Chronic Pain," 32.

23. Buchman, Ho, and Goldberg, "Investigating Trust, Expertise, and Epistemic Injustice in Chronic Pain," 32.

24. Sokolowski, "The Fiduciary Relationship and the Nature of Professions."

25. Rogers and Ballantyne, "Gender and Trust in Medicine," 49.

26. Pellegrino, "Trust and Distrust in Professional Ethics," 80.

27. Jessica Miller explains the vulnerability of exposing our bodies in physician offices: "Even during routine office visits, significant patient vulnerability attends disrobing, waiting in a clockless room, allowing near strangers access to one's body, and talking about bodily sensations or functions which are often intensely personal. Indeed, because our bodies are so central to our sense of self—our lived experience of being who we are here and now—the need for medical help to manage them in and of itself can create a sense of alienation and loss." Miller, "The Other Side of Trust in Health Care," 54.

In discussing the vulnerability of the patient "in the hands" of a clinician, Richard M. Zaner argues that trust in the clinician is grounded on trustworthiness of the clinician. Zaner, "Trust and the Patient-Physician Relationship," 47.

28. Buchman, Ho, and Goldberg, "Investigating Trust, Expertise, and Epistemic Injustice in Chronic Pain," 33; Ho, "Trusting Experts and Epistemic Humility in Disability," 105–107.

29. Buchman, Ho, and Goldberg, "Investigating Trust, Expertise, and Epistemic Injustice in Chronic Pain," 36.

30. Scrutton, "Epistemic Injustice and Mental Illness."

31. Carel and Kidd, "Epistemic Injustice in Healthcare"; Carel and Kidd, "Epistemic Injustice in Medicine and Healthcare"; Kidd and Carel, "Epistemic Injustice and Illness."

32. Buchman and Ho, "What's Trust Got to Do with It?," 3–4; Buchman, Ho, and Goldberg, "Investigating Trust, Expertise, and Epistemic Injustice in Chronic Pain," 38–39; Buchman, Ho, and Illes, "You Present Like a Drug Addict," 1402; Ho, "They Just Don't Get It!," 500; Ho, "Trusting Experts and Epistemic Humility in Disability," 115–117.

33. Zaner, "Trust and the Patient-Physician Relationship," 55 (italics original).

34. Miller, "The Other Side of Trust in Health Care," 53.

35. Rogers, "Is There a Moral Duty for Doctors to Trust Patients?," 77–78.

36. Rogers, "Is There a Moral Duty for Doctors to Trust Patients?," 77–78.

37. Klugman et al., "The Ethics of Smart Pills and Self-Acting Devices," 43–44; Rogers, "Is There a Moral Duty for Doctors to Trust Patients?," 77.

38. Buchman, Ho, and Illes, "You Present Like a Drug Addict," 1400.

39. Buchman, Ho, and Illes, "You Present Like a Drug Addict," 1400.

40. Miller, "The Other Side of Trust in Health Care," 53.

41. Browne et al., "The Relationship between the Therapeutic Alliance and Client Variables in Individual Treatment for Schizophrenia Spectrum Disorders and Early Psychosis," 52; Nienhuis et al., "Therapeutic Alliance, Empathy, and Genuineness in Individual Adult Psychotherapy," 593.

42. Hasson-Ohayon, Kravetz, and Lysaker, "The Special Challenges of Psychotherapy with Persons with Psychosis."

43. Browne et al., "The Relationship between the Therapeutic Alliance and Client Variables in Individual Treatment for Schizophrenia Spectrum Disorders and Early Psychosis," 52.

44. Fisher et al., "Communication and Decision-Making in Mental Health"; King et al., "Role of Patient Treatment Beliefs and Provider Characteristics in Establishing Patient-Provider Relationships"; Malin and Pos, "The Impact of Early Empathy on Alliance Building, Emotional Processing, and Outcome During Experiential Treatment of Depression."

45. Winick, *Civil Commitment*, 25–26.

46. Winick, *Civil Commitment*, 26.

47. Winick, *Civil Commitment*, 26.

48. Landeweer, Abma, and Widdershoven, "Moral Margins Concerning the Use of Coercion in Psychiatry"; Vuckovich and Artinian, "Justifying Coercion."

49. Winick, *Civil Commitment*, 45–46.

50. Bruce Winick refers to this as the police power justification. Winick, *Civil Commitment*, 43–44.

51. Beauchamp and Childress, *Principles of Biomedical Ethics*, 227–228.

52. Egonsson, "Hypothetical Approval in Prudence and Medicine," 245–252.

53. Beauchamp and Childress, *Principles of Biomedical Ethics*, 227.

54. Beauchamp and Childress, *Principles of Biomedical Ethics*, 228; Peele and Chodoff, "Involuntary Hospitalization and Deinstitutionalization," 218.

55. Egonsson, "Hypothetical Approval in Prudence and Medicine."

56. Verkerk, "A Care Perspective on Coercion and Autonomy."

57. Ryan, "One Flu Over the Cuckoo's Nest"; Tannsjo, "The Convention on Human Rights and Biomedicine and the Use of Coercion in Psychiatry," 42–43.

58. Other mental conditions besides mental incompetence may justify paternalistic approaches to treatment; for example, Craig Edwards argues that paternalism is justified in cases where the values and goals that comprise a person's character are not persistent and reflect some severance of character. But here we are concerned with the role that incompetence plays, when a person lacks the capacity to make meaningful decisions for themselves in some relevant area, here in terms of medical treatment. Edwards, "Beyond Mental Competence."

59. Winick, *Civil Commitment*, 27–31.

60. I owe this observation to an anonymous reviewer.

61. Winick, *Civil Commitment*, 27–31.

62. Winick, *Civil Commitment*, 32–34.

63. Jones, "Trust as an Affective Attitude," 22.

64. Jones, "Trust as an Affective Attitude," 22–23.

65. Jones, "Trust as an Affective Attitude," 23.

66. Pickard, "Responsibility without Blame: Empathy and the Effective Treatment of Personality Disorder."

67. Shabo, "Incompatibilism and Personal Relationships"; Shabo, "Where Love and Resentment Meet."

68. Winick, *Civil Commitment*, 174–175.

5 Empathy

1. Tichon, Loh, and King, "Psychology Student Opinion of Virtual Reality a Tool to Educate about Schizophrenia," 41.

2. Birchwood and Chadwick, "The Omnipotence of Voices: Testing the Validity of a Cognitive Model"; Chadwick and Birchwood, "The Omnipotence of Voices";

Chin, Hayward, and Drinnan, "'Relating' to Voices"; Close and Garety, "Cognitive Assessment of Voices"; Sayer, Ritter, and Gournay, "Beliefs about Voices and Their Effects on Coping Strategies"; van der Gaag, Hageman, and Birchwood, "Evidence for a Cognitive Model of Auditory Hallucinations."

3. Jenner et al., "Positive and Useful Auditory Vocal Hallucinations"; Moritz et al., "The Other Side of 'Madness'"; Thomas, "Can We Listen in a New Way to Those Who Listen to Voices?"
   Moritz and Larøi report that 78 percent of schizophrenic patients have positive hallucinatory experiences. Moritz and Larøi, "Differences and Similarities in the Sensory and Cognitive Signatures of Voice-Hearing, Intrusions and Thoughts," 104.

4. Studies show a range of experience of positive and negative voices; anywhere between a quarter to over a half of participants in various studies report hearing positive voices. Beavan and Read show that 58 percent of participants heard positive voices, 76 percent of participants heard negative voices, and 92 percent of participants heard neutral and/or ambiguous voices; Corstens and Longden report that 59 percent of participants heard solely negative voices, four participants heard solely positive voices, and 37 percent heard a mix of both; Jenner et al. find that 70 to 80 percent patients heard positive voices on a daily basis, with 10 to 25 percent reporting predominantly positive voices. Beavan and Read, "Hearing Voices and Listening to What They Say"; Corstens and Longden, "The Origins of Voices"; Jenner et al., "Positive and Useful Auditory Vocal Hallucinations," 241.

5. Martin, "Hearing Voices and Listening to Those That Hear Them"; Moritz et al., "The Other Side of 'Madness'"; Nixon, Hagen, and Peters, "Recovery From Psychosis," 630–631.

6. Beavan, "Towards a Definition of 'Hearing Voices'"; Benjamin, "Is Chronicity a Function of the Relationship between the Person and the Auditory Hallucination?"; Chin, Hayward, and Drinnan, "'Relating' to Voices"; Suri, "Making Sense of Voices."

7. Evans et al., "Simulation in Nursing Education," 510.

8. David and Leudar, "Head to Head," 256; Leudar and Thomas, *Voices of Reason, Voices of Insanity*, 137.

9. Leudar and Thomas, *Voices of Reason, Voices of Insanity*, 205.

10. Amy Coplan identifies seven definitions, while C. Daniel Batson gives eight. Batson, "These Things Called Empathy"; Coplan, "Understanding Empathy."

11. Betzler, "How to Clarify the Aims of Empathy in Medicine."

12. Coplan, "Understanding Empathy"; Simmons, "In Defense of the Moral Significance of Empathy."

13. Gelhaus, "The Desired Moral Attitude of the Physician: (I) Empathy."

14. Morgan, "Against Compassion."

15. Green, "Illocution and Empathy," 884.

16. For more on emotional matching, see Hatfield, Rapson, and Le, "Emotional Contagion and Empathy"; McFee, "Empathy"; and van Baaren et al., "Being Imitated."

17. Battaly, "Is Empathy a Virtue?"; Gelhaus, "The Desired Moral Attitude of the Physician: (I) Empathy."

18. Halpern, *From Detached Concern to Empathy*, 17.

19. Gelhaus, "The Desired Moral Attitude of the Physician: (I) Empathy." For more on this understanding of empathy as constructively imagining someone else's experience, see Emerick, "Empathy and a Life of Moral Endeavor"; Goldie, *The Emotions*, 178; Harvey, "Moral Solidarity and Empathetic Understanding"; Meyers, *Being Yourself*, 115; Simmons, "In Defense of the Moral Significance of Empathy"; Snow, "Empathy."

20. Halpern, *From Detached Concern to Empathy*, 50.

21. Halpern, *From Detached Concern to Empathy*, 72–74.

22. Gelhaus, "The Desired Moral Attitude of the Physician: (II) Compassion"; Newham, "The Emotion of Compassion and the Likelihood of Its Expression in Nursing Practice."

23. Gelhaus, "The Desired Moral Attitude of the Physician: (I) Empathy."

24. Goldie objects to other-oriented perspective-taking because we do not have access to other people's minds and so cannot give an adequate characterization of their motives such that we can truly take their perspective. Goldie, "Anti-Empathy." See also Slaby, "Empathy's Blind Spot."

25. Goldie, *The Emotions*, 199. For more on empathy as projecting one's own experiences onto the experiences of another person, see also Masto, "Empathy and Its Role in Morality," 76–77; and Nickerson, Butler, and Carlin, "Empathy and Knowledge Projection."

26. Goldie, *The Emotions*, 195 (italics original).

27. For more on the potential harm of empathy that involves self-oriented perspective-taking or emotional contagion, see Goldie, *The Emotions*, 215; Prinz, "Is Empathy Necessary for Morality?"; and Kaplan, "Empathy and Trauma Culture."

28. Boleyn-Fitzgerald, "Care and the Problem of Pity," 10–11.

29. Halpern, *From Detached Concern to Empathy*, 73.

30. Charon, "Narrative Medicine," 1897.

31. Arber and Gallagher, "Generosity and the Moral Imagination in the Practice of Teamwork."

32. Harvey, "Moral Solidarity and Empathetic Understanding"; Emerick, "Empathy and a Life of Moral Endeavor."

33. Davidson, *Living Outside Mental Illness*, 119.

34. Emerick, "Empathy and a Life of Moral Endeavor."

35. Bailey, "Empathy and Testimonial Trust."

36. Nickerson, Butler, and Carlin, "Empathy and Knowledge Projection," 45.

37. Burcher, "Beyond Empathy"; Frank, *The Renewal of Generosity*.

38. Jackson, "Patronizing Depression," 372.

39. Ratcliffe, "Phenomenology as a Form of Empathy"; Ratcliffe, "The Phenomenology of Depression and the Nature of Empathy."

40. Morgan, "Against Compassion," e12148.

41. Ratcliffe, "Phenomenology as a Form of Empathy"; Ratcliffe, "The Phenomenology of Depression and the Nature of Empathy."

42. Morgan, "Against Compassion," e12148; Arber and Gallagher, "Generosity and the Moral Imagination in the Practice of Teamwork."

43. Halpern, "From Idealized Clinical Empathy to Empathic Communication in Medical Care," 304.

44. Halpern, "From Idealized Clinical Empathy to Empathic Communication in Medical Care," 302.

45. Halpern, "From Idealized Clinical Empathy to Empathic Communication in Medical Care," 308.

46. Halpern, "From Idealized Clinical Empathy to Empathic Communication in Medical Care," 311. See also Halpern, *From Detached Concern to Empathy*, 131.

47. Halpern, *From Detached Concern to Empathy*, 101.

48. Halpern, *From Detached Concern to Empathy*, 107–110.

49. Halpern, *From Detached Concern to Empathy*, 114.

50. Halpern, *From Detached Concern to Empathy*, 105.

51. Halpern, *From Detached Concern to Empathy*, 105.

52. Halpern, *From Detached Concern to Empathy*, 106.

53. Halpern, *From Detached Concern to Empathy*, 104.

54. Halpern, *From Detached Concern to Empathy*, 112.

55. Kauppinen, "Empathy as the Moral Sense?"; Masto, "Empathy and Its Role in Morality"; Slote, "The Many Faces of Empathy"; Steinberg, "An Epistemic Case for Empathy."

56. Slote, "The Many Faces of Empathy," 844.

57. Smith, "What Is Empathy For?"

58. Masto, "Empathy and Its Role in Morality."

59. Steinberg, "An Epistemic Case for Empathy."

60. Slote, "The Many Faces of Empathy."

61. Frank, *The Wounded Storyteller*, 150.

62. Halpern, "From Idealized Clinical Empathy to Empathic Communication in Medical Care," 305.

63. Boleyn-Fitzgerald, "Care and the Problem of Pity"; Miller, "Empathy as the Only Hope for the Virtue of Compassion and as Support for a Limited Unity of the Virtues."

64. Svenaeus, "The Relationship between Empathy and Sympathy in Good Health Care."

65. Gelhaus, "The Desired Moral Attitude of the Physician: (II) Compassion," 400.

66. Crisp, "Compassion and Beyond," 240.

67. Carr, "Pity and Compassion as Social Virtues," 411.

68. Gelhaus, "The Desired Moral Attitude of the Physician: (II) Compassion"; Newham, "The Emotion of Compassion and the Likelihood of Its Expression in Nursing Practice."

69. Gelhaus, "The Desired Moral Attitude of the Physician: (II) Compassion," 401.

70. Gelhaus, "The Desired Moral Attitude of the Physician: (III) Care."

71. Boleyn-Fitzgerald, "Care and the Problem of Pity," 8–10; Gelhaus, "The Desired Moral Attitude of the Physician: (II) Compassion," 401.

72. Eisenberg and Eggum, "Empathic Responding."

73. Ted Zenzinger helped me to conceptualize this point more clearly.

6 Testimony

1. Potter, *The Virtue of Defiance and Psychiatric Engagement*, 143.

2. Potter, *The Virtue of Defiance and Psychiatric Engagement*, 143.

3. Potter, *The Virtue of Defiance and Psychiatric Engagement*, 143.

4. Tate, "Contributory Injustice in Psychiatry."

5. Potter, *The Virtue of Defiance and Psychiatric Engagement*, 144–147.

6. Frank, *The Wounded Storyteller*, 143–144. Quote is on 144.

7. Potter, "Voice, Silencing, and Listening Well." See also Crichton, Carel, and Kidd, "Epistemic Injustice in Psychiatry."

8. Carel and Kidd, "Epistemic Injustice in Healthcare," 535–536.

9. Blease, Carel, and Geraghty, "Epistemic Injustice in Healthcare Encounters," 552; Carel and Kidd, "Epistemic Injustice in Healthcare," 535; Scrutton, "Epistemic Injustice and Mental Illness," 351–353.

10. Scrutton, "Epistemic Injustice and Mental Illness," 351.

11. Tekin, "Patients as Experienced-Based Experts in Psychiatry," 88.

12. Marsh, "Trust, Testimony, and Prejudice in the Credibility Economy," 280–281.

13. Fricker, *Epistemic Injustice.*

14. Origgi, "Epistemic Injustice and Epistemic Trust."

15. Carel and Kidd, "Epistemic Injustice in Medicine and Healthcare," 339–340; Kidd and Carel, "Epistemic Injustice and Illness," 180.

16. Kurs and Grinshpoon, "Vulnerability of Individuals with Mental Disorders to Epistemic Injustice in Both Clinical and Social Domains"; Sanati and Kyratsous, "Epistemic Injustice in Assessment of Delusions."

17. Scientific studies have shown that people have more distrust toward people with mental illness than they do toward most other people. Rice, Richardson, and Kraemer, "Emotion Mediates Distrust of Persons with Mental Illnesses."

18. The obligation to prove one's credibility in contexts where one's credibility is automatically distrusted creates additional epistemic work for people who are already epistemically marginalized and who are positioned by virtue of their marginalization to have their testimony—and whatever reasons they can give in favor of being granted credibility—not be trusted. In some circumstances this burden can result in epistemic exploitation. Epistemic exploitation involves expecting people who are epistemically marginalized to educate people who have privilege about their privilege. Marginalized people are positioned in such a way that they can see relations of oppression more easily than those who are privileged, seeing both marginalized and the privileged perspectives. Privileged people have biases that prevent them from seeing their privilege and from seeing the way marginalized groups are marginalized. Gaile Pohlhaus Jr. calls this interest of epistemically privileged people to not see their own privilege "willful hermeneutical injustice." When people with mental illness feel obligated to draw on their own experience of marginalization to illuminate relations of power to those who have epistemic privilege, this constitutes epistemic exploitation. See Berenstain, "Epistemic Exploitation"; Pohlhaus, "Relational Knowing and Epistemic Injustice."

19. Sanati and Kyratsous, "Epistemic Injustice in Assessment of Delusions"

20. Fricker, *Epistemic Injustice*, 28.

21. Dotson, "In Search of Tanzania."

22. Pohlhaus, "Discerning the Primary Epistemic Harm in Cases of Testimonial Injustice," 104–107.

23. Scrutton, "Epistemic Injustice and Mental Illness," 349.

24. For example, the Psychosis Outside the Box project encourages people experiencing psychosis to describe their experiences on their own terms, in their own way, compiling these firsthand accounts into a document that demonstrates what psychosis looks like to the people who experience it. "Outside the Box."

25. Hookway, "Some Varieties of Epistemic Injustice: Reflections on Fricker," 157–158. See also Carel and Kidd, "Epistemic Injustice in Medicine and Healthcare," 339–340; and Kidd and Carel, "Epistemic Injustice and Illness," 180–181.

26. Carel and Kidd, "Epistemic Injustice in Medicine and Healthcare," 340–341; Kidd and Carel, "Epistemic Injustice and Illness," 181.

27. Powell and Clarke, "Information in Mental Health."

28. Hardwig, "Autobiography, Biography, and Narrative Ethics," 62.

29. Kurs and Grinshpoon, "Vulnerability of Individuals with Mental Disorders to Epistemic Injustice in Both Clinical and Social Domains," 342. Kristie Dotson describes this silencing as testimonial smothering. Dotson, "Tracking Epistemic Violence, Tracking Practices of Silencing."

30. Carel and Kidd, "Epistemic Injustice in Medicine and Healthcare," 342; Kidd and Carel, "Epistemic Injustice and Illness," 184–185.

31. Joan Houghton describes how this misinterpretation of behavior extends long after a hospital stay: "Former patients live in emotional straightjackets simply by the nature of their illness. To others, misplaced anger may be a sign of repressed violence. Tears, a state of sadness, may be misread as an impending state of depression. Laughter may be heard as mania. Emotional extremes create fear, especially in those who only know of our history rather than our personalities." Houghton, "Maintaining Mental Health in a Turbulent World," 89–90.

32. Steslow, "Metaphors in Our Mouths."

7 Meaning Making

1. Montmarquet, *Epistemic Virtue and Doxastic Responsibility*, 21.

2. Eflin, "Epistemic Presuppositions and Their Consequences."

3. Eflin, "Epistemic Presuppositions and Their Consequences," 49.

4. Kovach, "Epistemic Virtues and the Deliberative Frame of Mind."

5. Fricker, "Epistemic Injustice and a Role for Virtue in the Politics of Knowing."

6. Henderson, "Testimonial Beliefs and Epistemic Competence," 198.

7. Hookway, "Affective States and Epistemic Immediacy," 88.

8. Hookway, "Affective States and Epistemic Immediacy," 88.

9. Montmarquet, *Epistemic Virtue and Doxastic Responsibility*, 21.

10. Kwong, "Open-Mindedness as a Critical Virtue," 410.

11. Montmarquet, *Epistemic Virtue and Doxastic Responsibility*, 23.

12. Montmarquet, *Epistemic Virtue and Doxastic Responsibility*, 23.

13. Montmarquet, *Epistemic Virtue and Doxastic Responsibility*, 23.

14. Montmarquet, *Epistemic Virtue and Doxastic Responsibility*, 23.

15. Montmarquet, *Epistemic Virtue and Doxastic Responsibility*, 20–26.

16. Goldberg, "Self-Trust and Extended Trust: A Reliabilist Account."

17. Repper and Perkins, *Social Inclusion and Recovery*, 21–22.

18. Objecting to the idea that experience is authoritative, Joan Scott notes that experience, when shared in a testimonial context, is always an interpretation and must be examined and historicized as much as any other kind of evidence. Scott, "The Evidence of Experience."

19. Eisenacher and Zink, "Holding On to False Beliefs."

20. So et al., "Jumping to Conclusions, A Lack of Belief Flexibility and Delusional Conviction in Psychosis."

21. Colbert, Peters, and Garety, "Jumping to Conclusions and Perceptions in Early Psychosis."

22. Langdon and Coltheart, "The Cognitive Neuropsychology of Delusions."

23. Gold and Hohwy, "Rationality and Schizophrenic Delusion."

24. Moritz et al., "A Two-Stage Cognitive Theory of the Positive Symptoms of Psychosis."

25. So et al., "Jumping to Conclusions, A Lack of Belief Flexibility and Delusional Conviction in Psychosis."

26. Gawęda, Moritz, and Kokoszka, "Impaired Discrimination between Imagined and Performed Actions in Schizophrenia."
The different data may reflect a difference in the preponderance of symptoms of confusion and disorganization versus commitment to false beliefs. Patients who

feel confused about reality probably have lowered confidence in their ability to perceive and understand reality, while patients who feel committed to their view of the world probably have greater confidence in their perception and understanding of it.

27. Hewson, "Telling Stories and Re-Authoring Lives."

28. Lumsden, "Whole Life Narratives and the Self."

29. Tekin, "How Does the Self Adjudicate Narratives?"

30. Thornhill, Clare, and May, "Escape, Enlightenment and Endurance."

31. Frank, *The Wounded Storyteller*.

32. Cohen, *Mental Health User Narratives*, 150–153.

33. Gould, DeSouza, and Rebeiro-Gruhl, "And Then I Lost that Life."

34. Woesner and Kidd, "The Use of Personal Accounts in the Study of Severe Mental Illness."

35. Gould, DeSouza, and Rebeiro-Gruhl, "And Then I Lost that Life."

36. Woesner and Kidd, "The Use of Personal Accounts in the Study of Severe Mental Illness."

37. Cohen, *Mental Health User Narratives*; Gould, DeSouza, and Rebeiro-Gruhl, "And Then I Lost that Life"; Woesner and Kidd, "The Use of Personal Accounts in the Study of Severe Mental Illness."

38. Howes and Kapur, "The Dopamine Hypothesis of Schizophrenia"; Laruelle, Kegeles, and Abi-Dargham, "Glutamate, Dopamine, and Schizophrenia"; Stahl, "Beyond the Dopamine Hypothesis to the NMDA Glutamate Receptor Hypofunction Hypothesis of Schizophrenia"; Stone, Morrison, and Pilowsky, "Review: Glutamate and Dopamine Dysregulation in Schizophrenia."

39. Fatemi et al., "GABAergic Dysfunction in Schizophrenia and Mood Disorders as Reflected by Decreased Levels of Glutamic Acid Decarboxylase 65 and 67 kDa and Reelin Proteins in Cerebellum"; Guidotti et al., "GABAergic Dysfunction in Schizophrenia"; Wassef, Baker, and Kochan, "GABA and Schizophrenia."

40. Honea et al., "Regional Deficits in Brain Volume in Schizophrenia"; Vita et al., "Progressive Loss of Cortical Gray Matter in Schizophrenia"; Yue et al., "Regional Abnormality of Grey Matter in Schizophrenia."

41. Bernstein et al., "Glial Cells as Key Players in Schizophrenia Pathology"; Bernstein, Steiner, and Bogerts, "Glial Cells in Schizophrenia"; Takahashi and Sakurai, "Roles of Glial Cells in Schizophrenia."

42. Meyer, *Psychobiology*.

43. Midlands Psychology Group, "Manifesto for a Social Materialist Psychology of Distress"; Romme et al., *Living with Voices*; Romme and Morris, "The Recovery Process with Hearing Voices."

A high percentage of people who have schizophrenia have experienced trauma in their past. Pienkos et al., "Hallucinations Beyond Voices," S72. See also Bentall, *Madness Explained*, 477–484.

44. Midlands Psychology Group, "Manifesto for a Social Materialist Psychology of Distress"; Romme et al., *Living with Voices*; Romme and Morris, "The Recovery Process with Hearing Voices."

45. Bentall, *Madness Explained*, 420–428, 465–474; Johnstone, *Users and Abusers of Psychiatry*, 17–39.

46. Coles, "Meaning, Madness and Marginalisation"; Midlands Psychology Group, "Manifesto for a Social Materialist Psychology of Distress."

For example, the rate of schizophrenia is higher among immigrant and migrant populations than it is in the general public, especially among non-Western groups of people living in Western countries. This may be because of the difficulties of navigating cultural identity in a different country, where immigrants often feel disconnected both from their ethnic culture and from the culture where they now live. Bentall, *Madness Explained*, 474–476.

47. Coles, "Meaning, Madness and Marginalisation"; Midlands Psychology Group, "Manifesto for a Social Materialist Psychology of Distress."

People who are schizophrenic are also more likely to be poor. Kposowa, Tsunokai, and Butler, "The Effects of Race and Ethnicity on Schizophrenia."

48. Harper and Speed, "Uncovering Recovery"; Morrow and Weisser, "Towards a Social Justice Framework of Mental Health Recovery."

49. For example, Boyle, "The Persistence of Medicalisation."

In fact, stigma actually increases when people accept a biomedical explanation of mental illness because it reinforces negative stereotypes of people with mental illness as having an intrinsic permanent defect that is out of their control and of being incompetent and needing to be taken care of. The fact that acceptance of this model can lead to increased stigma is not a reason to abandon the model, however, particularly if it has scientific evidence to support it. Corrigan and Watson, "At Issue: Stop the Stigma"; Glannon, "The Blessing and Burden of Biological Psychiatry"; Read et al., "Prejudice and Schizophrenia"; Thachuk, "Stigma and the Politics of Biomedical Models of Mental Illness."

50. The feminine stereotype of women's weakness leading to illness is discussed in relation to hysteria in Shorter, *From Paralysis to Fatigue*; and Showalter, *Hystories*. The stereotype is discussed in relation to anxiety and depression in Herzberg, *Happy Pills in America*, 47–82.

51. Tekin, "Self-Insight in the Time of Mood Disorders."

52. Hoffman and Hansen, "Prozac or Prosaic Diaries?," 294.

53. The DSM culture creates a looping effect: the act of classifying people's experiences according to diagnostic categories can influence the people who are classified by transforming their self-awareness and self-understanding in relation to these diagnostic categories so that they learn to interpret their experiences in a certain way, according to DSM-identified symptoms. In changing their self-awareness and self-understanding, the act of classifying people's experiences changes how people experience their condition and thus ultimately it can transform the classification scheme as well. The DSM framework thus exerts epistemological and cultural power in transforming people's self-understanding and behavior to the point where changes in their behavior can in turn affect DSM classifications. Tekin, "Self-Concept through the Diagnostic Looking Glass."

54. Johnson, "Are We Prosaic Deep Inside?"

55. Bedrick, "Diagnosis and the Individual."

56. For example, John Stuart Mill was able to construct a narrative of his depression for himself that allowed him a way to move forward: by appreciating poetry and natural beauty. This prudential reaction to depression was resourceful in giving him tools to deal with his condition. Graham, "Melancholic Epistemology."

57. Tekin, "The Missing Self in Scientific Psychiatry."

58. Rashed, *Madness and the Demand for Recognition*, 190–191.

59. Chiu, "Historical, Religious, and Medical Perspectives of Possession Phenomenon"; Crabb et al., "Attitudes towards Mental Illness in Malawi"; Endrawes, O'Brien, and Wilkes, "Mental Illness and Egyptian Families"; Islam and Campbell, "Satan Has Afflicted Me!"; Kabir et al., "Perception and Beliefs about Mental Illness among Adults in Karfi Village, Northern Nigeria"; Mercer, "Deliverance, Demonic Possession, and Mental Illness"; Morrison and Thornton, "Influence of Southern Spiritual Beliefs on Perceptions of Mental Illness"; Razali, Khan, and Hasanah, "Belief in Supernatural Causes of Mental Illness among Malay Patients."

60. Rashed, *Madness and the Demand for Recognition*, 191–193.

61. The Icarus Project, "The Icarus Project."

62. The healing voices narrative is described by Mohammed Abouelleil Rashed. Rashed, *Madness and the Demand for Recognition*, 193–194. For more detail on how this narrative works, see Longden, Corsten, and Dillon, "Recovery, Discovery and Revolution"; McCarthy-Jones, *Hearing Voices*, 315–331; Romme et al., *Living with Voices*; Romme and Morris, "The Recovery Process with Hearing Voices."

63. Cohen, *Mental Health User Narratives*; Gould, DeSouza, and Rebeiro-Gruhl, "And Then I Lost that Life"; Thornhill, Clare, and May, "Escape, Enlightenment

and Endurance"; Woesner and Kidd, "The Use of Personal Accounts in the Study of Severe Mental Illness."

64. Mason, "Epistemic Restraint and the Vice of Curiosity."

65. Hardwig, "The Role of Trust in Knowledge."

66. Hardwig, "Toward an Ethics of Expertise."

67. McCraw, "The Nature of Epistemic Trust."

68. Tobin, "The Relevance of Trust for Moral Justification."

69. Hardwig, "Toward an Ethics of Expertise."

70. Goldberg, "Self-Trust and Extended Trust."

71. Origgi, "Epistemic Injustice and Epistemic Trust."

72. Goldberg, "Anonymous Assertions," 142; McKinnon, "Epistemic Injustice," 437.

73. Henderson, "Testimonial Beliefs and Epistemic Competence."

74. Shieber, "Against Credibility."

75. Origgi, "Epistemic Injustice and Epistemic Trust."

76. Shieber, "Against Credibility."

8 Choices

1. One study found the risk of relapse to be 28 to 54 percent of experiencing positive symptoms of psychosis after one to three years following a remitted psychotic episode and a hospital readmission rate of 26 to 83 percent after one to seven and a half years following a psychotic episode. Alvarez-Jimenez et al., "Risk Factors for Relapse Following Treatment for First Episode Psychosis," 125.

In another study, among patients who discontinued use of medication in less than a year's time, nearly half relapsed. Bowtell et al., "Rates and Predictors of Relapse Following Discontinuation of Antipsychotic Medication After a First Episode of Psychosis."

A further study found that patients who discontinued antipsychotic medications had a relapse rate of 77 percent after one year and a relapse rate of over 90 percent after two years, with a relapse rate of only 3 percent when patients took maintenance medications; these stark statistics prompted the authors to conclude that antipsychotic medications should not be discontinued following remission of psychosis. Zipursky, Menezes, and Streiner, "Risk of Symptom Recurrence with Medication Discontinuation in First-Episode Psychosis."

2. Bowtell et al., "Clinical and Demographic Predictors of Continuing Remission or Relapse Following Discontinuation of Antipsychotic Medication After a First Episodes of Psychosis."

3. Medication nonadherence used to be called "medication noncompliance," suggesting that adhering to treatment was an act of will where patients chose to obey their doctors or not. Today we have a more complicated understanding of nonadherence, recognizing that nonadherence is not always an act of will, that patients may have good reasons for not taking medication as prescribed, and that nonadherence should not be understood as a form of disobedience. The idea of compliance is thus connected to obedience and is usually the goal in involuntary treatment where coercion is used, while adherence involves being an active participant in one's treatment. In this chapter, I refer to the practice of not taking medication as prescribed, at least sometimes, as medication nonadherence. For more on compliance vs. adherence, see Vuckovich, "Compliance versus Adherence in Serious and Persistent Mental Illness."

4. Bright, "Measuring Medication Adherence in Patients with Schizophrenia," 99; Gibson et al., "Understanding Treatment Non-Adherence in Schizophrenia and Bipolar Disorder"; Yang et al., "Symptom Severity and Attitudes toward Medication."

5. Bowtell et al., "Rates and Predictors of Relapse Following Discontinuation of Antipsychotic Medication after a First Episode of Psychosis"; Breen and Thornhill, "Noncompliance with Medication for Psychiatric Disorders."

6. Boardman, McCann, and Kerr, "A Peer Support Programme for Enhancing Adherence to Oral Antipsychotic Medication in Consumers with Schizophrenia," 2294.

7. Elster, *Strong Feelings*, 141.

8. Elster, *Strong Feelings*, 141–145.

9. Gibson et al., "Understanding Treatment Non-Adherence in Schizophrenia and Bipolar Disorder"; and Roe et al., "Why and How People Decide to Stop Taking Prescribed Psychiatric Medication." See also Gray and Deane, "What Is It Like to Take Antipsychotic Medication?"; and Usher, "Taking Neuroleptic Medications as the Treatment for Schizophrenia."

10. Boardman, McCann, and Clark, "Accessing Health Care Professionals About Antipsychotic Medication Related Concerns"; Breen and Thornhill, "Noncompliance with Medication for Psychiatric Disorders"; Lieberman et al., "Effectiveness of Antipsychotic Drugs in Patients with Chronic Schizophrenia."

11. Gibson et al., "Understanding Treatment Non-Adherence in Schizophrenia and Bipolar Disorder"; Katz et al., "Retrospective Accounts of the Process of Using and Discontinuing Psychiatric Medication," 199; Roe et al., "Why and How People Decide to Stop Taking Prescribed Psychiatric Medication," 40.

12. Ansell et al., "Divergent Effects of First-Generation and Second-Generation Antipsychotics on Cortical Thickness in First-Episode Psychosis"; Lesh et al., "A Multimodal Analysis of Antipsychotic Effects on Brain Structure and Function in

First-Episode Schizophrenia"; Nesvåg et al., "Regional Thinning of the Cerebral Cortex in Schizophrenia."

13. Emsley, "Discontinuing Antipsychotic Treatment after a First-Episode of Psychosis."

14. Harrow and Jobe, "Long-Term Antipsychotic Treatment of Schizophrenia"; Yin et al., "Antipsychotic Induced Dopamine Supersensitivity Psychosis."

15. Rungruangsiripan et al., "Mediating Role of Illness Representation among Social Support, Therapeutic Alliance, Experience of Medication Side Effects, and Medication Adherence in Persons with Schizophrenia"; Sendt, Tracy, and Bhattacharyya, "A Systematic Review of Factors Influencing Adherence to Antipsychotic Medication in Schizophrenia-Spectrum Disorders"; Tham et al., "Factors Affecting Medication Adherence Among Adults with Schizophrenia."

16. Fenton, Blyler, and Heinssen, "Determinants of Medication Compliance in Schizophrenia," 642.

17. Fenton, Blyler, and Heinssen, "Determinants of Medication Compliance in Schizophrenia," 644.

18. Roe et al., "Why and How People Decide to Stop Taking Prescribed Psychiatric Medication," 38–46.

19. Vargas-Huicochea et al., "Taking or Not Taking Medications."

20. McCann et al., "Risk Profiles for Non-adherence to Antipsychotic Medications"; Rungruangsiripan et al., "Medicating Role of Illness Representation among Social Support, Therapeutic Alliance, Experience of Medication Side Effects, and Medication Adherence in Persons with Schizophrenia"; Tessier et al., "Medication Adherence in Schizophrenia."

21. In one study, more than half of patients stated they had not received adequate information about their diagnosis and treatment and almost half had not been given information about possible side effects of medications. Gray et al., "A Survey of Patient Satisfaction with and Subjective Experiences of Treatment with Antipsychotic Medication."

22. Fenton, Blyler, and Heinssen, "Determinants of Medication Compliance in Schizophrenia," 644; Kini, "Interventions to Improve Medication Adherence."

23. Sendt, Tracy, and Bhattacharyya, "A Systematic Review of Factors Influencing Adherence to Antipsychotic Medication in Schizophrenia-Spectrum Disorders"; Tattan and Creed, "Negative Symptoms of Schizophrenia and Compliance with Medication"; Tham et al., "Factors Affecting Medication Adherence Among Adults with Schizophrenia."

24. Tattan and Creed, "Negative Symptoms of Schizophrenia and Compliance with Medication."

25. Lear, *Radical Hope*.

26. Fenton, Blyler, and Heinssen, "Determinants of Medication Compliance in Schizophrenia," 644; Rofail, Heelis, and Gournay, "Results of a Thematic Analysis to Explore the Experiences of Patients with Schizophrenia Taking Antipsychotic Medication," 1491–1492; Usher, "Taking Neuroleptic Medications as the Treatment for Schizophrenia."

27. Fischer and Ravizza, *Responsibility and Control*, 210–211.

28. Ciurria, "Mental Illness, Agency, and Responsibility."

29. Eschleman, "Being is Not Believing"; Judisch, "Responsibility, Manipulation and Ownership."

30. Fischer and Ravizza, *Responsibility and Control*, 220–223.

31. Radden, *Divided Minds and Successive Selves*, 121, 146.

32. Radden, *Divided Minds and Successive Selves*, 112–113.

33. Watson, "Two Faces of Responsibility," 271.

Conclusion

1. See, for instance, Schreber, *Memoirs of My Nervous Illness*, where Schreber chronicles his retreat into a psychotic inner world of his own, but from the perspective of someone who believes that he is sane and that his delusions are true.

2. Baril argues that only people who have been suicidal in the past (but not presently suicidal) are able to speak with authority and credibility in a way that gets their voices heard, for those who are presently suicidal often are not taken seriously as having something legitimate to say about suicide. Similarly, only people who have participated in recovery from psychosis are able to speak with credibility about the experience of psychosis. Baril is critical of the assumption that presently suicidal people do not have credibility to speak about suicide, but I am not critical of this assumption made about presently psychotic people, because people in the midst of psychosis do not have enough insight about their condition and cannot take a step back from their condition enough to be able to reflect critically and evaluate it. Baril, "Suicidism."

3. I discuss the importance of subjecting first-person testimony to critical engagement in order for such testimony to have philosophical value in philosophical discourse in Gosselin, "Philosophizing from Experience."

Bibliography

Alvarez-Jimenez, M., A. Priede, S. E. Hetrick, S. Bendall, E. Killackey, A. G. Parker, P. D. McGorry, and J. F. Gleeson. "Risk Factors for Relapse Following Treatment for First Episode Psychosis: A Systematic Review and Meta-Analysis of Longitudinal Studies." *Schizophrenia Research* 139 (2012): 116–128.

American Psychiatric Association. *Diagnostic and Statistical Manual of Mental Disorders, Fifth Edition (DSM-5)*. Washington, DC: American Psychiatric Publishing, 2013.

Amundson, Ron, and Shari Tresky. "Bioethics and Disability Rights: Conflicting Values and Perspectives." *Bioethical Inquiry* 5 (2008): 111–123.

Ansell, B. R., D. B. Dwyer, S. J. Wood, E. Bora, W. J. Brewer, T. M. Proffitt, D. Velakoulis, P. D. McGorry, and C. Pantelis. "Divergent Effects of First-Generation and Second-Generation Antipsychotics on Cortical Thickness in First-Episode Psychosis." *Psychological Med* 45, no. 3 (February 2015): 515–527.

Arber, Anne, and Ann Gallagher. "Generosity and the Moral Imagination in the Practice of Teamwork." *Nursing Ethics* 16, no. 6 (2009): 775–785.

Aristotle, *Nicomachean Ethics*. Translated by Robert C. Bartlett and Susan D. Collins. Chicago: University of Chicago Press, 2011.

Baier, Annette. "Trust and Antitrust." *Ethics* 96, no. 2 (January 1986): 231–260.

Bailey, Olivia. "Empathy and Testimonial Trust." *Royal Institute of Philosophy Supplement* 84 (2018): 139–160.

Baril, Alexandre. "Suicidism: A New Theoretical Framework to Conceptualize Suicide from an Anti-Oppressive Perspective." *Disability Studies Quarterly* 40, no. 3 (2020). Accessed May 31, 2021. https://dsq-sds.org/article/view/7053/5711.

Barnes, Elizabeth. "Disability, Minority, and Difference." *Journal of Applied Philosophy* 26, no. 4 (2009): 337–355.

Barnes, Elizabeth. "Valuing Disability, Causing Disability." *Ethics* 125, no. 1 (October 2014): 88–113.

Batson, C. Daniel. "These Things Called Empathy: Eight Related but Distinct Phenomena." In *The Social Neuroscience of Empathy*, edited by Jean Decety and William Ickes, 3–15. Cambridge, MA: MIT Press, 2009.

Battaly, Heather D. "Is Empathy a Virtue?" In *Empathy: Philosophical and Psychological Perspectives*, edited by Amy Coplan and Peter Goldie, 277–301. Oxford: Oxford University Press, 2011.

Beauchamp, Tom L., and James F. Childress. *Principles of Biomedical Ethics, Seventh Edition*. Oxford: Oxford University Press, 2013.

Beaulaurier, Richard L., and Samuel H. Taylor. "Social Work Practice With Disabilities in the Era of Disability Rights." In *The Psychological and Social Impact of Illness and Disability, Fifth Edition*, edited by Arthur E. Dell Orto and Paul W. Power, 53–74. New York: Springer, 2007.

Beavan, Vanessa. "Towards a Definition of 'Hearing Voices': A Phenomenological Approach." *Psychosis* 3, no. 1 (2001): 63–73.

Beavan, Vanessa, and John Read. "Hearing Voices and Listening to What They Say: The Importance of Voice Content in Understanding and Working with Distressing Voices." *The Journal of Nervous and Mental Disease* 198, no. 3 (March 2010): 201–205.

Bedrick, Jeffrey. "Diagnosis and the Individual." *Philosophy Psychiatry & Psychology* 21, no. 2 (June 2014): 157–159.

Benjamin, Lorna Smith. "Is Chronicity a Function of the Relationship between the Person and the Auditory Hallucination?" *Schizophrenia Bulletin* 15, no. 2 (1989): 291–310.

Bentall, Richard P. *Madness Explained: Psychosis and Human Nature*. New York: Penguin, 2003.

Berenstain, Nora. "Epistemic Exploitation." *Ergo* 33, no. 2 (2016): 569–590.

Bernstein, H. G., J. Steiner, and B. Bogerts. "Glial Cells in Schizophrenia: Pathophysiological Significance and Possible Consequences for Therapy." *Expert Review of Neurotherapeutics* 9, no. 7 (July 2009): 1059–1071.

Bernstein, H. G., J. Steiner, P. C. Guest, H. Dobrowolny, and B. Bogerts. "Glial Cells as Key Players in Schizophrenia Pathology: Recent Insights and Concepts of Therapy." *Schizophrenia Research* 161, no. 1 (January 2015): 4–18.

Betzler, Riana J. "How to Clarify the Aims of Empathy in Medicine." *Medicine, Health Care and Philosophy* 21 (2018): 569–582.

Birchwood, Max, and Paul Chadwick. "The Omnipotence of Voices: Testing the Validity of a Cognitive Model." *Psychological Medicine* 27 (1997): 1345–1353.

Blease, Charlotte, Havi Carel, and Keith Geraghty. "Epistemic Injustice in Healthcare Encounters: Evidence from Chronic Fatigue Syndrome." *Journal of Medical Ethics* 43 (2017): 549–557.

Boardman, Gayelene H., Terence V. McCann, and Eileen Clark. "Accessing Health Care Professionals About Antipsychotic Medication Related Concerns." *Issues in Mental Health Nursing* 29, no. 7 (2008): 739–754.

Boleyn-Fitzgerald, Patrick. "Care and the Problem of Pity." *Bioethics* 17, no. 1 (2003): 1–20.

Bolton, Derek. *What is Mental Disorder? An Essay in Philosophy, Science, and Values.* Oxford: Oxford University Press, 2008.

Bowtell, Meghan, Aswin Ratheesh, Patrick McGorry, Eoin Killackey, and Brian O'Donoghue. "Clinical and Demographic Predictors of Continuing Remission or Relapse Following Discontinuation of Antipsychotic Medication After a First Episodes of Psychosis: A Systematic Review." *Schizophrenia Research* 197 (2018): 9–18.

Bowtell, Meghan, Scott Eaton, Kristen Thien, Melissa Bardell-Williams, Linglee Downey, Aswin Ratheesh, Eoin Killackey, Patrick McGorry, and Brian O'Donoghue. "Rates and Predictors of Relapse Following Discontinuation of Antipsychotic Medication After a First Episode of Psychosis." *Schizophrenia Research* 195 (2018): 231–236.

Boyle, Mary. "The Persistence of Medicalisation: Is the Presentation of Alternatives Part of the Problem?" In *Madness Contested: Power and Practice*, edited by Steven Coles, Sarah Keenan, and Bob Diamond, 3–22. Ross-on-Wye, UK: PCCS Books, 2013.

Breen, Robert, and Joshua T. Thornhill. "Noncompliance with Medication for Psychiatric Disorders." *CNS Drugs* 9, no. 6 (June 1998): 457–471.

Bright, Cordellia E. "Measuring Medication Adherence in Patients with Schizophrenia: An Integrative Review." *Archives of Psychiatric Nursing* 31 (2017): 99–110.

Brock, Dan. "Paternalism and Promoting the Good." In *Paternalism*, edited by Rolf Sartorius, 237–260. Minneapolis: University of Minnesota Press, 1983.

Brosnan, Liz. "Power and Participation: An Examination of the Dynamics of Mental Health Service-User Involvement in Ireland." *Studies in Social Justice* 6, no. 1 (2012): 45–66.

Brown, Jeffrey. "Is Disability a Neutral Condition?" *Journal of Social Philosophy* 47, no. 2 (Summer 2016): 188–210.

Browne, Julia, Arundati Nagendra, Matthew Kurtz, Katherine Berry, and David L. Penn. "The Relationship between the Therapeutic Alliance and Client Variables in Individual Treatment for Schizophrenia Spectrum Disorders and Early Psychosis: Narrative Review." *Clinical Psychology Review* 71 (2019): 51–62.

Buchman, Daniel Z., and Anita Ho. "What's Trust Got to Do with It? Revisiting Opioid Contracts." *Journal of Medical Ethics* (2013): 1–4.

Buchman, Daniel Z., Anita Ho, and Daniel S. Goldberg. "Investigating Trust, Expertise, and Epistemic Injustice in Chronic Pain." *Bioethical Inquiry* 14 (2017): 31–42.

Buchman, Daniel Z, Anita Ho, and Judy Illes. "You Present Like a Drug Addict: Patient and Clinician Perspectives on Trust and Trustworthiness in Chronic Pain Management." *Pain Medicine* 17 (2016): 1394–1406.

Burcher, Paul. "Beyond Empathy: Teaching Alterity." *Canadian Journal of Bioethics* 1, no. 2 (2018): 18–21.

Carel, Havi, and Ian James Kidd. "Epistemic Injustice in Healthcare: A Philosophical Analysis." *Medicine, Heath Care, and Philosophy* 17 (2014): 529–540.

Carel, Havi, and Ian James Kidd. "Epistemic Injustice in Medicine and Healthcare." In *The Routledge Handbook of Epistemic Injustice*, edited by Ian James Kidd, Jose Medina, and Gaile Pohlhaus Jr., 336–346. London: Routledge, 2017.

Carr, Brian. "Pity and Compassion as Social Virtues." *Philosophy* 74 (1999): 411–429.

Catala, Amandine. "Metaepistemic Injustice and Intellectual Disability: A Pluralist Account of Epistemic Agency." *Ethical Theory and Moral Practice* 23 (2020): 755–776.

Chadwick, Paul, and Max Birchwood. "The Omnipotence of Voices: A Cognitive Approach to Auditory Hallucinations." *British Journal of Psychiatry* 164 (1994): 190–201.

Chamberlin, Judi. "User-Run Services." In *Models of Madness: Psychological, Social and Biological Approaches to Schizophrenia*, edited by John Read, Loren R. Mosher, and Richard P. Bentall, 283–290. Hove, UK: Brunner-Routledge, 2004.

Chapman, Robert. "Neurodiversity Theory and Its Discontents: Autism, Schizophrenia, and the Social Model of Disability." In *The Bloomsbury Companion to Philosophy of Psychiatry*, edited by Şerife Tekin and Robyn Bluhm, 371–389. London: Bloomsbury Academic, 2019.

Charon, Rita. "Narrative Medicine: A Model for Empathy, Reflection, Profession, and Trust." *The Journal of the American Medical Association* 286, no. 15 (October 2001): 1897–1902.

Chin, Jasmine T., Mark Hayward, and Ange Drinnan. "'Relating' to Voices: Exploring the Relevance of This Concept to People Who Hear Voices." *Psychology and Psychotherapy: Theory, Research and Practice* 82 (2009): 1–17.

Chiu, S. N. "Historical, Religious, and Medical Perspectives of Possession Phenomenon." *Hong Kong Journal of Psychiatry* 10, no. 1 (March 2000), 1–14.

Ciurria, Michelle. "Mental Illness, Agency, and Responsibility." In *The Bloomsbury Companion to Philosophy of Psychiatry*, edited by Şerife Tekin and Robyn Bluhm, 325–345. London: Bloomsbury Academic, 2019.

Close, Helen, and Philippa Garety. "Cognitive Assessment of Voices: Further Developments in Understanding the Emotional Impact of Voices." *British Journal of Clinical Psychology* 37 (1998): 173–188.

Cohen, Bruce M. Z. *Mental Health User Narratives: New Perspectives on Illness and Recovery*. New York: Palgrave MacMillan, 2008.

Colbert, Susannah May, Emmanuelle Peters, and Philippa Garety. "Jumping to Conclusions and Perceptions in Early Psychosis: Relationship with Delusional Beliefs." *Cognitive Neuropsychiatry* 15, no. 4 (2010): 422–440.

Cole, Philip. "The Body Politic: Theorising Disability and Impairment." *Journal of Applied Philosophy* 24, no. 2 (2007): 169–176.

Coles, Steven. "Meaning, Madness and Marginalisation." In *Madness Contested: Power and Practice*, edited by Steven Coles, Sarah Keenan, and Bob Diamond, 42–55. Ross-on-Wye, UK: PCCS Books, 2013.

Collins, Amy B., and Marvin D. Kuehn. "The Construct of Hope in the Rehabilitation Process." In *The Psychological and Social Impact of Illness and Disability, Fifth Edition*, edited by Arthur E. Dell Orto and Paul W. Power, 427–440. New York: Springer, 2007.

Conrad, Peter. "Medicalization and Social Control." *Annual Review of Sociology* 18 (1992): 209–232.

Coplan, Amy. "Understanding Empathy: Its Features and Effects." In *Empathy: Philosophical and Psychological Perspectives*, edited by Amy Coplan and Peter Goldie, 3–18. Oxford: Oxford University Press, 2011.

Corrigan, Patrick W., and Amy C. Watson. "At Issue: Stop the Stigma: Call Mental Illness a Brain Disease." *Schizophrenia Bulletin* 30, no. 3 (2004): 477–479.

Corrigan, Patrick W., and Petra Kleinlein. "The Impact of Mental Illness Stigma." In *On the Stigma of Mental Illness: Practical Strategies for Research and Social Change*, edited by Patrick W. Corrigan, 11–44. Washington, DC: American Psychological Association, 2005.

Corstens, Dirk, and Eleanor Longden. "The Origins of Voices: Links Between Life History and Voice Hearing in a Survey of 100 Cases." *Psychosis: Psychological, Social and Integrative Approaches* 5, no. 3 (2013): 275–208.

Cox, Leonie G., and Alan Simpson. "Cultural Safety, Diversity and the Service User and Carer Movement in Mental Health Research." *Nursing Inquiry* 22, no. 4 (2015): 306–316.

Crabb, Jim, Robert C. Stewart, Demoubly Kokota, Neil Masson, Sylvester Chabunya, and Rajeev Krishnadas. "Attitudes towards Mental Illness in Malawi: A Cross-Sectional Survey." *BMC Public Health* 12 (2012): article 541. Accessed September 2, 2019. https://bmcpublichealth.biomedcentral.com/articles/10.1186/1471-2458-12-541.

Crichton, Paul, Havi Carel, and Ian James Kidd. "Epistemic Injustice in Psychiatry." *British Journal of Psychiatry Bulletin* 41 (2017): 65–70.

Crisp, Roger. "Compassion and Beyond." *Ethical Theory and Moral Practice* 11 (2008): 233–246.

Darwall, Stephen. "The Value of Autonomy and Autonomy of the Will." *Ethics* 116 (January 2006): 263–284.

Das, A. K., A. Malik, and P. M. Haddad. "A Qualitative Study of the Attitudes of Patients in an Early Intervention Service Towards Antipsychotic Long-Acting Injections." *Therapeutic Advances in Psychopharmacology* 4, no. 5 (October 2014): 179–185.

David, Tony, and Ivan Leudar. "Head to Head: Is Hearing Voices a Sign of Mental Illness?" *The Psychologist* 14 (May 2001): 256–259.

Davidson, Larry. *Living Outside Mental Illness: Qualitative Studies of Recovery in Schizophrenia*. New York: New York University Press, 2003.

De Mamani, A. Weisman, K. Gurak, J. Maura, A. Martinez De Andino, M. J. Weintraub, and M. Mejia. "Free Will Perceptions and Psychiatric Symptoms in Patients Diagnosed with Schizophrenia." *Journal of Psychiatric and Mental Health Nursing* 23 (2016): 156–162.

Demarco, Joseph P. "Competence and Paternalism." *Bioethics* 16, no. 3 (2002): 231–245.

DeVidi, David, and Catherine Klausen. "No Mere Difference." *Dialogue* 56 (2017): 357–379.

Diller, Lawrence H. "The Run on Ritalin: Attention Deficit Disorder and Stimulant Treatment in the 1990s." *Hastings Center Report* 26, no. 2 (March–April 1996): 12–18.

Dotson, Kristie. "In Search of Tanzania: Are Effective Epistemic Practices Sufficient for Just Epistemic Practices?" *The Southern Journal of Philosophy* 46 (2008), 52–64.

Dotson, Kristie. "Tracking Epistemic Violence, Tracking Practices of Silencing." *Hypatia* 26, no. 2 (2011): 236–257.

Dworkin, Gerald. "Paternalism: Some Second Thoughts." In *Paternalism*, edited by Rolf Sartorius, 105–111. Minneapolis: University of Minnesota Press, 1983.

Dworkin, Gerald. *The Theory and Practice of Autonomy*. Cambridge: Cambridge University Press, 1988.

Earley, Pete. *Crazy: A Father's Search through America's Mental Health Madness*. New York: Berkley Books, 2006.

Edwards, Craig. "Beyond Mental Competence." *Journal of Applied Philosophy* 27, no. 3 (2010): 273–289.

Eflin, Juli. "Epistemic Presuppositions and Their Consequences." In *Moral and Epistemic Virtues*, edited by Michael Brady and Duncan Pritchard, 47–66. Malden, MA: Blackwell, 2003.

Egonsson, Dan. "Hypothetical Approval in Prudence and Medicine." *Medicine, Health Care and Philosophy* 10 (2007): 245–252.

Eisenacher, Sarah, and Mathias Zink. "Holding On to False Beliefs: The Bias Against Disconfirmatory Evidence Over the Course of Psychosis." *Journal of Behavior Therapy and Experimental Psychiatry* 56 (2017): 79–89.

Eisenberg, Nancy, and Natalie D. Eggum. "Empathic Responding: Sympathy and Personal Distress." In *The Social Neuroscience of Empathy*, edited by Jean Decety and William Ickes, 71–83. Cambridge, MA: MIT Press, 2009.

Elster, Jon. *Strong Feelings: Emotion, Addiction, and Human Behavior (The 1997 Jean Nicod Lectures)*. Cambridge, MA: MIT Press, 1999.

Emerick, Barrett. "Empathy and a Life of Moral Endeavor." *Hypatia* 31, no. 2 (Winter 2016): 171–186.

Eminson, Mary. "Personal Responses to a Lack of Shared Perception." In *Every Family in the Land: Understanding Prejudice and Discrimination Against People with Mental Illness, Revised Edition*, edited by Arthur H. Crisp, 123–128. London: The Royal Society of Medicine Press, 2004.

Emsley, Robin. "Discontinuing Antipsychotic Treatment after a First-Episode of Psychosis: Who, When and How?" *Schizophrenia Research* 197 (2018): 59–60.

Endrawes, Gihane, Louise O'Brien, and Lesley Wilkes. "Mental Illness and Egyptian Families." *International Journal of Mental Health Nursing* 16, no. 3 (May 2007). https://doi.org/10.1111/j.1447-0349.2007.00465.x.

Eriksen, Kristin Ådnøy, Maria Arman, Larry Davidson, Bengt Sundfør, and Bengt Karlsson. "Challenges in Relating to Mental Health Professionals: Perspectives of Persons with Severe Mental Illness." *International Journal of Mental Health Nursing* 23 (2014): 110–117.

Eschleman, Andrew S. "Being is Not Believing: Fischer and Ravizza on Taking Responsibility." *Australasian Journal of Philosophy* 79, no. 4 (December 2001): 479–490.

Evans, Jennifer, Sue Webster, Susan Gallagher, Peter Brown, and John Sinclair. "Simulation in Nursing Education: iPod As a Teaching Tool for Undergraduate Nurses." *Issues in Mental Health Nursing* 36, no. 7 (2015): 505–512.

Fatemi, S. Hossein, Joel M. Stary, Julie A. Earle, Mohsen Araghi-Niknam, and Elisabeth Eagan. "GABAergic Dysfunction in Schizophrenia and Mood Disorders as

Reflected by Decreased Levels of Glutamic Acid Decarboxylase 65 and 67 kDa and Reelin Proteins in Cerebellum." *Schizophrenia Research* 72, no. 2–3 (January 2005): 109–122.

Feinberg, Joel. *Harm to Self: The Moral Limits of the Criminal Law.* Oxford: Oxford University Press, 1986.

Feinberg, Joel. "Legal Paternalism." In *Paternalism*, edited by Rolf Sartorius, 3–18. Minneapolis: University of Minnesota Press, 1983.

Fenton, Wayne S., Crystal R. Blyler, and Robert K. Heinssen. "Determinants of Medication Compliance in Schizophrenia: Empirical and Clinical Findings." *Schizophrenia Bulletin* 23, no. 4 (1997): 637–651.

Fischer, John Martin, and Mark Ravizza. *Responsibility and Control: A Theory of Moral Responsibility.* Cambridge: Cambridge University Press, 1998.

Fisher, Alana, Vijaya Manicavasagar, Felicity Kiln, and Ilona Juraskova. "Communication and Decision-Making in Mental Health: A Systematic Review Focusing on Bipolar Disorder." *Patient Education & Counseling* 99, no. 7 (July 2016): 1106–1120.

Flanagan, Owen. "Identity and Addiction: What Alcoholic Memoirs Teach." In *The Oxford Handbook of Philosophy and Psychiatry*, edited by K. W. M. Fulford, Martin Davies, Richard G. T. Gipps, George Graham, John Z. Sadler, Giovanni Stanghellini, and Tim Thornton, 1–29. Oxford: Oxford University Press, September 2013.

Frank, Arthur W. *The Renewal of Generosity: Illness, Medicine, and How to Live.* Chicago: University of Chicago Press, 2004.

Frank, Arthur W. *The Wounded Storyteller: Body, Illness, and Ethics.* Chicago: University of Chicago Press, 1995.

Frankfurt, Harry G. "Freedom of the Will and the Concept of a Person." In *Free Will, Second Edition*, edited by Gary Watson, 322–336. Oxford: Oxford University Press, 2003.

Fricker, Miranda. *Epistemic Injustice: Power and the Ethics of Knowing.* Oxford: Oxford University Press, 2007.

Fricker, Miranda. "Epistemic Injustice and a Role for Virtue in the Politics of Knowing." *Metaphilosophy* 34, no. 1–2 (January 2003): 154–173.

Gawęda, Łukasz, Steffen Moritz, and Andrzej Kokoszka. "Impaired Discrimination between Imagined and Performed Actions in Schizophrenia." *Psychiatry Research* 195 (2012): 1–8.

Gaylin, Willard, and Bruce Jennings. *The Perversion of Autonomy: The Proper Uses of Coercion and Constraints in a Liberal Society.* New York: Free Press, 1996.

Gelhaus, Petra. "The Desired Moral Attitude of the Physician: (I) Empathy." *Medicine, Health Care and Philosophy* 15 (2012): 103–113.

Gelhaus, Petra. "The Desired Moral Attitude of the Physician: (II) Compassion." *Medicine, Health Care and Philosophy* 15 (2012): 397–410.

Gelhaus, Petra. "The Desired Moral Attitude of the Physician: (III) Care." *Medicine, Health Care and Philosophy* 16 (2013): 125–139.

Gibson, Susanne, Sarah L. Brand, Sarah Burt, Zoë V. R. Boden, and Outi Benson. "Understanding Treatment Non-Adherence in Schizophrenia and Bipolar Disorder: A Survey of What Service Users Do and Why." *BMC Psychiatry* 13, no. 153 (2013): 1–12.

Gill, Carol J., Donald G. Kewman, and Ruth W. Brannon. "Transforming Psychological Practice and Society: Policies That Reflect the New Paradigm." In *The Psychological and Social Impact of Illness and Disability, Fifth Edition*, edited by Arthur E. Dell Orto and Paul W. Power, 37–53. New York: Springer, 2007.

Glannon, Walter. "The Blessing and Burden of Biological Psychiatry." *Journal of Ethics in Mental Health* 3, no. 2 (2008): 1–4.

Goffman, Erving. *Asylums: Essays on the Social Situation of Mental Patients and Other Inmates*. New York: Anchor Books, 1961.

Gold, Ian, and Jakob Hohwy. "Rationality and Schizophrenic Delusion." In *Pathologies of Belief*, edited by Max Coltheart and Martin Davies, 145–165. Oxford: Cambridge University Press, 2000.

Goldberg, Sandy. "Self-Trust and Extended Trust: A Reliabilist Account." *Res Philosophica* 90, no. 2 (April 2013), 277–292.

Goldberg, Sanford C. "Anonymous Assertions." *Episteme* 10, no. 2 (2013): 135–151.

Goldie, Peter. "Anti-Empathy." In *Empathy: Philosophical and Psychological Perspectives*, edited by Amy Coplan and Peter Goldie, 308–316. Oxford: Oxford University Press, 2011.

Goldie, Peter. *The Emotions: A Philosophical Exploration*. Oxford: Clarendon Press, 2000.

Gosselin, Abigail. "Global Gender Injustice and Mental Disorders." In *Global Gender Justice*, edited by Alison M. Jaggar, 100–118. Cambridge: Polity Press, 2014.

Gosselin, Abigail. *Humanizing Mental Illness: Enhancing Agency through Social Interaction*. Montreal: McGill-Queen's University Press, 2021.

Gosselin, Abigail. "Mental Illness Stigma and Epistemic Credibility." *Social Philosophy Today* 34 (2018): 77–94.

Gosselin, Abigail. "Philosophizing from Experience: First-Person Accounts and Epistemic Justice." *The Journal of Social Philosophy* 50, no. 1 (Spring 2019): 45–68.

Gould, Alicia, Sharon DeSouza, and Karen I. Rebeiro-Gruhl. "And Then I Lost that Life: A Shared Narrative of Four Young Men with Schizophrenia." *British Journal of Occupational Therapy* 68, no. 10 (October 2005): 467–473.

Graham, George. "Melancholic Epistemology." *Synthese* 82, no. 3 (1990): 399–422.

Gray, R., and K. Deane. "What Is It Like to Take Antipsychotic Medication? A Qualitative Study of Patients with First-Episode Psychosis." *Journal of Psychiatric and Mental Health Nursing* 23 (2016): 108–115.

Gray, Richard, Diana Rofail, Jon Allen, and Tim Newey. "A Survey of Patient Satisfaction with and Subjective Experiences of Treatment with Antipsychotic Medication." *Journal of Advanced Nursing* 52, no. 1 (2005): 31–37.

Green, Mitchell. "Illocution and Empathy." *Philosophia* 45 (2017): 881–893.

Guidotti, Alessandro, James Auta, John M. Davis, Erbo Dong, Dennis R. Grayson, Marin Veldic, Xianquan Zhang, and Erminio Costa. "GABAergic Dysfunction in Schizophrenia: New Treatment Strategies on the Horizon." *Psychopharmacology* 180, no. 2 (July 2005): 191–205.

Hall, Mark A. "The Importance of Trust for Ethics, Law, and Public Policy." *Cambridge Quarterly of Healthcare Ethics* 14 (2005): 156–167.

Halpern, Jodi. *From Detached Concern to Empathy: Humanizing Medical Practice.* Oxford: Oxford University Press, 2001.

Halpern, Jodi. "From Idealized Clinical Empathy to Empathic Communication in Medical Care." *Medicine, Health Care and Philosophy* 17 (2014): 301–311.

Hamm, Jay A., Benjamin Buck, and Paul H. Lysaker. "Reconciling the Ipseity-Disturbance Model with the Presence of Painful Affect in Schizophrenia." *Philosophy, Psychiatry, and Psychology* 22, no. 3 (September 2015): 197–208.

Hannan, Barbara. "Depression, Responsibility, and Criminal Defenses." *International Journal of Law and Psychiatry* 28 (2005): 321–333.

Hardwig, John. "Autobiography, Biography, and Narrative Ethics." In *Stories and Their Limits: Narrative Approaches to Bioethics,* edited by Hilde Lindemann Nelson, 50–64. New York: Routledge, 1997.

Hardwig, John. "The Role of Trust in Knowledge." *The Journal of Philosophy* 88, no. 12 (1991): 693–708.

Hardwig, John. "Toward an Ethics of Expertise." In *Professional Ethics and Social Responsibility,* edited by Daniel E. Wueste, 83–101. Lanham, MD: Rowman & Littlefield, 1994.

Harper, David, and Ewen Speed. "Uncovering Recovery: The Resistible Rise of Recovery and Resilience." *Studies in Social Justice* 6, no. 1 (2012): 9–25.

Harre, Rom. "The Logical Basis of Psychiatric Meta-Narratives." In *Reconceiving Schizophrenia,* edited by Man Cheung Chung, K. W. M. (Bill) Fulford, and George Graham, 295–305. Oxford: Oxford University Press, 2007.

Harrow, Martin, and Thomas H. Jobe. "Long-Term Antipsychotic Treatment of Schizophrenia: Does It Help or Hurt Over a 20-Year Period?" *World Psychiatry* 17, no. 2 (June 2018): 162–163.

Harvey, Jean. "Moral Solidarity and Empathetic Understanding." *Journal of Social Philosophy* 38, no. 1 (Spring 2007): 22–37.

Hasson-Ohayon, Ilanit, Shlomo Kravetz, and Paul H. Lysaker. "The Special Challenges of Psychotherapy with Persons with Psychosis: Intersubjective Metacognitive Model of Agreement and Shared Meaning." *Clinical Psychology and Psychotherapy* 24 (2017): 428–440.

Hatfield, Elaine, Richard L. Rapson, and Yen-Chi L. Le. "Emotional Contagion and Empathy." In *The Social Neuroscience of Empathy*, edited by Jean Decety and William Ickes, 19–30. Cambridge, MA: MIT Press, 2009.

Hauptman, Robert. "Justice without Moral Responsibility?" *Journal of Information Ethics* 28, no. 1 (Spring 2019), 1–27.

Hawley, Katherine. "Trust, Distrust and Commitment." *Noûs* 48, no. 1 (2014): 1–20.

Heard, Heidi L., and Michaela A. Swales. *Changing Behavior in DBT: Problem Solving in Action*. New York: Guildford Press, 2016.

Henderson, David. "Testimonial Beliefs and Epistemic Competence." *Noûs* 42, no. 2 (2008): 190–221.

Herzberg, David L. *Happy Pills in America: From Miltown to Prozac*. Baltimore: Johns Hopkins University Press, 2009.

Hewson, Helen. "Telling Stories and Re-Authoring Lives: A Narrative Approach to Individuals with Psychosis." In *Innovations in Psychosocial Interventions for Psychosis: Working with the Hard to Reach*, edited by Alan Meaden and Andrew Fox, 147–163. London: Routledge, 2015.

Ho, Anita. "'They Just Don't Get It!' When Family Disagrees with Expert Opinion." *Journal of Medical Ethics* 35 (2009): 497–501.

Ho, Anita. "Trusting Experts and Epistemic Humility in Disability." *The International Journal of Feminist Approaches to Bioethics* 4, no. 2 (Fall 2011): 102–123.

Hoffman, Ginger A., and Jennifer L. Hansen. "Prozac or Prosaic Diaries?: The Gendering of Psychiatric Disability in Depression Memoirs." *Philosophy, Psychiatry & Psychology* 24, no. 4 (December 2017): 285–298.

Holyrod, Jules. "Relational Autonomy and Paternalistic Interventions." *Res Publica* 15 (2009): 321–336.

Honea, R., T. J. Crow, D. Passingham, and C. E. Mackay. "Regional Deficits in Brain Volume in Schizophrenia: A Meta-Analysis of Voxel-Based Morphometry Studies." *American Journal of Psychiatry* 162, no. 12 (December 2005): 2233–2245.

Hookway, Christopher. "Affective States and Epistemic Immediacy." In *Moral and Epistemic Virtues*, edited by Michael Brady and Duncan Pritchard, 75–92. Malden, MA: Blackwell, 2003.

Hookway, Christopher. "Some Varieties of Epistemic Injustice: Reflections on Fricker." *Episteme* 7, no. 2 (2010), 151–163.

Houghton, Joan F. "Maintaining Mental Health in a Turbulent World." In *Psychological and Social Aspects of Psychiatric Disability*, edited by LeRoy Spaniol, Cheryl Gagne, and Martin Koehler, 86–91. Boston: Center for Psychiatric Rehabilitation (Boston University), 1997.

Howes, Oliver D., and Shitij Kapur. "The Dopamine Hypothesis of Schizophrenia: Version III—The Final Common Pathway." *Schizophrenia Bulletin* 35, no. 3 (2009): 549–562.

The Icarus Project. "The Icarus Project." Accessed September 3, 2019. https://theicarusproject.net/.

Islam, F., and R. A. Campbell. "'Satan Has Afflicted Me!': Jinn-Possession and Mental Illness in the Qur'an." *Journal of Religion and Health* 53, no. 1 (February 2014): 229–243.

Iyer, S., N. Banks, M. A. Roy, P. Tibbo, R. Williams, R. Manchanda, P. Chue, and A. Malla. "A Qualitative Study of Experiences With and Perceptions Regarding Long-Acting Injectable Antipsychotics: Part I-Patient Perspectives." *Canadian Journal of Psychiatry* 58 (5 Suppl 1) (May 2013): 14S–22S.

Jackson, Jake. "Patronizing Depression: Epistemic Injustice, Stigmatizing Attitudes, and the Need for Empathy." *Journal of Social Philosophy* 48, no. 3 (Fall 2017): 359–376.

Jenner, J. A., S. Rutten, J. Beuckens, N. Boonstra, and S. Sytema. "Positive and Useful Auditory Vocal Hallucinations: Prevalence, Characteristics, Attributions, and Implications for Treatment." *Acta Psychiatrica Scandinavia* 118 (2008): 238–245.

Johnson, Anne E. "Are We Prosaic Deep Inside? Depression Memoirs, Resourceful Narratives, and the Biomedical Model of Depression." *Philosophy, Psychiatry & Psychology* 24, no. 4 (December 2017): 299–301.

Johnstone, Lucy. *Users and Abusers of Psychiatry: A Critical Look at Psychiatric Practice.* London: Routledge, 2000.

Jones, Karen. "Trust as an Affective Attitude." *Ethics* 107 (October 1996): 4–25.

Judisch, Neal. "Responsibility, Manipulation and Ownership." *Philosophical Explorations* 8, no. 2 (June 2005): 115–130.

Jutel, Annemarie Goldstein. *Putting a Name to It: Diagnosis in Contemporary Society.* Baltimore: Johns Hopkins Press, 2011.

Kabir, Mohammed, Zubair Iliyasu, Isa S. Abubakar, and Muktar H. Aliyu. "Perception and Beliefs about Mental Illness among Adults in Karfi Village, Northern Nigeria." *BMC International Health and Human Rights* 4, no. 3 (August 2004). Accessed September 1, 2019. https://bmcinthealthhumrights.biomedcentral.com/articles/10 .1186/1472-698X-4-3.

Kaplan, E. Ann. "Empathy and Trauma Culture: Imaging Catastrophe." In *Empathy: Philosophical and Psychological Perspectives*, edited by Amy Coplan and Peter Goldie, 255–276. Oxford: Oxford University Press, 2011.

Kapur, Shitij. "Psychosis as a State of Aberrant Salience: A Framework Linking Biology, Phenomenology, and Pharmacology in Schizophrenia." *American Journal of Psychiatry* 160 (2003): 12–23.

Kapur, Shitij, Romina Mizrahi, and Ming Li. "From Dopamine to Salience to Psychosis—Linking Biology, Pharmacology and Phenomenology of Psychosis." *Schizophrenia Research* 79 (2005): 59–68.

Katz, Shimon, Hadass Goldblatt, Ilanit Hasson-Ohayon, and David Roe. "Retrospective Accounts of the Process of Using and Discontinuing Psychiatric Medication." *Qualitative Health Research* 29, no. 2 (2019): 198–210.

Kauppinen, Antti. "Empathy as the Moral Sense?" *Philosophia* 45 (2017): 867–879.

Kidd, Ian James, and Havi Carel. "Epistemic Injustice and Illness." *Journal of Applied Philosophy* 34, no. 2 (February 2017): 172–190.

Kim, Scott Y. H. "The Place of Ability to Value in the Evaluation of Decision-Making Capacity." In *Philosophy and Psychiatry: Problems, Intersections, and New Perspectives*, edited by Daniel D. Moseley and Gary Gala, 189–203. New York: Routledge: 2016.

King, Matt, and Joshua May. "Moral Responsibility and Mental Illness: A Call for Nuance." *Neuroethics* 11 (2018): 11–22.

King, Patricia A. Lee, Julie A. Cederbaum, Seth Kurzban, Timony Norton, Steven C. Palmer, and James C. Coyne. "Role of Patient Treatment Beliefs and Provider Characteristics in Establishing Patient-Provider Relationships." *Family Practice* 32, no. 2 (April 2015): 224–231.

Kini, Vinay. "Interventions to Improve Medication Adherence: A Review." *Journal of the American Medical Association* 320, no. 23 (December 18, 2018): 2461–2473.

Klugman, Craig M., Laura B. Dunn, Jack Schwartz, and I. Glenn Cohen. "The Ethics of Smart Pills and Self-Acting Devices: Autonomy, Truth-Telling, and Trust at the Dawn of Digital Medicine." *The American Journal of Bioethics* 18, no. 9 (2018): 38–47.

Knaapen, Loes, and George Weisz. "The Biomedical Standardization of Premenstrual Syndrome." *Studies in History and Philosophy of Biological and Biomedical Sciences* 39 (2008): 120–134.

Kovach, Adam. "Epistemic Virtues and the Deliberative Frame of Mind." *Social Epistemology* 20, no. 1 (2006): 105–115.

Kozuch, Benajmin, and Michael McKenna. "Free Will, Moral Responsibility, and Mental Illness." In *Philosophy and Psychiatry: Problems, Intersections, and New Perspectives*, edited by Daniel D. Moseley and Gary Gala, 89–113. New York: Routledge, 2016.

Kposowa, Augustine J., Glenn T. Tsunokai, and Edgar W. Butler. "The Effects of Race and Ethnicity on Schizophrenia: Individual and Neighborhood Contexts." *Race, Gender & Class* 9, no. 1 (2001): 33–54.

Kurs, Rena, and Alexander Grinshpoon. "Vulnerability of Individuals with Mental Disorders to Epistemic Injustice in Both Clinical and Social Domains." *Ethics & Behavior* 28, no. 4 (2018): 336–346.

Kwong, Jack M. C. "Open-Mindedness as a Critical Virtue." *Topoi* 35 (2016): 403–411.

Landeweer, Elleke G. M., Tineke A. Abma, and Guy A. M. Widdershoven. "Moral Margins Concerning the Use of Coercion in Psychiatry." *Nursing Ethics* 18, no. 3 (2011): 304–316.

Langdon, Robyn, and Max Coltheart. "The Cognitive Neuropsychology of Delusions." In *Pathologies of Belief*, edited by Max Coltheart and Martin Davies, 183–216. Oxford: Cambridge University Press, 2000.

Laruelle, Marc, Lawrence S. Kegeles, and Anissa Abi-Dargham. "Glutamate, Dopamine, and Schizophrenia: From Pathophysiology to Treatment." *Annuals of the New York Academy of Sciences* 1003 (2003): 138–158.

Lear, Jonathan. *Radical Hope: Ethics in the Face of Cultural Devastation*. Cambridge, MA: Harvard University Press, 2006.

Lesh, Tyler A., Costin Tanase, Benjamin R. Geib, Tara A. Niendam, Jong H. Yoon, Michael J. Minzenberg, J. Daniel Ragland, Marjorie Solomon, and Camerson S. Carter. "A Multimodal Analysis of Antipsychotic Effects on Brain Structure and Function in First-Episode Schizophrenia." *JAMA Psychiatry* 72, no. 3 (March 2015): 226–234.

Leudar, Ivan, and Philip Thomas. *Voices of Reason, Voices of Insanity: Studies of Verbal Hallucinations*. London: Routledge, 2000.

Lieberman, Jeffrey A., T. Scott Stroup, Joseph P. McEvoy, Marvin S. Swartz, Robert A. Rosenheck, Diana O. Perkins, Richard S. E. Keefe et al. "Effectiveness of Antipsychotic Drugs in Patients with Chronic Schizophrenia." *The New England Journal of Medicine* 353, no. 12 (September 22, 2005): 1209–1223.

Longden, Eleanor, Dirk Corsten, and Jacqui Dillon. "Recovery, Discovery and Revolution: The Work of Intervoice and the Hearing Voices Movement." In *Madness Contested: Power and Practice*, edited by Steven Coles, Sarah Keenan, and Bob Diamond, 161–180. Ross-on-Wye, UK: PCCS Books, 2013.

Lumsden, David. "Whole Life Narratives and the Self." *Philosophy, Psychiatry & Psychology* 20, no. 1 (March 2013): 1–10.

Lutz, Barbara J., and Barbara J. Bowers. "Understanding How Disability is Defined and Conceptualized in the Literature." In *The Psychological and Social Impact of Illness and Disability, 5th Edition*, edited by Arthur E. Dell Orto and Paul W. Power, 11–21. New York: Springer, 2007.

Malin, Ashley J., and Alberta E. Pos. "The Impact of Early Empathy on Alliance Building, Emotional Processing, and Outcome During Experiential Treatment of Depression." *Psychotherapy Research* 25, no. 4 (July 2015): 445–459.

Marsh, Gerald. "Trust, Testimony, and Prejudice in the Credibility Economy." *Hypatia* 26, no. 2 (Spring 2011): 280–293.

Martin, P. J. "Hearing Voices and Listening to Those That Hear Them." *Journal of Psychiatric and Mental Health Nursing* 7 (2000): 135–141.

Mason, Neil C. "Epistemic Restraint and the Vice of Curiosity." *Philosophy* 87 (2012): 239–259.

Masto, Meghan. "Empathy and Its Role in Morality." *The Southern Journal of Philosophy* 53, no. 1 (March 2015): 74–96.

Mauritz, Maria, and Berno van Meijel. "Loss and Grief in Patients with Schizophrenia: On Living in Another World." *Archives of Psychiatric Nursing* 23, no. 3 (June 2009): 251–260.

McCann, T. V., G. Boardman, E. Clark, and S. Lu. "Risk Profiles for Non-adherence to Antipsychotic Medications." *Journal of Psychiatric and Mental Health Nursing* 15 (2008): 622–629.

McCarthy-Jones, Simon. *Hearing Voices: The Histories, Causes and Meanings of Auditory Verbal Hallucinations*. Cambridge: Cambridge University Press, 2012.

McCraw, Benjamin W. "The Nature of Epistemic Trust." *Social Epistemology: A Journal of Knowledge, Culture and Policy* 29, no. 4 (2015): 413–430.

McFee, Graham. "Empathy: Interpersonal vs Artistic?" In *Empathy: Philosophical and Psychological Perspectives*, edited by Amy Coplan and Peter Goldie, 185–210. Oxford: Oxford University Press, 2011.

McWade, Brigit, Damian Milton, and Peter Beresford. "Mad Studies and Neurodiversity: A Dialogue." *Disability & Society* 30, no. 2 (2015): 305–309.

Mercer, Jean. "Deliverance, Demonic Possession, and Mental Illness: Some Considerations for Mental Health Professionals." *Mental Health, Religion & Culture* 16, no. 6 (2013): 595–611.

Meyer, Adolf. *Psychobiology*. Springfield, IL: Charles C. Thomas, 1957.

Meyers, Diana Tietjens. *Being Yourself: Essays on Identity, Action, and Social Life.* Lanham, MD: Rowman & Littlefield, 2004.

Midlands Psychology Group. "Manifesto for a Social Materialist Psychology of Distress." In *Madness Contested: Power and Practice*, edited by Steven Coles, Sarah Keenan, and Bob Diamond, 121–140. Ross-on-Wye, UK: PCCS Books, 2013.

Miller, Christian. "Empathy as the Only Hope for the Virtue of Compassion and as Support for a Limited Unity of the Virtues." *Philosophy, Theology and the Sciences* 2, no. 1 (2015): 89–113.

Miller, Jessica. "The Other Side of Trust in Health Care: Prescribing Drugs with the Potential for Abuse." *Bioethics* 21, no. 1 (2007): 51–60.

Minett, R. J. "User Participation in Mental Health Care: A Literature Review." *British Journal of Therapy & Rehabilitation* 9, no. 2 (February 2002): 52–55.

Moncrieff, Joanna. "Neoliberalism and Biopsychiatry: A Marriage of Convenience." In *Liberatory Psychiatry: Philosophy, Politics, and Mental Health*, edited by Carl I. Cohen and Sami Timimi, 235–255. Cambridge: Cambridge University Press, 2008.

Montmarquet, James A. *Epistemic Virtue and Doxastic Responsibility*. Lanham, MD: Rowman and Littlefield, 1993.

Morgan, Alastair. "Against Compassion: In Defence of a 'Hybrid' Concept of Empathy." *Nursing Philosophy* 18 (2017): e12148. Accessed December 28, 2019. https://doi .org/10.1111/nup12148.

Moritz, Steffen, and Frank Larøi. "Differences and Similarities in the Sensory and Cognitive Signatures of Voice-Hearing, Intrusions and Thoughts." *Schizophrenia Research* 102 (2008): 96–107.

Moritz, Steffen, Gerit Pfuhl, Thies Lüdtke, Mahesh Menon, Ryan P. Balzan, and Christina Andreou. "A Two-Stage Cognitive Theory of the Positive Symptoms of Psychosis: Highlighting the Role of Lowered Decision Thresholds." *Journal of Behavior Therapy and Experimental Psychiatry* 56 (2017): 12–20.

Moritz, Steffen, Liz Rietschel, Ruth Veckenstedt, Francesca Bohn, Brooke C. Schneider, Tania M. Lincoln, and Anne Karow. "The Other Side of 'Madness': Frequencies of Positive and Ambivalent Attitudes Towards Prominent Positive Symptoms in Psychosis." *Psychosis: Psychological, Social and Integrative Approaches* 7, no. 1 (2015): 14–24.

Morris, Jenny. "Impairment and Disability: Constructing an Ethics of Care That Promotes Human Rights." *Hypatia* 16, no. 4 (Fall 2001): 1–16.

Morrison, Eileen F., and Karen A. Thornton. "Influence of Southern Spiritual Beliefs on Perceptions of Mental Illness." *Issues in Mental Health Nursing* 20, no. 5 (1999): 443–458.

Morrow, Marina, and Julia Weisser. "Towards a Social Justice Framework of Mental Health Recovery." *Studies in Social Justice* 6, no. 1 (2012): 27–43.

Nelson, Barnaby, Josef Parnas, and Louis A. Sass. "Disturbance of Minimal Self (Ipseity) in Schizophrenia: Clarification and Current Status." *Schizophrenia Bulletin* 40, no. 3 (2014): 479–482.

Nemec, Patricia B., and Cheryl J. Gagne. "Recovery from Psychiatric Disabilities." In *The Psychological and Social Impact of Illness and Disability, Fifth Edition*, edited by Arthur E. Dell Orto and Paul W. Power, 596–610. New York: Springer, 2007.

Nesvåg, Ragnar, Gleen Lawyer, Katarina Varnäs, Anders M. Fjell, Kristine B. Walhovd, Arnoldo Frigessi, Erik G. Jönsson, and Ingrid Agartz. "Regional Thinning of the Cerebral Cortex in Schizophrenia: Effects of Diagnosis, Age and Antipsychotic Medication." *Schizophrenia Research* 98, no. 1–3 (January 2008): 16–28.

Newham, Roger Alan. "The Emotion of Compassion and the Likelihood of Its Expression in Nursing Practice." *Nursing Philosophy* 18 (2017): 1–6, e12163. Accessed January 3, 2020. https://doi.org/10.1111/nup12163.

Nickerson, Raymond S., Susan F. Butler, and Michael Carlin. "Empathy and Knowledge Projection." In *The Social Neuroscience of Empathy*, edited by Jean Decety and William Ickes, 43–56. Cambridge, MA: MIT Press, 2009.

Nienhuis, Jacob B., Jesse Owen, Jeffrey C. Valentine, Stephanie Winkeljohn Black, Tyler C. Halford, Stephanie E. Parazak, Stephanie Budge, and Mark Hilsenroth. "Therapeutic Alliance, Empathy, and Genuineness in Individual Adult Psychotherapy: A Meta-Analytic Review." *Psychotherapy Research* 28, no. 4 (2018): 593–605.

Nixon, Gary, Brad Hagen, and Tracey Peters. "Recovery From Psychosis: A Phenomenological Inquiry." *International Journal of Mental Health and Addiction* 8 (2010): 620–635.

Nordenfelt, Lennart. *On the Nature of Health: An Action-Theoretic Approach, Second Revised and Enlarged Edition*. Dordrecht: Kluwer Academic Publishers, 1995.

Nordenfelt, Lennart. *Rationality and Compulsion: Applying Action Theory to Psychiatry*. Oxford: Oxford University Press, 2007.

Origgi, Gloria. "Epistemic Injustice and Epistemic Trust." *Social Epistemology: A Journal of Knowledge, Culture and Policy* 26, no. 2 (2012): 221–235.

Oshana, Marina. "How Much Should We Value Autonomy?" *Social Philosophy & Policy* (2003): 99–126.

Oshana, Marina. "The Misguided Marriage of Responsibility and Autonomy." *The Journal of Ethics* 6 (2002): 261–280.

"Outside the Box." *Rethink Psychosis*. Accessed June 9, 2021. https://rethinkpsychosis
.weebly.com/outside-the-box.html.

Parsons, Talcott. *The Social System: The Major Exposition of the Author's Conceptual Scheme for the Analysis of the Dynamics of the Social System*. London: Free Press of Glencoe (Collier-MacMillan), 1951.

Patel, M. X., N. de Zoysa, M. Bernadt, J. Bindman, and A. S. David. "Are Depot Antipsychotics More Coercive than Tablets? The Patient's Perspective." *Journal of Psychopharmacology* 24, no. 10 (October 2010): 1483–1489.

Peele, Roger, and Paul Chodoff. "Involuntary Hospitalization and Deinstitutionalization." In *Psychiatric Ethics, Fourth Edition*, edited by Sydney Bloch and Stephen A. Green, 211–228. Oxford: Oxford University Press, 2009.

Pellegrino, Edmund D. "Trust and Distrust in Professional Ethics." In *Ethics, Trust, and the Professions: Philosophical and Cultural Aspects*, edited by Edmund D. Pellegrino, Robert M. Veatch, and John P. Langan, 69–89. Washington, DC: Georgetown University Press, 1991.

Pepper-Smith, Robert, William R. Harvey, and M. Silberfield. "Competency and Practical Judgment." *Theoretical Medicine* 17 (1996): 135–150.

Perry, Alexandra. "Neuropluralism." *Journal of Ethics in Mental Health* 6 (2011): 1–4.

Pfeiffer, David. "The Categorization and Control of People with Disabilities." *Disability and Rehabilitation* 21, no. 3 (1999): 106–107.

Pickard, Hanna. "Responsibility without Blame: Empathy and the Effective Treatment of Personality Disorder." *Philosophy, Psychiatry, & Psychology* 18, no. 3 (September 2011): 209–224.

Pienkos, Elizabeth, Anne Giersch, Marie Hansen, Clara Humpston, Simon McCarthy-Jones, Aaron Mishara, Barnaby Nelson et al. "Hallucinations Beyond Voices: A Conceptual Review of the Phenomenology of Altered Perception in Psychosis." *Schizophrenia Bulletin* 45, suppl. no. 1 (2019): S67–S77.

Pilgrim, David, and Richard Bentall. "The Medicalisation of Misery: A Critical Realist Analysis of the Concept of Depression." *Journal of Mental Health* 8, no. 3 (1999): 261–274.

Pitt, Liz, Martina Kilbride, Mary Welford, Sarah Nothard, and Anthony P. Morrison. "Impact of a Diagnosis of Psychosis: User-Led Qualitative Study." *Psychiatric Bulletin* 33 (2009): 419–423.

Pohlhaus, Gaile, Jr. "Discerning the Primary Epistemic Harm in Cases of Testimonial Injustice." *Social Epistemology* 28, no. 2 (2014): 99–114.

Pohlhaus, Gaile, Jr. "Relational Knowing and Epistemic Injustice: Toward a Theory of *Willful Hermeneutical Ignorance*." *Hypatia* 27, no. 4 (Fall 2012): 715–735.

Potter, Nancy Nyquist. *The Virtue of Defiance and Psychiatric Engagement*. Oxford: Oxford University Press, 2016.

Potter, Nancy Nyquist. "Voice, Silencing, and Listening Well: Socially Located Patients, Oppressive Structures, and an Invitation to Shift the Epistemic Terrain." In *The Bloomsbury Companion to Philosophy of Psychiatry*, edited by Şerife Tekin and Robyn Bluhm, 305–324. London: Bloomsbury Academic, 2019.

Powell, John, and Aileen Clarke. "Information in Mental Health: Qualitative Study of Mental Health Service Users." *Health Expectations* 9 (2006): 359–365.

Prinz, Jesse J. "Is Empathy Necessary for Morality?" In *Empathy: Philosophical and Psychological Perspectives*, edited by Amy Coplan and Peter Goldie, 211–229. Oxford: Oxford University Press, 2011.

Radden, Jennifer. *Divided Minds and Successive Selves: Ethical Issues in Disorders of Identity and Personality*. Cambridge, MA: MIT Press, 1996.

Rashed, Mohammed Abouelleil. *Madness and the Demand for Recognition: A Philosophical Inquiry into Identity and Mental Health Activism*. Oxford: Oxford University Press, 2019.

Ratcliffe, Matthew. "Phenomenology as a Form of Empathy." *Inquiry: An Interdisciplinary Journal of Philosophy* 55, no. 5 (2012): 473–495.

Ratcliffe, Matthew. "The Phenomenology of Depression and the Nature of Empathy." *Medicine, Health Care and Philosophy* 17 (2014): 269–280.

Razali, S. M., U. A. Khan, and C. I. Hasanah. "Belief in Supernatural Causes of Mental Illness among Malay Patients: Impact on Treatment." *Acta Psychiatrica Scandinavica* 94, no. 4 (October 1996): 229–233.

Read, J., N. Haslam, L. Sayce, and E. Davies. "Prejudice and Schizophrenia: A Review of the 'Mental Illness is an Illness Like Any Other' Approach." *Acta Psychiatrica Scandinavica* 114 (2006): 303–318.

Regan, Donald H. "Paternalism, Freedom, Identity, and Commitment." In *Paternalism*, edited by Rolf Sartorius, 113–138. Minneapolis: University of Minnesota Press, 1983.

Reiheld, Alison. "Patient Complains of . . . : How Medicalization Mediates Power and Justice." *International Journal of Feminist Approaches to Bioethics* 3, no. 1 (Spring 2010): 72–98.

Repper, Julie, and Rachel Perkins. *Social Inclusion and Recovery: A Model for Mental Health Practice*. Edinburgh: Ballière Tindall, 2003.

Reyre, Aymeric, Raphaël Jeannin, Myriam Larguèche, Emmanuel Hirsch, Thierry Baubet, Marie Rose Moro, and Olivier Taïeb. "Care and Prejudice: Moving Beyond

Mistrust in the Care Relationship with Addicted Patients." *Medicine, Health Care and Philosophy* 17 (2014): 183–190.

Rice, Stephen, Jessica Richardson, and Keegan Kraemer. "Emotion Mediates Distrust of Persons with Mental Illnesses." *International Journal of Mental Health* 43, no. 1 (Spring 2014): 3–29.

Roe, David, Hadass Goldblatt, Vered Baloush-Klienman, Margaret Swarbrick, and Larry Davidson. "Why and How People Decide to Stop Taking Prescribed Psychiatric Medication: Exploring the Subjective Process of Choice." *Psychiatric Rehabilitation Journal* 33, no. 1 (2009): 38–46.

Roe, David, and Larry Davidson. "Destinations and Detours of the Users' Movement." *Journal of Mental Health* 14, no. 5 (October 2005): 429–433.

Rofail, Diana, Rebecca Heelis, and Kevin Gournay. "Results of a Thematic Analysis to Explore the Experiences of Patients with Schizophrenia Taking Antipsychotic Medication." *Clinical Therapeutics* 31 (2009): 1488–1496.

Rogers, W. A. "Is There a Moral Duty for Doctors to Trust Patients?" *Journal of Medical Ethics* 28 (2002): 77–80.

Rogers, Wendy, and Angela Ballantyne. "Gender and Trust in Medicine: Vulnerabilities, Abuses, and Remedies." *International Journal of Feminist Approaches to Bioethics* 1, no. 1 (Spring 2008): 48–66.

Romme, Marius, and Mervyn Morris. "The Recovery Process with Hearing Voices: Accepting as well as Exploring Their Emotional Background through a Supported Process." *Psychosis: Psychological, Social and Integrative Approaches* 5, no. 3 (2013): 259–269.

Romme, Marius, Sandra Escher, Jacqui Dillon, Dirk Costens, and Mervyn Morris. *Living with Voices: 50 Stories of Recovery*. Monmouth, UK: PCCS Books, 2009.

Rudnick, Abraham. "What Is a Psychiatric Disability?" *Health Care Analysis* 22 (2014): 105–113.

Rungruangsiripan, Malatee, Yajai Sitthimongkol, Wantana Maneesriwongul, Sandra Talley, and Thavatchai Vorapongsathorn. "Medicating Role of Illness Representation among Social Support, Therapeutic Alliance, Experience of Medication Side Effects, and Medication Adherence in Persons with Schizophrenia." *Archives of Psychiatric Nursing* 25, no. 4 (August 2011): 269–283.

Rusch, Nicolas, Matthias C. Angermeyer, and Patrick W. Corrigan. "Mental Illness Stigma: Concepts, Consequences, and Initiatives to Reduce Stigma." *European Psychiatry* 20 (2005): 529–539.

Rush, B. "Mental Health Service User Involvement in England: Lessons from History." *Journal of Psychiatric and Mental Health Nursing* 11 (2004): 313–318.

Ryan, Christopher James. "One Flu Over the Cuckoo's Nest: Comparing Legislated Coercive Treatment for Mental Illness with that for Other Illness." *Bioethical Inquiry* 8 (2011): 87–93.

Saks, Elyn R. *The Center Cannot Hold: My Journey through Madness.* New York: Hyperion, 2007.

Sanati, Abdi, and Michalis Kyratsous. "Epistemic Injustice in Assessment of Delusions." *Journal of Evaluation in Clinical Practice* 21 (2015): 479–485.

Sass, Louis. "Self-Disturbance and Schizophrenia: Structure, Specificity, Pathogenesis (Current Issues, New Directions)." *Schizophrenia Research* 152 (2014): 5–11.

Sayce, Liz. *From Psychiatric Patient to Citizen: Overcoming Discrimination and Social Exclusion.* New York: St. Martin's Press, 2000.

Sayer, Jane, Susan Ritter, and Kevin Gournay. "Beliefs about Voices and Their Effects on Coping Strategies." *Journal of Advanced Nursing* 31, no. 5 (2000): 1199–1205.

Schermer, Maartje. "The Dynamics of the Treatment-Enhancement Distinction: ADHD as a Case Study." *Philosophica* 79 (2007): 25–37.

Schreber, Daniel Paul. *Memoirs of My Nervous Illness.* New York: New York Review Books Classics, 2000.

Scoccia, Danny. "In Defense of Hard Paternalism." *Law and Philosophy* 27 (2008): 351–381.

Scoccia, Danny. "Paternalism and Respect for Autonomy." *Ethics* 100, no. 2 (January 1990): 318–334.

Scott, Joan W. "The Evidence of Experience." *Critical Inquiry* 17, no. 4 (Summer 1991): 773–797.

Scrutton, Anastasia Philippa. "Epistemic Injustice and Mental Illness." In *The Routledge Handbook of Epistemic Injustice*, edited by Ian James Kidd, Jose Medina, and Gaile Pohlhaus Jr., 347–355. London: Routledge, 2017.

Sendt, Kyra-Verena, Derek Kenneth Tracy, and Sagnik Bhattacharyya. "A Systematic Review of Factors Influencing Adherence to Antipsychotic Medication in Schizophrenia-Spectrum Disorders." *Psychiatry Research* 225 (2015): 14–30.

Shabo, Seth. "Incompatibilism and Personal Relationships: Another Look at Strawson's Objective Attitude." *Australasian Journal of Philosophy* 90, no. 1 (March 2012): 131–147.

Shabo, Seth. "Where Love and Resentment Meet: Strawson's Intrapersonal Defense of Compatibilism." *Philosophical Review* 121, no. 1 (2012): 95–124.

Shattock, Lucy, Katherine Berry, Amy Degnan, and Dawn Edge. "Therapeutic Alliance in Psychological Therapy for People with Schizophrenia and Related Psychoses: A Systematic Review." *Clinical Psychology & Psychotherapy* 25 (2018): e60–e85.

Shaw, Rhonda. "Towards Disability Ethics: A Social Science Perspective." *New Zealand Bioethics Journal* 4, no. 2 (2003): 7–14.

Shieber, Joseph. "Against Credibility." *Australasian Journal of Philosophy* 90, no. 1 (March 2012): 1–18.

Shorter, Edward. *From Paralysis to Fatigue: A History of Psychosomatic Illness in the Modern Era.* New York: Free Press, 1992.

Showalter, Elaine. *Hystories: Hysterical Epidemics and Modern Media.* New York: Columbia University Press, 1997.

Simmons, Aaron. "In Defense of the Moral Significance of Empathy." *Ethical Theory and Moral Practice* 17 (2014): 97–111.

Slaby, Jan. "Empathy's Blind Spot." *Medicine, Health Care and Philosophy* 17 (2014): 249–258.

Slade, Mike. *Personal Recovery and Mental Illness: A Guide for Mental Health Professionals.* Cambridge: Cambridge University Press, 2009.

Slote, Michael. "The Many Faces of Empathy." *Philosophia* 45 (2017): 843–855.

Smart, Julie F., and David W. Smart. "Models of Disability: Implications for the Counseling Profession." In *The Psychological and Social Impact of Illness and Disability, Fifth Edition*, edited by Arthur E. Dell Orto and Paul W. Power, 75–100. New York: Springer, 2007.

Smith, Joel. "What Is Empathy For?" *Synthese* 194 (2017): 709–722.

Snow, Nancy. "Empathy." *American Philosophical Quarterly* 37, no. 1 (2000): 65–78.

So, Suzanne H., Daniel Freeman, Graham Dunn, Shitij Kapur, Elizabeth Kupers, Paul Bebbington, David Fowler, and Philippa A. Garety. "Jumping to Conclusions, A Lack of Belief Flexibility and Delusional Conviction in Psychosis: A Longitudinal Investigation of the Structure, Frequency, and Relatedness of Reasoning Biases." *Journal of Abnormal Psychology* 121, no. 1 (2012): 129–139.

Sokolowski, Robert. "The Fiduciary Relationship and the Nature of Professions." In *Ethics, Trust, and the Professions: Philosophical and Cultural Aspects*, edited by Edmund D. Pellegrino, Robert M. Veatch, and John P. Langan, 23–43. Washington, DC: Georgetown University Press, 1991.

Speed, Ewen. "Patients, Consumers and Survivors: A Case Study of Mental Health Service User Discourses." *Social Science & Medicine* 62 (2006): 28–38.

Stahl, Stephen M. "Beyond the Dopamine Hypothesis to the NMDA Glutamate Receptor Hypofunction Hypothesis of Schizophrenia." *CNS Spectrums* 12, no. 4 (April 2007): 265–268.

Steinberg, Justin. "An Epistemic Case for Empathy." *Pacific Philosophical Quarterly* 95 (2014): 47–71.

Stephens, G. Lynn, and George Graham. *When Self-Consciousness Breaks: Alien Voices and Inserted Thoughts*. Cambridge, MA: MIT Press, 2000.

Steslow, K. "Metaphors in Our Mouths: The Silencing of the Psychiatric Patient." *The Hastings Center Report* 40, no. 4 (2010): 30–33.

Stone, James M., Paul D. Morrison, and Lyn S. Pilowsky. "Review: Glutamate and Dopamine Dysregulation in Schizophrenia—A Synthesis and Selective Review." *Psychopharmacology* 21, no. 4 (June 2007): 440–452.

Suri, Rochelle. "Making Sense of Voices: An Exploration of Meaningfulness in Auditory Hallucinations in Schizophrenia." *Journal of Humanistic Psychology* 51, no. 2 (2011): 152–171.

Svenaeus, Fredrik. "The Relationship between Empathy and Sympathy in Good Health Care." *Medicine, Health Care and Philosophy* 18 (2015): 267–277.

Szmukler, George. "Coercion in Psychiatric Treatment and Its Justifications." In *Philosophy and Psychiatry: Problems, Intersections, and New Perspectives*, edited by Daniel D. Moseley and Gary Gala, 125–146. New York: Routledge: 2016.

Szmukler, George. "When Psychiatric Diagnosis Becomes an Overworked Tool." *Journal of Medical Ethics* 40, no. 8 (August 2014): 517–520.

Takahashi, Nagahide, and Takeshi Sakurai. "Roles of Glial Cells in Schizophrenia: Possible Targets for Therapeutic Approaches." *Neurobiology of Disease* 53 (May 2013): 49–60.

Tannsjo, T. "The Convention on Human Rights and Biomedicine and the Use of Coercion in Psychiatry." *Journal of Medical Ethics* 30 (2004): 430–434.

Tate, Alex James Miller. "Contributory Injustice in Psychiatry." *Journal of Medical Ethics* 45 (2019): 97–100.

Tattan, Theresa M. G., and Francis H. Creed. "Negative Symptoms of Schizophrenia and Compliance with Medication." *Schizophrenia Bulletin* 27, no. 1 (2001): 149–155.

Tekin, Şerife. "How Does the Self Adjudicate Narratives?" *Philosophy, Psychiatry & Psychology* 20, no. 1 (March 2013): 25–28.

Tekin, Şerife. "Looking for the Self in Psychiatry: Perils and Promises of Phenomenology-Neuroscience Partnership in Schizophrenia Research." In *Extraordinary Science and Psychiatry: Responses to the Crisis in Mental Health Research*, edited by Jeffrey Poland and Şerife Tekin, 249–266. Cambridge, MA: MIT Press, 2017.

Tekin, Şerife. "The Missing Self in Scientific Psychiatry." *Synthese* 196 (2019): 2197–2215.

Tekin, Şerife. "Patients as Experienced-Based Experts in Psychiatry: Insights from the Natural Method." In *The Natural Method: Essays on Mind, Ethics, and Self in Honor of Owen Flanagan*, edited by Eddy Nahmias, Thomas W. Polger, and Wenqing Zhao, 79–97. Cambridge, MA: MIT Press, 2020.

Tekin, Şerife. "Self-Concept through the Diagnostic Looking Glass: Narratives and Mental Disorder." *Philosophical Psychology* 24, no. 3 (June 2011): 357–380.

Tekin, Şerife. "Self-Insight in the Time of Mood Disorders: After the Diagnosis, Beyond the Treatment." *Philosophy Psychiatry & Psychology* 21, no. 2 (June 2014): 139–155.

Terzi, Lorella. "The Social Model of Disability: A Philosophical Critique." *Journal of Applied Philosophy* 21, no. 2 (2004): 141–157.

Tessier, Arnaud, Laurent Boyer, Mathilde Husky, Franck Baylé, Pierre-Michel Llorca, and David Misdrahi. "Medication Adherence in Schizophrenia: The Role of Insight, Therapeutic Alliance and Perceived Trauma Associated with Psychiatric Care." *Psychiatry Research* 257 (2017): 315–321.

Thachuk, Angela K. "Stigma and the Politics of Biomedical Models of Mental Illness." *International Journal of Feminist Approaches to Bioethics* 4, no. 1 (Special Issue: Feminist Perspectives on Ethics in Psychiatry) (Spring 2011): 140–163.

Tham, Xiang Cong, Huiting Xie, Cecilia Mui Lee Chng, Xin Yi Seah, Violeta Lopez, and Piyanee Klainin-Yobas. "Factors Affecting Medication Adherence Among Adults with Schizophrenia: A Literature Review." *Archives of Psychiatric Nursing* 30 (2016): 797–809.

Thomas, Sandra P. "Can We Listen in a New Way to Those Who Listen to Voices?" *Issues in Mental Health Nursing* 33, no. 8 (2012): 449.

Thornhill, Hermione, Linda Clare, and Rufus May. "Escape, Enlightenment and Endurance: Narratives of Recovery from Psychosis." *Anthropology & Medicine* 11, no. 2 (August 2004): 181–199.

Tichon, Jennifer, Jennifer Loh, and Robert King. "Psychology Student Opinion of Virtual Reality a Tool to Educate about Schizophrenia." *International Journal on e-Learning* (October–December 2004): 40–46.

Timimi, Sami. "Children's Mental Health and the Global Market: An Ecological Analysis." In *Liberatory Psychiatry: Philosophy, Politics, and Mental Health*, edited by Carl I. Cohen and Sami Timimi, 163–182. Cambridge: Cambridge University Press, 2008.

Tobin, Theresa Weynand. "The Relevance of Trust for Moral Justification." *Social Theory and Practice* 37, no. 4 (October 2011): 599–628.

Tremain, Shelley. "On the Government of Disability." *Social Theory and Practice* 27, no. 4 (October 2001): 617–636.

Usher, Kim. "Taking Neuroleptic Medications as the Treatment for Schizophrenia: A Phenomenological Study." *Australian and New Zealand Journal of Mental Health Nursing* 10 (2001): 145–155.

Ussher, Jane. "Are We Medicalizing Women's Misery? A Critical Review of Women's Higher Rates of Reported Depression." *Feminism & Psychology* 20, no. 9 (2010): 9–35.

van Baaren, Rick B., Jean Decety, Ap Dijksterhuis, Andries van der Leij, and Matthijs L. van Leeuwen. "Being Imitated: Consequences of Nonconsciously Showing Empathy." In *The Social Neuroscience of Empathy*, edited by Jean Decety and William Ickes, 31–42. Cambridge, MA: MIT Press, 2009.

van der Gaag, Mark, Marie Claire Hageman, and Max Birchwood. "Evidence for a Cognitive Model of Auditory Hallucinations." *The Journal of Nervous and Mental Disease* 191, no. 8 (August 2003): 542–545.

Vargas-Huicochea, I., L. Huicochea, C. Berlanga, and A. Fresán. "Taking or Not Taking Medications: Psychiatric Treatment Perceptions in Patients Diagnosed with Bipolar Disorder." *Journal of Clinical Pharmacy and Therapeutics* 39 (2014): 673–679.

Verkerk, Marian. "A Care Perspective on Coercion and Autonomy." *Bioethics* 13, no. 3–4 (1999): 358–368.

Vita, A., L. De Peri, G. Deste, and E. Sacchetti. "Progressive Loss of Cortical Gray Matter in Schizophrenia: A Meta-Analysis and Meta-Regression of Longitudinal MRI Studies." *Translational Psychiatry* 2, no. 11 (November 2012): e190. Accessed August 28, 2019. https://www.ncbi.nlm.nih.gov/pmc/articles/PMC3565772/.

Vuckovich, Paula K. "Compliance versus Adherence in Serious and Persistent Mental Illness." *Nursing Ethics* 17, no. 1 (2010): 77–85.

Vuckovich, Paula K., and Barbara M. Artinian. "Justifying Coercion." *Nursing Ethics* 12, no. 4 (2005): 370–380.

Wardrope, Alistair. "Medicalization and Epistemic Injustice." *Medicine, Health Care, and Philosophy* 18 (2015): 341–352.

Wassef, Adel, Jeffrey Baker, and Lisa Kochan. "GABA and Schizophrenia: A Review of Basic Science and Clinical Studies." *Journal of Clinical Psychopharmacology* 23, no. 6 (December 2003): 601–640.

Watson, Gary. "Free Agency." In *Free Will, Second Edition*, edited by Gary Watson, 337–351. Oxford: Oxford University Press, 2003.

Watson, Gary. "Two Faces of Responsibility." In *Agency and Answerability: Selected Essays*, 260–288. Oxford: Clarendon Press, 2004.

Watson, Gary. "Volitional Necessities." In *Agency and Answerability: Selected Essays*, 88–122. Oxford: Clarendon Press, 2004.

Westlund, Andrea C. "Rethinking Relational Autonomy." *Hypatia* 24, no. 4 (Fall 2009): 26–49.

Widdershoven, Guy A. M., Andrea Ruissen, Anton J. L. M. van Balkom, and Gerben Meynen. "Competence in Chronic Mental Illness: The Relevance of Practical Wisdom." *Journal of Medical Ethics* 43 (2017): 374–378.

Wikler, Daniel. "Persuasion and Coercion for Health: Ethical Issues in Government Efforts to Change Life-Styles." In *Paternalism*, edited by Rolf Sartorius, 35–59. Minneapolis: University of Minnesota Press, 1983.

Winick, Bruce J. *Civil Commitment: A Therapeutic Jurisprudence Model*. Durham, NC: Carolina Academic Press, 2005.

Woesner, Mary, and Christian Kidd. "The Use of Personal Accounts in the Study of Severe Mental Illness." *Einstein Journal of Biology and Medicine* 29, no. 1–2 (2013): 40–45.

Yang, Jaewon, Young-Hoon Ko, Jong-Woo Paik, Moon-Soo Lee, Changsu Han, Sook-Haeng Joe, In-Kwa Jung, Hyun-Gang Jung, and Seung-Hyun Kim. "Symptom Severity and Attitudes toward Medication: Impacts on Adherence in Outpatients with Schizophrenia." *Schizophrenia Research* 134 (2012): 226–231.

Yin, J., A. M. Barr, A. Ramos-Miguel, and R. M. Procyshyn. "Antipsychotic Induced Dopamine Supersensitivity Psychosis: A Comprehensive Review." *Current Neuropharmacology* 15, no. 1 (2017): 174–183.

Yue, Ying, Li Kong, Jijun Wang, Chunbo Li, Ling Tan, Hui Su, and Yifeng Xu. "Regional Abnormality of Grey Matter in Schizophrenia: Effect from the Illness of Treatment?" *PLoS One* 11, no. 1 (2016): e0147204. Accessed August 28, 2019. https://www.ncbi.nlm.nih.gov/pmc/articles/PMC4720276/.

Zaner, Richard M. "Trust and the Patient-Physician Relationship." In *Ethics, Trust, and the Professions: Philosophical and Cultural Aspects*, edited by Edmund D. Pellegrino, Robert M. Veatch, and John P. Langan, 45–67. Washington, DC: Georgetown University Press, 1991.

Zipursky, Robert B., Natasja M. Menezes, and David L. Streiner. "Risk of Symptom Recurrence with Medication Discontinuation in First-Episode Psychosis: A Systematic Review." *Schizophrenia Research* 152 (2014): 408–414.

Index

Basic Bioethics

Arthur Caplan, editor

Books Acquired under the Editorship of Glenn McGee and Arthur Caplan

Peter A. Ubel, *Pricing Life: Why It's Time for Health Care Rationing*

Mark G. Kuczewski and Ronald Polansky, eds., *Bioethics: Ancient Themes in Contemporary Issues*

Suzanne Holland, Karen Lebacqz, and Laurie Zoloth, eds., *The Human Embryonic Stem Cell Debate: Science, Ethics, and Public Policy*

Gita Sen, Asha George, and Piroska Östlin, eds., *Engendering International Health: The Challenge of Equity*

Carolyn McLeod, *Self-Trust and Reproductive Autonomy*

Lenny Moss, *What Genes Can't Do*

Jonathan D. Moreno, ed., *In the Wake of Terror: Medicine and Morality in a Time of Crisis*

Glenn McGee, ed., *Pragmatic Bioethics, 2nd edition*

Timothy F. Murphy, *Case Studies in Biomedical Research Ethics*

Mark A. Rothstein, ed., *Genetics and Life Insurance: Medical Underwriting and Social Policy*

Kenneth A. Richman, *Ethics and the Metaphysics of Medicine: Reflections on Health and Beneficence*

David Lazer, ed., *DNA and the Criminal Justice System: The Technology of Justice*

Harold W. Baillie and Timothy K. Casey, eds., *Is Human Nature Obsolete? Genetics, Bioengineering, and the Future of the Human Condition*

Robert H. Blank and Janna C. Merrick, eds., *End-of-Life Decision Making: A Cross-National Study*

Norman L. Cantor, *Making Medical Decisions for the Profoundly Mentally Disabled*

Margrit Shildrick and Roxanne Mykitiuk, eds., *Ethics of the Body: Post-Conventional Challenges*

Alfred I. Tauber, *Patient Autonomy and the Ethics of Responsibility*

David H. Brendel, *Healing Psychiatry: Bridging the Science/Humanism Divide*

Jonathan Baron, *Against Bioethics*

Michael L. Gross, *Bioethics and Armed Conflict: Moral Dilemmas of Medicine and War*

Karen F. Greif and Jon F. Merz, *Current Controversies in the Biological Sciences: Case Studies of Policy Challenges from New Technologies*

Deborah Blizzard, *Looking Within: A Sociocultural Examination of Fetoscopy*

Ronald Cole-Turner, ed., *Design and Destiny: Jewish and Christian Perspectives on Human Germline Modification*

Holly Fernandez Lynch, *Conflicts of Conscience in Health Care: An Institutional Compromise*

Mark A. Bedau and Emily C. Parke, eds., *The Ethics of Protocells: Moral and Social Implications of Creating Life in the Laboratory*

Jonathan D. Moreno and Sam Berger, eds., *Progress in Bioethics: Science, Policy, and Politics*

Eric Racine, *Pragmatic Neuroethics: Improving Understanding and Treatment of the Mind-Brain*

Martha J. Farah, ed., *Neuroethics: An Introduction with Readings*

Jeremy R. Garrett, ed., *The Ethics of Animal Research: Exploring the Controversy*

Books Acquired under the Editorship of Arthur Caplan

Sheila Jasanoff, ed., *Reframing Rights: Bioconstitutionalism in the Genetic Age*

Christine Overall, *Why Have Children? The Ethical Debate*

Yechiel Michael Barilan, *Human Dignity, Human Rights, and Responsibility: The New Language of Global Bioethics and Bio-Law*

Tom Koch, *Thieves of Virtue: When Bioethics Stole Medicine*

Timothy F. Murphy, *Ethics, Sexual Orientation, and Choices about Children*

Daniel Callahan, *In Search of the Good: A Life in Bioethics*

Robert Blank, *Intervention in the Brain: Politics, Policy, and Ethics*

Gregory E. Kaebnick and Thomas H. Murray, eds., *Synthetic Biology and Morality: Artificial Life and the Bounds of Nature*

Dominic A. Sisti, Arthur L. Caplan, and Hila Rimon-Greenspan, eds., *Applied Ethics in Mental Healthcare: An Interdisciplinary Reader*

Barbara K. Redman, *Research Misconduct Policy in Biomedicine: Beyond the Bad-Apple Approach*

Russell Blackford, *Humanity Enhanced: Genetic Choice and the Challenge for Liberal Democracies*

Nicholas Agar, *Truly Human Enhancement: A Philosophical Defense of Limits*

Bruno Perreau, *The Politics of Adoption: Gender and the Making of French Citizenship*

Carl Schneider, *The Censor's Hand: The Misregulation of Human-Subject Research*

Lydia S. Dugdale, ed., *Dying in the Twenty-First Century: Towards a New Ethical Framework for the Art of Dying Well*

John D. Lantos and Diane S. Lauderdale, *Preterm Babies, Fetal Patients, and Childbearing Choices*

Harris Wiseman, *The Myth of the Moral Brain*

Arthur L. Caplan and Jason Schwartz, eds., *Vaccine Ethics and Policy: An Introduction with Readings*

Tom Koch, *Ethics in Everyday Places: Mapping Moral Stress, Distress, and Injury*

Nicole Piemonte, *Afflicted: How Vulnerability Can Heal Medical Education and Practice*

Abigail Gosselin, *Mental Patient: Psychiatric Ethics from a Patient's Perspective*